OXFORD STATISTICAL SCIENCE SERIES
SERIES EDITORS
A. C. ATKINSON   R. J. CARROLL   J. B. COPAS
D. J. HAND   D. A. PIERCE   M. J. SCHERVISH
R. L. SMITH   D. M. TITTERINGTON

OXFORD STATISTICAL SCIENCE SERIES

1. A. C. Atkinson: *Plots, transformations, and regression*
2. M. Stone: *Coordinate-free multivariable statistics*
3. W. J. Krzanowski: *Principles of multivariate analysis: a user's perspective*
4. M. Aitkin, D. Anderson, B. Francis, and J. Hinde: *Statistical modelling in GLIM*
5. Peter J. Diggle: *Time series: a biostatistical introduction*
6. Howell Tong: *Non-linear time series: a dynamical system approach*
7. V. P. Godambe: *Estimating functions*
8. A. C. Atkinson and A. N. Donev: *Optimum experimental designs*
9. U. N. Bhat and I. V. Basawa: *Queuing and related models*
10. J. K. Lindsey: *Models for repeated measurements*
11. N. T. Longford: *Random coefficient models*
12. P. J. Brown: *Measurement, regression, and calibration*
13. Peter J. Diggle, Kung-Yee Liang, and Scott L. Zeger: *Analysis of longitudinal data*
14. J. I. Ansell and M. J. Phillips: *Practical methods for reliability data analysis*
15. J. K. Lindsey: *Modelling frequency and count data*
16. J. L. Jensen: *Saddlepoint approximations*
17. Steffen L. Lauritzen: *Graphical models*
18. A. W. Bowman and A. Azzalini: *Applied smoothing methods for data analysis*
19. J. K. Lindsey: *Models for repeated measurements* second edition
20. Michael Evans and Tim Swartz: *Approximating integrals via Monte Carlo and deterministic methods*
21. D. F. Andrews and J. E. Stafford: *Symbolic computation for statistical inference*
22. T. A. Severini: *Likelihood methods in statistics*
23. W. J. Krzanowski: P*rinciples of multivariate analysis: a user's persepective* updated edition
24. J. Durbin and S. J. Koopman: *Time series analysis by state space models*
25. Peter J. Diggle, Patrick Heagerty, Kung-Yee Liang, and Scott L. Zeger: *Analysis of longitudinal data* second edition
26. J. K. Lindsey: *Nonlinear models in medical statistics*

Nonlinear Models in Medical Statistics

J. K. LINDSEY
Limburgs Universitair Centrum
Diepenbeek, Belgium

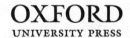

OXFORD
UNIVERSITY PRESS

Great Clarendon Street, Oxford OX2 6DP
Oxford University Press is a department of the University of Oxford.
It furthers the University's objective of excellence in research, scholarship,
and education by publishing worldwide in
Oxford New York

Athens Auckland Bangkok Bogotá Buenos Aires Cape Town
Chennai Dar es Salaam Delhi Florence Hong Kong Istanbul Karachi
Kolkata Kuala Lumpur Madrid Melbourne Mexico City Mumbai Nairobi
Paris São Paulo Shanghai Singapore Taipei Tokyo Toronto Warsaw
with associated companies in Berlin Ibadan

Oxford is a registered trade mark of Oxford University Press
in the UK and in certain other countries

Published in the United States
by Oxford University Press Inc., New York

© J. K. Lindsey, 2001

The moral rights of the author have been asserted
Database right Oxford University Press (maker)

First published 2001

All rights reserved. No part of this publication may be reproduced,
stored in a retrieval system, or transmitted, in any form or by any means,
without the prior permission in writing of Oxford University Press,
or as expressly permitted by law, or under terms agreed with the appropriate
reprographics rights organization. Enquiries concerning reproduction
outside the scope of the above should be sent to the Rights Department,
Oxford University Press, at the address above

You must not circulate this book in any other binding or cover
and you must impose this same condition on any acquirer

British Library Cataloguing in Publication Data
Data available

Library of Congress Cataloging in Publication Data
Data available
ISBN 0 19 850812 3

1 3 5 7 9 10 8 6 4 2

Typeset by the author using LaTex
Printed in Great Britain
on acid-free paper by Biddles Ltd, Guildford & King's Lynn

Preface

Much of statistics is dominated by linear models, a legacy of the pre-computer era. However, nonlinear models provide many advantages in modelling scientific data and only a few technical disadvantages. Usually, the idea is to construct a *mechanistic* model to attempt to *explain* how the responses are being produced. This goal can rarely be attained using linear models.

Mechanistic nonlinear models have many advantages. Parameters often have a natural physical interpretation. If such models do describe the data-generating mechanism adequately, they should provide better predictions outside the range of observed data than would a linear model. As well, in many situations, nonlinear models require fewer parameters than corresponding linear ones that fit equally closely to the data. On the other hand, nonlinear models usually involve more complex estimation techniques that require initial estimates of parameters to be supplied.

This text attempts to provide an introduction to the use of such nonlinear models in medical statistics. It assumes a basic level of knowledge of statistical modelling such as that provided by Lindsey (1995a) and some familiarity with generalized linear models (Lindsey, 1997). Acquaintance with repeated measurements (Lindsey, 1999a) would also be helpful. Access to the statistical software, R, will make practical applications easier. Otherwise, the reader must be prepared to do considerable programming because most of the models considered are not available in standard software packages.

This is meant to be a practical, not a theoretical, text. For some of the theory behind nonlinear modelling, at least when a (multivariate) normal distribution is assumed, the reader may like to consult Bates and Watts (1988), Davidian and Giltinan (1995), Ross (1990), Seber and Wild (1989), and Vonesh and Chinchilli (1997). Note, however, that the normality assumption is rarely entertained in this text, except for assays in Chapter 9.

Thus, in contrast to most publications on nonlinear modelling, here I concentrate on models involving non-normal response distributions. In many medical applications, the nonlinear relationships are studied simultaneously for a number of individuals, often over time, whether in epidemiology or in clinical trials. In such situations, it is also necessary to use multivariate distributions to take into account the dependency among the repeated responses on each subject. Appendix B provides information on various possible dependency structures for use in such models.

Nonlinear modelling does require some knowledge of fairly advanced mathematics and statistics. The need for multivariate distributions has just been mentioned. The nonlinear regression curves themselves often must be derived by the solution of differential equations. Complex numerical methods are required for optimizing and subsequently studying the form of the likelihood function for the model.

The first three chapters provide a general introduction to nonlinear modelling. The following chapters are organized around a number of the most important areas of medical research: epidemiology, clinical trials, pharmacokinetics, molecular biology, and so on. Various applications of nonlinear models are given in each area, based on actual research studies. This, however, does not imply that the examples presented here are the only applications of nonlinear modelling in a given area. Nor does it mean that the models illustrated in a given area are not widely used in many other areas. Indeed, for example, growth curves in various forms reappear in several chapters.

All of the examples in this text were analysed using functions written in the freely available software, R, a fast clone of S-Plus developed by Ross Ihaka, Robert Gentleman, and the R core group (Ihaka and Gentleman, 1996; Gentleman and Ihaka, 2000). These libraries of R functions, required for replicating the modelling, are available at www.luc.ac.be/~jlindsey.

The original data sets come from a wide number of sources. The references to those from the literature are given when they are used; the authors are to be thanked for making them publicly available. Dan Heitjan kindly provided the clinical trial data in Section 5.2, Luc Duchateau the quality of life data in Section 6.5, Bill Byrom the pharmacokinetic data in Section 7.2, and John Stephens the pharmacodynamic data in Section 8.3.

The large data sets analysed in the examples are not reproduced in the text. They are available at the same site, along with the R code to perform the analyses of all the examples and reproduce the results in the text. On the other hand, the data for the exercises are given in Appendix C so that the reader can see more easily what is involved. (They are also available electronically at the above site.)

My thanks go to the many people who helped me in this work, including those mentioned above. The PKPD analyses in Chapter 7 were done in collaboration with Byron Jones. Patrick Lindsey helped with the analysis of the ordinal data in Chapter 6, including furnishing the computer code for hidden Markov models for ordinal responses, and with the copulas.

Troels Ring and Jan van den Broek provided useful comments on earlier versions of the manuscript and on the analysis of some of the examples; Pat Altham pointed out a number of errors in the text. My students in the Biostatistics Programme provided stimulation over the past two years to make my presentation clearer. Niko Speybroeck and Roel Straetemans were especially diligent in finding errors in the text and in the R code.

Diepenbeek J.K.L.
March, 2001

Contents

1 Basic concepts — 1
  1.1 Statistical modelling — 1
    1.1.1 Data-generating mechanisms — 1
    1.1.2 Probability models — 3
    1.1.3 Distributions — 5
    1.1.4 Regression functions — 7
  1.2 Limitations of generalized linear models — 9
    1.2.1 Definition — 10
    1.2.2 Choice of distribution — 11
    1.2.3 Regression functions — 12
    1.2.4 Dependent observations — 13
    1.2.5 Inference — 14
  1.3 Definitions of nonlinearity — 15
    1.3.1 Distribution and regression functions — 15
    1.3.2 Models with a linear part — 16
    1.3.3 Transformable linearity — 16
    1.3.4 Intrinsic and parameter-effects nonlinearity — 17
  1.4 Developing regression functions — 18
    1.4.1 Descriptive versus mechanistic models — 18
    1.4.2 Solving differential equations — 19
  1.5 Exercises — 22

2 Practical aspects — 23
  2.1 Data — 23
    2.1.1 Response variables — 23
    2.1.2 Covariates — 25
  2.2 Specifying models — 27
    2.2.1 Software — 27
    2.2.2 Model components — 27
  2.3 Calculating the likelihood — 29
    2.3.1 Nonlinear optimization — 29
    2.3.2 Parametrizations — 30
    2.3.3 Initial estimates — 31
    2.3.4 Checking convergence — 32
  2.4 Inference — 33

		2.4.1	Model selection	34
		2.4.2	Likelihood regions	34
		2.4.3	Goodness of fit	35
	2.5	Exercises		36

3 Families of nonlinear regression functions — 37
- 3.1 Growth curves — 37
  - 3.1.1 Polynomials — 37
  - 3.1.2 Exponential forms — 38
  - 3.1.3 Sigmoidal curves — 39
- 3.2 Sums of exponentials — 42
  - 3.2.1 Compartment models — 42
  - 3.2.2 Diffusion models — 44
- 3.3 Other nonlinear functions — 45
  - 3.3.1 Power functions — 45
  - 3.3.2 Cyclic functions — 45
  - 3.3.3 Change-point models — 46
- 3.4 Exercises — 47

4 Epidemiology — 49
- 4.1 Studying natural populations — 49
  - 4.1.1 Goals — 49
  - 4.1.2 Designs — 50
  - 4.1.3 Ecological regression — 50
- 4.2 Growth curves — 51
  - 4.2.1 Richards curve — 51
  - 4.2.2 Weight gains of pregnant women — 52
  - 4.2.3 Differences among women — 53
- 4.3 Death rates — 55
  - 4.3.1 Log linear models — 55
  - 4.3.2 Malignant neoplasms — 55
  - 4.3.3 Overdispersion — 56
- 4.4 Change points — 57
  - 4.4.1 Poisson process — 57
  - 4.4.2 The hæmolytic uræmic syndrome study — 58
  - 4.4.3 Detecting a change point — 58
  - 4.4.4 A dynamic model — 60
- 4.5 Recurrent epidemics — 60
  - 4.5.1 Epidemic models — 63
  - 4.5.2 Childhood infections — 65
- 4.6 Infectious disease outbreaks — 67
  - 4.6.1 Micro-organism subtyping — 67
  - 4.6.2 Typing model — 68
  - 4.6.3 The Maine tuberculosis outbreak — 69

		4.7	Exercises	69
5	**Clinical trials**			73
	5.1		Evaluating a new medication	73
		5.1.1	Goals	73
		5.1.2	Designs	74
		5.1.3	Validity	74
		5.1.4	Models	75
	5.2		Response decline to a stable state	75
		5.2.1	The azathioprine study	75
		5.2.2	Asymptotic and polynomial curves	76
		5.2.3	Conclusions	82
	5.3		Exercises	83
6	**Quality of life**			85
	6.1		Effects of medical treatment	85
		6.1.1	Goals	85
		6.1.2	Constructing event history models	85
		6.1.3	Models for ordinal variables	86
	6.2		Recurrent events	88
		6.2.1	The bladder cancer study	88
		6.2.2	Birth processes	88
	6.3		Change of state	90
		6.3.1	The adenosine deaminase study	90
		6.3.2	Time-varying covariates	91
	6.4		Transition probabilities	93
		6.4.1	The peptic œsophagitis study	93
		6.4.2	Ordinal regression	95
		6.4.3	Random walks	95
	6.5		Analysis of diary cards	96
		6.5.1	The seasonal rhinitis study	97
		6.5.2	Spells	97
	6.6		Exercises	101
7	**Pharmacokinetics**			105
	7.1		Studying drug concentrations in the body	105
		7.1.1	Goals	105
		7.1.2	Compartment models	106
		7.1.3	Statistical models	110
	7.2		Parent drug and metabolite	113
		7.2.1	The flosequinan study	113
		7.2.2	Modelling the parent drug	114
		7.2.3	Modelling the metabolite	119
		7.2.4	Simultaneous modelling	121

		7.2.5	Serial dependence	126
		7.2.6	Conclusions	130
	7.3	Repeated dosing		131
		7.3.1	The propoxyphene study	131
		7.3.2	Tracking patients	132
	7.4	Exercises		135
8	**Pharmacodynamics**			**141**
	8.1	Studying the effects of drugs on the body		141
		8.1.1	Goals	141
		8.1.2	Response variables	142
	8.2	Continuous response		142
		8.2.1	The gastric pH study	142
		8.2.2	Regression functions	143
		8.2.3	Gaussian copulas	143
	8.3	Count response		146
		8.3.1	The capsaicin cough challenge study	146
		8.3.2	Overdispersed autoregression	150
		8.3.3	Analysing the challenge–response curve	151
		8.3.4	Conclusions	153
	8.4	Exercises		155
9	**Assays and formulations**			**157**
	9.1	Assays		157
		9.1.1	Goals	157
		9.1.2	Methods	158
	9.2	Colorimetric enzyme assay		159
		9.2.1	Assay methodology	159
		9.2.2	Michaëlis–Menten function	159
		9.2.3	Analysis of the acid phosphatase assay	160
	9.3	DNase assay		161
		9.3.1	Generalized Michaëlis–Menten function	161
		9.3.2	Analysis of the rat serum	163
	9.4	Ames *Salmonella* microsome assay		164
		9.4.1	Assay methodology	164
		9.4.2	Mechanistic models	166
		9.4.3	The International Programme on Chemical Safety study	168
	9.5	Determining formulations		169
		9.5.1	Developing delivery systems	169
		9.5.2	Transport models	171
		9.5.3	Pill dissolution rates	172
	9.6	Exercises		174

10	**Molecular genetics**		179
	10.1 Sequence analysis		179
		10.1.1 Basic DNA structure	179
		10.1.2 Sequencing methods	180
		10.1.3 Alignment	181
	10.2 Finding genes and their exons		182
		10.2.1 The β-globin gene	183
		10.2.2 Locating the gene	184
		10.2.3 Locating the exons	185
	10.3 Detecting locations of mutations		187
		10.3.1 Mitochondrial DNA	187
		10.3.2 Modelling mutation rates	188
	10.4 Exercises		190

APPENDICES

A	**Data and model examples from R**		193
	A.1 Data		193
		A.1.1 Data objects	193
		A.1.2 Data methods	196
	A.2 Models		198
		A.2.1 Software	198
		A.2.2 Probability distribution	198
		A.2.3 Covariate dependence	199
		A.2.4 General nonlinear specification	200
	A.3 Likelihoods		202
		A.3.1 A simple example	202
		A.3.2 More complex cases	203
B	**Stochastic dependence structures**		205
	B.1 Random effects		205
		B.1.1 Mixture models	205
		B.1.2 Conjugate distributions	207
		B.1.3 Other mixtures	207
	B.2 Time dependence		208
		B.2.1 Ordered dependence	208
		B.2.2 Autoregression	209
	B.3 Multivariate distributions with correlation matrices		211
		B.3.1 Multivariate Student t distribution	211
		B.3.2 Multivariate power-exponential distribution	212
		B.3.3 Copulas	213
	B.4 Dynamic models		214
		B.4.1 Dynamic generalized linear models	214

		B.4.2	General dynamic nonlinear models	215
	B.5	Markov processes		219
		B.5.1	Markov chains	219
		B.5.2	Hidden Markov models	220
	B.6	Duration data		221
		B.6.1	Survival and intensity functions	222
		B.6.2	Counting processes	224
		B.6.3	Important special cases	227
C	**Data tables for the exercises**			229
	C.1	Gastric half-emptying times		229
	C.2	Bacteriuria infections		230
	C.3	Cases of lung cancer		231
	C.4	Case–control study of asbestos		232
	C.5	Rectal polyps		233
	C.6	Recurrence of kidney infections		237
	C.7	Mammary tumours		238
	C.8	Skin papilloma in mice		240
	C.9	LeukÆmia clinical trial		241
	C.10	LeukÆmia patients		242
	C.11	Breast cancer		243
	C.12	Prednisolone concentrations		244
	C.13	Indomethicin concentrations		245
	C.14	Ephedrine concentrations		245
	C.15	Blood glucose levels		246
	C.16	Theophylline concentrations		248
	C.17	Declomycin concentrations		249
	C.18	Propoxyphene concentrations		250
	C.19	Phenylbiguanide and blood pressure		251
	C.20	ELISA for anticoronavirus		251
	C.21	Cortisol radioimmunological assay		252
	C.22	ELISA for allergens		252
	C.23	Penicillin G and theophylline		253

Bibliography 255

Author index 263

Subject index 266

1
Basic concepts

Nonlinear modelling is one of the more sophisticated areas of modern statistics. It involves advanced statistical concepts from a wide variety of areas, from inference to repeated measurements. In this chapter, I shall review some of the most important ones. Those for stochastic dependencies are outlined in Appendix B. Still others will be introduced throughout the following chapters, as required.

1.1 Statistical modelling

Statisticians often seem most fascinated by inference: how to draw general conclusions from specific, limited observations. Here, I concentrate on a different aspect of the statistical approach: how best to represent the 'reality' of what has been observed, both its systematic and its random aspects.

1.1.1 DATA-GENERATING MECHANISMS

A *model* is a simplifying representation of some *data-generating mechanism*. The latter is some complex process of interest whereby empirical observations can actually be produced. Usually, we are not interested in all of the complexities of the process that produces what is observed. Instead, we want to isolate certain pertinent aspects; these will depend on the goal of the study, that is, on the problem to be solved, and should still be present if observations were made in other similar circumstances. This is an important simplifying role of models.

Components of models Generally, in a model, we distinguish between *systematic* and *random*, or stochastic, variability, where the former describes the patterns of the phenomenon in which we are particularly interested. Thus, the distinction between the two depends on the phenomenon under study and on the particular questions being asked. Random variability can be described by a probability distribution, perhaps multivariate, or by a stochastic process, whereas the systematic part generally involves one or more regression functions.

Thus, in statistical modelling, we are interested in discovering what we can learn about systematic patterns from empirical data containing a random component. Although we suppose that some complex data-generating mechanism has produced the observations, we try to describe it by some simpler, but still realistic, model that highlights the specific aspects of interest. Thus, by definition, scientific models are never 'true' in any sense.

The type of data-generating mechanism that we consider to be operating will depend on the level of analysis of interest in the problem at hand. We can expect differing results when we construct the corresponding models to work at the levels of the atom, molecule, cell, organ, living being, or community.

In many situations, all of the factors not directly accounted for in the model cannot be controlled; they may vary over time. We must be assured that those aspects of the data-generating mechanism of interest are acting stably throughout and that they are not distorted by the process of data collection.

Types of mechanisms Two quite distinct types of data-generating mechanism commonly occur and should be clearly distinguished. In the natural sciences, such as physics and chemistry, and in engineering, deterministic scientific laws may be assumed to underlie many processes and can be expected to operate in any suitable circumstances. An important example in medical statistics is the analysis of assays (Chapter 9). The random variability in empirical studies, in such cases, may be assumed to arise purely from the production and observation process of the study. They may truly be called measurement 'errors'.

On the other hand, in studies involving living organisms, and especially human beings who have language, memory, and a will of their own, each individual has an enormous amount of built-in variability, due to genetic, environmental, and other factors. Thus, here the systematic 'laws' to be studied must include a random part or be *stochastic*. Measurement error is proportionally minor as compared to other sources of variation. In studies of living beings, most variability is (hopefully) *not* due to 'errors'!

Roles of models When scientists speak (loosely) of a scientific law, or a model, as being 'correct', they mean that any known deviations from it are sufficiently minor so as to be irrelevant for present practical purposes. The best *available* law or model will be used for scientific prediction, even given such discrepancies. Statistics has an important role to play in determining which is currently best.

Models, thus, serve to summarize, explain, and transmit available theoretical knowledge within the scientific community, making it unnecessary for the whole body of empirical observation to be directly available to every member. If a model can be completely specified beforehand, which is rarely the case, then data collection will serve only to check its validity. More usually, some parameters in the model have unknown values and data will also serve to provide information about them. The actual functional form of the model may not even be known with certainty so that several are in competition.

Some idea about possible values of the unknown parameter may be available but this is generally extremely difficult to quantify and rarely has the general agreement of the scientific community in the way that choice of models does.

1.1. STATISTICAL MODELLING

Thus, scientific data collection concentrates on obtaining empirical information about the functional form and validity of models and about values of unknown parameters in them.

A stochastic model must

(1) be in accordance with previous theoretical knowledge and empirical information;
(2) specify the probability distribution of all observations included in the data, taken as a typical sample;
(3) include, as parameters, all unknown constants to be estimated;
(4) not be contradicted in any relevant way by the newly collected data.

(Fisher, 1955)

Sample size In the study of deterministic data-generating mechanisms, increasing the number of observations should reduce the overall error in the parameters of interest, and, with enough observations, we should obtain the true values of the parameters in the model. Such circumstances are only available in tightly controlled laboratory conditions, and often not even then. However, in the study of human beings, we are faced with a dynamic situation that can never be exactly reproduced. Increasing the number of observations above a certain minimum will not usually yield more precise estimates of the parameters of a simple model but will, instead, force us to change to a more complex model.

Thus, as the number of observations increases, more complex models may be fitted, perhaps closer to the data-generating mechanism. Conversely, if enough observations are collected, any model with a fixed, finite number of unknown parameters can usually be shown to be untenable. If only simple models are of interest, then the *sample size* should be kept reasonably small. It should be just large enough for the aspect of the phenomenon of interest to be detectable; otherwise, time and money will be wasted.

1.1.2 PROBABILITY MODELS

The first step in the model-building procedure will involve the selection of one or more appropriate probability distributions to describe the random generation of some *response variable*, say Y, to be observed. These should be chosen to describe, in an informative way, some underlying data-generating mechanism which is of interest. Thus, a model is some more or less reasonable simple mathematical approximation to the reality of the data-generating mechanism that may help us in understanding the functioning of that mechanism. A model *smoothes* the observed data a chosen amount; this may help us to see patterns in them and to understand them. *No model is true.*

Types of randomness Following our discussion to now, we can distinguish three types of randomness in data generation:

(1) the stochastic process leading to the specific observed response(s) of an individual—this is the data-generating mechanism that the scientist wishes to study;
(2) random measurement errors in generating and observing the response;
(3) randomness introduced into the design of the observation scheme to ensure that the desired data-generating mechanism is actually being observed.

In all cases, the design described in point (3) should highlight the data-generating mechanism and not distort it. Its role is as guarantor that the data collection process has been correctly accomplished.

Point (2) above, measurement error, is an unavoidable side effect of all empirical observation. If this is judged to be important, it may need to be included in the model describing the data-generating mechanism. Often such errors can be modelled by a normal distribution. However, in most contexts outside of deterministic models, such variability will (hopefully!) be minor as compared to that created by the data-generating mechanism.

Describing individual variability   Suppose that we are interested in some large, but finite, clearly definable *population* of individuals. One fruitful, but simplistic, way to think of the data-generating mechanism in point (1) above is as some process that allocates each individual to one of a number of discrete classes defined by the values of some variable. This is the response to be observed, the data to be generated.

The categories can be assumed discrete, for the moment, because any existing measuring instrument has finite precision, called the *unit of measurement*. Then, if all individuals in the population, however conceived, could be observed, a histogram of the population frequencies could be constructed for that variable. Owing to the random elements in this generation process, described above, no simple mathematical function could ever be expected to describe it exactly. In fact, the larger is the population, the more difficult the task would be! However, certain systematic features should be present.

When a sample is collected from the population, we can actually construct a histogram. In spite of the random variation, we hope to be able to discern the same systematic features as would be present in the population histogram and to be able to describe them by a simple model, not depending on sample size. If the sample is too small, only random fluctuation will be present. But increasing it beyond some reasonable size will not generally augment knowledge about those aspects of the data-generating mechanism, that is, the pattern, of interest. Rather, the uninteresting irregularities of the population will become more apparent. The simple model for the pattern of interest will not converge to some 'true' data-generating mechanism; instead, the complexity of the model would need to be allowed to increase with the sample size for the data to be adequately described.

1.1. STATISTICAL MODELLING

Parameters Often the model describing the data-generating mechanism is only specified up to some unknown constants, called parameters, indexing a family of distributions. (When statisticians interact with scientists, this can be confusing because the latter generally refer to observable, and controllable, quantities as parameters: the statistician's variables.) In other words, one or more mathematical functions are proposed as descriptions of the pertinent features of the histogram.

Each probability distribution corresponds to some aspects of one or more possible data-generating mechanisms. Thus, the appropriate distribution should be chosen in light of knowledge about this mechanism.

This simplified description of model building has limited usefulness because it supposes that the population is static, whereas it will often be in dynamic evolution, perhaps even during the time in which a sample can be collected.

1.1.3 DISTRIBUTIONS

Let us now summarize the preceding developments.

Random component In the simplest cases, we observe some *response variable* on a number of independent subjects under conditions that we assume homogeneous in all aspects of interest. Certain responses will appear more frequently than others as the result of some stochastic data-generating mechanism that we imagine might have produced them. Our model, then, is some *probability distribution*, hopefully corresponding in pertinent ways to this mechanism, and one that we expect might represent adequately the frequencies with which the various possible responses are observed.

The hypothesized data-generating mechanism, and the corresponding candidate statistical models to describe it, are scientific or technical constructs. They are used to gain insight into the process under study, but are generally vast simplifications of reality. In a more descriptive context, a model is just smoothing the random irregularities in the data; in this way, we are attempting to detect patterns in them.

Location and dispersion parameters A probability distribution will usually have one or more unknown parameters that can be estimated from the data, allowing it to be fitted to them. Often, one parameter will represent the average response, or some transformation of it. This determines the *location* of the distribution on the axis of the responses. If there are other parameters, they will describe, in various ways, the *variability* or *dispersion* of the responses. They determine the *shape* of the distribution, although the location parameter will usually also play an important role in this, the shape almost always changing with its location.

Choice of an appropriate location parameter can be very important, especially if the dispersion is not constant. A model with a simple relationship of, say, the geometric mean to covariates can induce a very complex relationship of the arithmetic mean to those covariates. See Section 1.3.3.

Types of response variables Responses may generally be classified into three broad types:

(1) measurements that can take any real value, positive or negative;
(2) measurements that can take only positive values;
(3) records of the frequency of occurrence of one or more kinds of events.

Let us consider them in turn.

Continuous responses The first type of response is well known because elementary statistics courses concentrate on normal theory models: linear regression and analysis of variance. However, such responses are probably the rarest of the three types actually encountered in practice. Response variables that have positive probability for negative values are rather difficult to find, making such models generally unrealistic, except as a rough approximation. This approximation will generally be best when all response values are large (far from zero). Such models have certain nice mathematical properties, but, for this very reason, the characteristics of these models are unrepresentative and quite misleading when we try to generalize to more realistic models.

Positive responses When responses are measurements, they most often can only take positive values (length, area, volume, weight, time, and so on). The distribution of the responses will usually be skewed, especially if many of these values tend to be relatively close to zero.

One type of positive response of special interest in medical statistics is the measurement of the duration time to some event (Section B.6): infection, illness, recovery, death, and so on. Because the length of time during which observations can be made is usually limited, an additional problem may be present: the response time may not be completely observed—it is censored if the event has not yet occurred; we only know that it is at least as long as the observation time.

Events Many responses are simple records of the occurrence of events. (In fact, *any* observation can be thought of as the record of an event.) If the event is repeatable, we shall often be interested in the *intensity* with which the events occur on each subject. If only one type of event is being recorded, summary data may take the form of *counts*: the number of times the event has occurred to a given subject (usual at least implicitly within some fixed interval of time). If more than one type of response event is possible, we have categorical data, with one category corresponding to each event type. If several such events are being recorded on each subject, we may still have counts, but now as many types on each subject as there are categories (some may be zero counts).

The categories may simply be nominal, or they may be ordered. If only one event is recorded on each subject, similar events may be aggregated across subjects to form *frequencies* in a *contingency table*. When covariates distinguish among events on the same subject, the situation becomes even more complex.

1.1. STATISTICAL MODELLING

Duration time responses are closely connected to event responses, because times are measured between events. Thus, many of the models for these two types of responses are closely related.

1.1.4 REGRESSION FUNCTIONS

Covariates A data-generating mechanism will generally not be identical for all subjects observed and, indeed, may change over time for the same individual. In the simple situation described so far, the variability in response outcomes was accounted for by the randomness in the probability distribution. However, in nonlinear modelling, we are usually interested in *systematic* changes in variability among distinguishable subgroups of the population and/or with the changing conditions of each individual, described by *explanatory variables* or *covariates*, including time. We, then, want to discover how the probability distribution of the random response variable changes shape among these different groups and conditions, a conditional distribution. In terms of our histograms above, we wish to see how they change form under the different conditions.

Models are intended to influence our future expectations about observations not already made. A scientific study must be designed to provide information about such generalizations. Obviously, if enough conditions (covariates) were specified, each individual observed in the study would be uniquely identified, that is, would have a unique data-generating mechanism. The model would be deterministic, and of little use. It would mean that the observed individuals were uninformative about those not observed and generalization could not be made. In empirical studies, probability statements rarely refer to individuals, except as typical members of some population. One important exception is the problem of predicting the future response of an individual based on a series of previously observed responses.

In a stochastic model, any variability that is not of direct interest should usually be allowed to be random. Thus, covariates are only used to describe the systematic effects of interest, within the data-generating mechanism, while the random or stochastic part of the model, the probability distribution, must describe the remaining variability. This is illustrated, for simple linear regression, in Figure 1.1. This is an extreme special case: the normal distribution, of constant shape because the variance is assumed constant, is being displaced to follow the straight regression line as the covariate changes.

Systematic component In simple cases, with only one response value per individual (however, see Section 2.1), we can denote the conditions specified by the covariates using a matrix, say **X**, called the *design matrix*. Here, each column, indexed by j, specifies a different type of fixed condition, and each row, indexed by i, a different individual. Thus, an entry in the matrix gives the (static) situation of the ith individual for the jth type of condition. This matrix defines a *design space* describing the conditions in which the study was conducted. Stating that conditions are fixed, and not stochastic, is arbitrary, but is generally done because, at

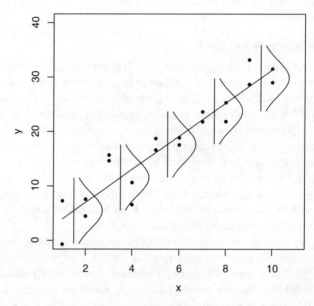

Fig. 1.1. A graphical representation of a simple linear normal regression showing the linear form of the regression function and the constant shape of the distribution about it.

least in simple cases, we are not interested in how they arise or do not have information about this; we are only interested in how they relate to the data-generating mechanism, and hence to the response.

Most often, a further simplifying assumption has been made: that only one parameter, say μ, in the probability distribution, describing the mean response, or some function of it, changes with the conditions of the individual. Thus, only the *location* of the histogram is changing. We might choose functions such that

$$g(\mu_i) = h(\mathbf{x}_i, \boldsymbol{\beta}) \tag{1.1}$$

Here, the function $h(\mathbf{x}_i, \boldsymbol{\beta})$ is called the systematic component of the model. Because the function $g(\cdot)$ links this component to the random or stochastic component, the probability distribution, through the mean value, it is called the *link function*.

We may note two important points in passing.

(1) There is no reason why only the mean parameter should change with the conditions: other parameters, such as the variance, or other shape and dispersion parameters, can also be made dependent on the covariates (see Sections 1.2.3 and 2.2.2).

(2) If both $g(\cdot)$ and $h(\cdot)$ are nonlinear, then they can be combined as

1.2. LIMITATIONS OF GENERALIZED LINEAR MODELS

$$\begin{aligned}\mu_i &= g^{-1}[h(\mathbf{x}_i, \boldsymbol{\beta})] \\ &= h^*(\mathbf{x}_i, \boldsymbol{\beta})\end{aligned} \quad (1.2)$$

without loss of generality.

In many situations, the systematic component, $h(\cdot)$, has been assumed, for mathematical simplicity, to be a linear function of the unknown parameters, $\boldsymbol{\beta}$,

$$h(\mathbf{x}_i, \boldsymbol{\beta}) = \boldsymbol{\beta}^\mathrm{T} \mathbf{x}_i \quad (1.3)$$

called the *linear structure* or *linear predictor*. Notice that this emphasis and terminology contrasts with the interests of scientists who are concerned with the linearity of the response in relation to $\mathbf{X}$.

When this linear function is equated to a link function for the mean, we have a *linear regression model*. One important family of such models is called the *generalized linear model* (Section 1.2; see also Nelder and Wedderburn, 1972, or Lindsey, 1997). Of course, in this text, we shall rather be interested in systematic components that are nonlinear functions.

Parameters index a family of models. In certain situations, especially when a model is not mechanistic, they may have no intrinsic interest, serving primarily to determine the shape of the probability distribution and of the systematic part. Then, they usually can be specified in a number of different, but equivalent, ways.

Simplifying assumptions We may now summarize some of the possible simplifying assumptions in model building suggested up until this point:

- observations can be made independently of each other;
- the data-generating mechanism is stable enough over time (and space) so that a small selection of observations from a long series will provide useful information about patterns of interest;
- the random part of the process can be described usefully by some simple probability function;
- this function is the same under all conditions, with only (some of) its parameters changing value;
- the systematic part involves only changes in the mean of that distribution; and
- these changes in the mean (or some function of it) are linearly (in the parameters) related to the conditions of interest.

As I have already indicated, most of these are simplistic but useful approximations that should be abandoned when necessary in any particular setting. One goal of this book is to illustrate ways in which this can be done.

1.2 Limitations of generalized linear models

Generalized linear models were the first class of nonlinear models to become widely available. For this reason, it is useful to look at them briefly.

These models have provided a unified approach to many of the common classical statistical procedures used in applied statistics. They established a first step towards making nonlinear models widely available, by relaxing certain of the strong assumptions of the classical linear normal model. In the years since the term was first introduced by Nelder and Wedderburn in 1972, they have slowly become more well known and more widely used.

The introduction of such models in the early 1970s had a significant impact on the way applied statistics has been carried out. In the beginning, their use was primarily restricted to fairly advanced statisticians because the only explanatory material and software available were addressed to them. One had to wait up to 20 years for generalized linear modelling procedures to be made more widely available in general-purpose computer packages such as Genstat, R, S-Plus, SAS, Stata, or XLisp-Stat.

However, we must now face the fact that such an approach is decidedly outdated, not in the sense that it is no longer useful, but in its limiting restrictions as compared to the kinds of statistical models that are needed with today's complex data sets and possible with modern computing power. What are now required, and feasible, are nonlinear models, often with dependence structures among responses.

Many of the restrictions imposed by generalized linear models arise from the powerful algorithm widely used in their estimation, iterated weighted least squares (IWLS): these are linearity of the regression function, need for a link function, limited choice among distributions.

1.2.1 DEFINITION

Let me first quickly review how generalized linear models are defined.

Response distribution Suppose that Y_i ($i = 1, \ldots, N$) are independent random variables, with means μ_i and observed values $y_i = \mu_i + \varepsilon_i$, where the ε_i are the residuals or 'errors'. These random variables share the same distribution from the exponential (dispersion) family

$$f[y_i; \theta(\mu_i), \phi] = \exp\left[\frac{y_i \theta(\mu_i) - b[\theta(\mu_i)]}{a(\phi)} + c(y_i, \phi)\right] \tag{1.4}$$

where $\theta(\cdot)$, $a(\cdot)$, $b(\cdot)$, and $c(\cdot)$ are known functions. This probability model for the data is the random or stochastic component.

Linear predictor Suppose now that a set of P (usually) unknown parameters, $\boldsymbol{\beta} = [\beta_1, \ldots, \beta_P]^T$, and the corresponding set of known covariates, $\mathbf{X}_{N \times P} = [\mathbf{x}_1, \ldots, \mathbf{x}_N]^T$, the design or model matrix, are such that Equation (1.3) holds:

$$h(\mathbf{x}_i, \boldsymbol{\beta}) = \mathbf{x}_i^T \boldsymbol{\beta}$$

As we have seen, these define the linear predictor. This describes how the location of the response distribution changes with the covariates. This *location regression*

1.2. LIMITATIONS OF GENERALIZED LINEAR MODELS

function for the data defines the systematic component. In more general cases of interest, outside the generalized linear model context, the structure describing change in location will be nonlinear, although it may contain linear components (Section 1.3.2).

Link function The relationship between the mean of the ith response and its *linear* predictor is given by the link function, $g_i(\cdot)$:

$$g_i(\mu_i) = \mathbf{x}_i^T \boldsymbol{\beta} \tag{1.5}$$

If $\theta(\mu_i) = g_i(\mu_i)$, this is known as the canonical link function.

The link function introduces the nonlinearity of the regression function in generalized linear models. The function must be monotonic and differentiable. Usually the same link function is used for all observations. A link function is only useful when there is a *linear* predictor; it serves no role for completely nonlinear models, as shown by Equation (1.2).

Generalized linear models may be fitted using a generalization of the 'least squares' procedure, IWLS. This is particularly interesting because, in contrast to most other nonlinear models, initial values of the parameters are not required. It has been implemented in such programs as Genstat, GLIM, R, S-Plus, Stata, and XLisp-Stat.

However, in modern statistics, there is no reason to constrain one's choice to this particular family. This is severely limiting because it only involves essentially linear regression models and only distributions from the exponential (dispersion) family. It is possible to combine any probability distribution with a location regression function; indeed, any parameter, not just the location parameter, can depend on covariates. In this way, we can obtain truly flexible statistical models to describe and to understand our data.

1.2.2 CHOICE OF DISTRIBUTION

Exponential dispersion family Generalized linear models are widely stated to be based on the exponential family of distributions. This is only correct if the dispersion parameter has a known value. More accurately and more generally, they are based on the exponential dispersion family (Tweedie, 1947; Jørgensen, 1987).

The standard models in this family involve the binomial, Poisson, normal, gamma, and inverse Gaussian distributions. Certain other useful members of the exponential family have long been excluded from practical applications because of an intractable normalizing constant. These include the multiplicative binomial distribution (Altham, 1978), the double exponential family (Efron, 1986), and a family of multivariate distributions (Marshall and Olkin, 1988). With modern computing power, these can now easily be handled.

Other distributions Certain parametric regression models, such as Weibull regression, that are not members of the generalized linear model family are fairly widely used. But why not also have a choice among the Student t, Laplace, and stable (Section 1.2.5) distributions, and three-parameter extensions of the gamma (Section 7.1.3), logistic, inverse Gaussian, or Weibull distributions, as well as the exponential dispersion family? With modern computing power and efficient nonlinear optimization algorithms, there is no longer any reason why generalized modelling procedures should not include such a vast array of possibilities.

Another collection of models that is not widely enough used is finite mixtures (see, for example, Wang *et al.*, 1996). Mixtures of two groups are especially important, where one of them involves a specific response value. Examples include zero-inflated Poisson data (see Lambert, 1992) and right-censored duration data where some subjects will never have the event (Farewell, 1982; Schmidt and Witte, 1988; Lindsey, 1998).

Censoring In the early days of generalized linear models, intricate procedures were invented in order to fit censored data (Aitkin and Clayton, 1980; Whitehead, 1980), even for distributions that are not generalized linear models. Now such techniques, although still widely used, are no longer necessary with modern computing power. Many programmable statistical software packages have available functions for the common cumulative probability distributions so that the likelihood functions for models involving censored data can easily be constructed and maximized (Section 2.3).

Alternatively, by means of the counting process approach, the intensity functions for common models can be fitted using Poisson regression, automatically handling censoring (Lindsey, 1995b). With nonlinear Poisson regression available, any intensity function can be fitted (Section B.6.2). This approach is especially important when time-varying covariates are present (Section 6.3.2).

Interval censoring is another widely discussed problem. However, in fact, all *observable* data are interval censored. In other words, the likelihood function, defined as the probability of the observed data, must allow for this. Thus, for example, using the probability functions mentioned above, one can program these exact likelihood functions for any data, as the product (for independent observations) of differences of such functions.

1.2.3 REGRESSION FUNCTIONS

Nonlinearity Linear regression has been a mainstay of statistics for centuries. A course concentrating on it remains at the centre of any respectable statistics programme. And yet linearity, in most problems, can only be a local approximation. To a large extent, generalized linear models retain the linearity requirement. Their innovation was to allow the mean to be a nonlinear function of this linear regression.

Nonlinear modelling with a normal distribution is now fairly well known; some rather sophisticated models have appeared (Heitjan, 1991a, 1991b). However, little work has been done for non-normal distributions with nonlinear regression functions.

1.2. LIMITATIONS OF GENERALIZED LINEAR MODELS

Nonconstant dispersion One of the fundamental postulates of classical linear regression is that the variance remains constant. Generalized linear models essentially retain this assumption, only relaxing it slightly. The *variance* is no longer constant, becoming a *fixed* function of the mean, but this is only a parameter of direct importance for the normal distribution. On the other hand, the dispersion parameter of each distribution is held constant.

In a generalized linear model, other than those based on the normal distribution, the shape, and not just the location, of the distribution depends on the covariates in the regression function. However, there is no reason not to let other parameters than the mean also vary, depending on some second, or third, regression function in the same model. Dispersion varying with the covariates is surprisingly common, considering that it is so often ignored (or attempts made to transform it away). However, in certain circumstances, it is standard practice. For example, pharmacokinetic models (Section 7.1.3) generally require a separate regression function for the dispersion parameter.

Statisticians have a fetish for analysing means, sometimes without any idea as to what distribution (if any) they refer. When comparing responses to different values of covariates, whether experimental treatments or observational values, it is totally unrealistic to assume that only location, and not the shape, of the distribution will change. Differences in overall shape of the distribution, and not just one measure of location, should be central to most scientific questions.

1.2.4 DEPENDENT OBSERVATIONS

The complexity of data sets has been rapidly increasing over time, as adequate means of collecting and managing large bodies of data have become available. Much of these data concern clustered or longitudinal observations so that the responses involve interdependencies (Appendix B). Although a fair number of useful models have been proposed, virtually no standard software is available, outside of the multivariate normal case. Much of this concentrates on random effects, with little attention to serial dependence.

For longitudinal data that may be serially dependent, a common method is to condition on previous responses in the regression function. However, this is generally only appropriate if the times are equally spaced and there is no problem with missing data. In other more complex situations, dynamic models using generalizations of the Kalman filter are now being developed (Lindsey, 1999a; see Section B.4).

For uniform dependence structures among clustered observations, the standard approach is to use a mixture distribution based on a random effects model as an artificial construct to generate a multivariate distribution. Certain such procedures have a reasonably long history, especially for overdispersion in count data and for split-plot designs. Fairly complex exact model-building procedures are now available, usually involving numerical integration.

Various approximations for mixture models have also been proposed, but some have the unfortunate characteristic that they do not specify the complete distributional assumptions about the responses. This can often be the most important aspect of the systematic differences among treatments, rather than simply how means change.

1.2.5 INFERENCE

Estimation Maximum likelihood estimates of the linear regression parameters in a generalized linear model can quickly and easily be obtained by the IWLS algorithm. Major advantages of this procedure include the facts that it is very stable and trustworthy and that initial estimates need not be supplied but can be obtained from the data.

However, use of this procedure greatly restricts the number of models that can be considered. Fast and efficient nonlinear optimization algorithms are now available that calculate first and second derivatives numerically (Dennis and Schnabel, 1983) so that these need not be supplied by the user.

Many theoretically useful families of distributions exist outside the exponential (dispersion) family. As one example, consider the four-parameter family of stable distributions that is important because of the often expressed concern for robustness and accommodation of 'outliers'. For this family, the density and cumulative distributions are not analytically available, except for three cases (including the normal distribution); it is most often defined by its characteristic function,

$$\phi(u) = \exp\{i\mu u - \sigma |u|^\alpha [1 + i\beta \, \text{sign}(u) \, \omega(u, \alpha)]\} \qquad (1.6)$$

$$\text{where} \quad \omega(u, \alpha) = \begin{cases} \tan(\pi\alpha/2) & \text{if } \alpha \neq 1 \\ \frac{2}{\pi} \log|u| & \text{if } \alpha = 1 \end{cases}$$

and μ, σ, β, and α are, respectively, parameters controlling the location, dispersion, skewness, and thickness of tails of the distribution. Nevertheless, it is now possible to fit regression functions for this family interactively, even though this involves numerical inversion of the characteristic function for each observation at each step in the iteration in order to construct the likelihood function (Lambert and Lindsey, 1999).

Sufficient statistics With a known dispersion parameter and a canonical link function, this family has an important feature for certain inference procedures: all regression parameters have sufficient statistics. However, the weight of this advantage was already considerably weakened from the time when generalized linear models were introduced because noncanonical link functions were allowed. These do not have sufficient statistics for the regression parameters.

Deviance Historically, inference procedures for generalized linear models have been based on the (scaled) deviance: in simple cases, twice the negative log likelihood ratio. The factor of two indicates that it as an asymptotic frequentist procedure. In addition, when the distribution contains a scale parameter, it is factored out, so that the deviance no longer corresponds directly to a likelihood. This has

1.3. DEFINITIONS OF NONLINEARITY

led to confusion in the literature because many writers, especially outside the generalized linear model context, call any $-2\log$ likelihood a deviance (what a GLIM user calls a scaled deviance).

A major disadvantage of founding inferences on deviances is that these are not comparable for different distributions. Generalized linear models provide us with a choice of distributions, but neither frequentists nor Bayesians have given us any simple statistical tools for choosing among them for a given data set. For skewed data, how do we choose among the log normal, gamma, and inverse Gaussian distributions (without mentioning those outside the family of generalized linear models)?

Model selection Use of the complete likelihood, including all constants, makes such inferences possible. However, if different numbers of parameters are involved in the models to be compared, the $-\log$ likelihood should be correspondingly penalized in some way. Model selection criteria, such as the AIC (Section 2.4.1), add the number of estimated parameters to the $-\log$ likelihood (in this text, not multiplied by two), although other penalties for complexity will be more reasonable in specific contexts. Smaller values indicate more preferable models.

Indeed, the ability to make such comparisons allows us, among other things, to resolve, once and for all, the dilemma as to whether or not to transform any given response variable. Transformations of response variables, in fact, create new distributions, as with the log normal from the normal or the Weibull from the exponential. Hence, for example, we may judge whether a logarithmic transformation of the responses or a log link is more appropriate for a given data set. See Section 1.3.3 for further discussion.

1.3 Definitions of nonlinearity

As we have seen, most of the classical models used in statistics are linear. We have noted that this implies linearity in the parameters, not the variables, although the latter is what will be of scientific interest. Thus, a function is nonlinear in its parameters if at least one of its derivatives with respect to the parameters in it depends on at least one of those parameters. If the derivative does not exist, as for change-point problems (Section 3.3.3), the model will also be said to be nonlinear.

1.3.1 DISTRIBUTION AND REGRESSION FUNCTIONS

In the strict sense, only the classical linear model—linear regression (including analysis of variance) involving the normal distribution with an identity link function—is linear: the maximum likelihood estimates may be obtained directly, without iteration, by solving the linear 'least squares' equations.

The extension of linear regression models to other distributions immediately implies nonlinearity in that the maximum likelihood estimates can only be obtained iteratively: the score equations are nonlinear. This, however, is not the usual sense in which the term, nonlinear models, is used. It generally refers only

16 [degrees of linearity] BASIC CONCEPTS

to a regression function that is nonlinear in its parameters, but still assuming a normal distribution. Hence, these provide two distinct departures from linearity: a non-normal distribution and/or a nonlinear regression function. In this book, I shall most often be interested in both occurring simultaneously.

1.3.2 MODELS WITH A LINEAR PART

As we have seen (Section 1.2.1), generalized linear models are a special case of nonlinear models that is particularly easy to handle. The models (except for the normal distribution with an identity link function) are nonlinear in the first sense above. However, the maximum likelihood estimates can be obtained by a simple extension of 'least squares' (IWLS) by iterating, playing on the linear part of the model. In terms of the canonical parameter of the exponential dispersion family, the models can be linear in the second sense (if the canonical link function is used). However, they are not linear, in the second sense, in terms of the mean parameter. Here, any link function, except the identity, introduces the nonlinearity.

Implementing models with a linear part outside the exponential dispersion family does not generally yield simple procedures for estimation so that they have not been widely investigated. We must cope with all of the problems of complete nonlinearity.

However, even in situations of 'complete' nonlinearity, it very often occurs that some 'linear part' exists in the model. Thus, in some standard nonlinear regression function, such as a logistic growth curve (Section 3.1.3) or a compartment model (Section 3.2.1), some physically interpretable parameter may vary in an additive way among subgroups of the population. Unfortunately, no simple methods are available that allow the nonlinear estimation problem to be simplified based on this partial linearity.

1.3.3 TRANSFORMABLE LINEARITY

Certain regression functions are *transformably* linear (sometimes called intrinsically linear, but see Section 1.3.4) in that a parameter transformation allows them to take a linear form.

Link functions One of the best known examples is the Michaëlis–Menten model for enzyme kinetics relating reaction velocity (y) to substrate concentration (x),

$$\mu_y(x) = \frac{\theta_1 x}{\theta_2 + x} \tag{1.7}$$

where θ_1 is the maximum velocity and θ_2 is the rate constant. This can be rewritten as

$$\frac{1}{\mu_y(x)} = \frac{1}{\theta_1} + \frac{\theta_2}{\theta_1}\frac{1}{x}$$
$$= \beta_0 + \beta_1 \frac{1}{x} \tag{1.8}$$

involving a reciprocal link function.

1.3. DEFINITIONS OF NONLINEARITY

Response transformations A possible alternative to using such a link function, often advocated, is to transform the response variable by taking reciprocals:

$$\mu_{1/y}(x) = \frac{1}{\theta_1} + \frac{\theta_2}{\theta_1}\frac{1}{x} \tag{1.9}$$

now with an identity link function. The results of such a procedure should be made clear to the user.

This response transformation modifies the skew of the distribution; if only measurement error is involved (Section 1.1.1), as in an assay (Chapter 9), this may not be a good idea because a normal distribution will often be most appropriate for the measured response, y, and not for its reciprocal, $1/y$. However, it also implies that the mean or location parameter is for the transformed (here, reciprocal) response scale; after such a transformation, it is generally difficult to obtain an expression for the mean on the original measurement scale.

In many applications, the log response has been assumed to have a normal distribution, or the response to have a log normal distribution, so that $\log(\mu)$ refers to the mean of the former quantity, estimated by $\sum \log(y_i)/N = \log(\prod y_i^{1/N})$. Hence, in such a model, μ is the geometric mean of response. The arithmetic mean for the log normal distribution is then given by $\exp[\log(\mu) + \sigma^2/2]$, where σ^2 is the variance.

Thus, when log response is used (with any distribution), the location regression parameters can only be interpreted in terms of the geometric mean of the response. The arithmetic mean will depend not only on these parameters but also on those in the variance (or dispersion) function. The situation is even more complex with other response transformations.

1.3.4 INTRINSIC AND PARAMETER-EFFECTS NONLINEARITY

Nonlinearity of the regression function can be investigated by studying its second derivatives (Bates and Watts, 1988, pp. 232–253; Seber and Wild, 1989, pp. 128–174). With P parameters, these $P \times P$ matrices can be evaluated at each set of covariate values. This can be considered to be a collection of, at most, $P(P+1)/2$ N-dimensional vectors. The latter can be decomposed into components normal (orthogonal) and tangent to the regression surface.

The degree to which these vectors lie outside the tangent plane, the normal component, measures how much the regression curve differs from linearity, called the *intrinsic nonlinearity* (not to be confused with the similar term in the literature sometimes referring to transformably linear; see Section 1.3.3). The tangent component depends on the parametrization, called *parameter-effects nonlinearity*. As such, these measures depend on the scaling of the data and the parameters (Section 2.3.2). Thus, relative curvatures should be calculated by dividing by the squared length of the tangent vector.

Intrinsic curvature is the reciprocal of the radius of the circle best approximating the regression surface in that direction. Its practical effects will be very small if there are sufficient data and the model being fitted is appropriate for them.

Reparametrization can only modify the parameter-effects nonlinearity. Certain transformations may reduce the effect for one data set and increase it for another.

One major disadvantage of such measures is that they describe the worst possible curvatures in any given direction. As well, because they have limited interest outside least squares estimation, further details are not given here.

1.4 Developing regression functions

Modern statistics can play many roles in the analysis of data containing random variability. Nonlinear models have a special place, especially in aiding scientific understanding. Usually, their development and use require close collaboration between the statisticians and the scientists, with their complementary areas of knowledge.

1.4.1 DESCRIPTIVE VERSUS MECHANISTIC MODELS

Much of modern statistics is primarily concerned with attempting to provide adequate *descriptions* of observed data, without trying to understand them. Major examples include nonparametric procedures such as splines and kernel density estimation, but also most applications of multiple regression and even some simple cases of analysis of variance. This approach has a major strength in that it allows the same basic techniques to be applied in a wide variety of disciplines. However, it provides little or no *understanding* of the process under study, of its data-generating mechanism (Section 1.1.1). In this sense, it may be said to be pre- or even anti-scientific. Such a statistical mentality arises because most statisticians are trained as mathematicians; they have little or no scientific background and are most at ease working with abstractions ('new statistical techniques looking for suitable data sets').

Most applications of nonlinear models provide a contrast to this in that they attempt to delve into the mechanics of data generation. Thus, they may be called mechanistic models because their users try to understand as much as possible of the mechanics of the process under study. Because of their complexity and their specificity, such models cannot be applied indiscriminately in just any context. Choosing or developing appropriate mechanistic nonlinear models demands close cooperation between scientists and statisticians.

Thus, for example, consider a study that records concentrations of a drug in the blood over time in a number of subjects under two treatments (see Chapter 7). On the one hand, one may simply look at differences in total drug available in the body (bioavailability) under the two treatments, perhaps measured by the 'area under the curve' (AUC). This might properly be handled by a classical analysis of variance. However, it tells us nothing about where and why that drug is available within the body. On the other hand, a pharmacokinetic analysis of drug concentration in the body over time generally requires a mechanistic nonlinear model, often a compartment model (Section 3.2.1), describing how concentration is changing over time. This, then, can inform us, for example, as to whether or

1.4. DEVELOPING REGRESSION FUNCTIONS

not differences between treatments arise from differences in absorption rates or in elimination rates, and so on.

If the scientists cannot suggest an appropriate mechanistic model, a literature search should be made to see if such models have been proposed in similar contexts. If none can be found, the scientists and statisticians will need to collaborate closely to develop a new one.

1.4.2 SOLVING DIFFERENTIAL EQUATIONS

If the phenomenon under study involves *rates* of change, then a model can often most easily be defined in terms of differential equations. These usually can only easily be solved if they are linear. In other cases, if the regression function involves nonlinear differential equations or integral equations, values can only be obtained numerically for a specified set of parameter values.

Direct solution In the simplest case of one linear equation, the result can be obtained by direct integration. Suppose, for example, that the change in the rate of a function is proportional to its size:

$$\frac{d\mu(t)}{dt} = -k\mu(t) \tag{1.10}$$

where the parameter, k, is called a *rate constant*. Then, integration yields the exponential (negative) growth curve,

$$\mu(t) = \mu(0)e^{-kt} \tag{1.11}$$

where $\mu(0)$ is the initial condition at $t = 0$.

Matrix exponentiation Consider now a system of linear differential equations such as

$$\frac{d\boldsymbol{\mu}(t)}{dt} = \mathbf{A}\boldsymbol{\mu}(t) + \mathbf{b}(t) \tag{1.12}$$

where $\boldsymbol{\mu}(t)$ is a vector of length P, $\mathbf{A}$ is a transfer matrix containing rate constants of movement between states in the system, and $\mathbf{b}(t)$ defines the inputs to the system. The general solution is

$$\boldsymbol{\mu}(t) = \boldsymbol{\mu}(0)e^{\mathbf{A}t} + \int_0^t e^{\mathbf{A}(t-u)}\mathbf{b}(u)du \tag{1.13}$$

where matrix exponentiation is defined by

$$e^{\mathbf{A}t} = \mathbf{I} + \frac{\mathbf{A}t}{1!} + \frac{(\mathbf{A}t)^2}{2!} + \cdots \tag{1.14}$$

and integration is component-wise.

However, a preferable way to calculate the exponential is by spectral decomposition. If $\mathbf{V}$ is a column matrix of the eigenvectors of $\mathbf{A}$ and $\mathbf{D}$ is a diagonal matrix containing the corresponding eigenvalues, then

$$\mathbf{A} = \mathbf{V}\mathbf{D}\mathbf{V}^{-1} \qquad (1.15)$$

and

$$e^{\mathbf{A}t} = \mathbf{V}e^{\mathbf{D}t}\mathbf{V}^{-1} \qquad (1.16)$$

In simple cases, Equation (1.13) can be solved symbolically, but often only a numerical solution can be obtained.

Example Consider the case where $P = 2$ and there are no inputs so that $\mathbf{b}(t) = 0$. Suppose that

$$\mathbf{A} = \begin{pmatrix} -k_1 - k_{12} & k_{12} \\ k_{21} & -k_2 - k_{21} \end{pmatrix} \qquad (1.17)$$

where k_{ij} is the rate of transfer between states i and j and k_i is the rate of output of state i from the system. $\mathbf{A}$ has eigenvalues $E_i = -[k_1 + k_2 + k_{12} + k_{21} \pm \sqrt{(k_1 - k_2 + k_{12} - k_{21})^2 + 4k_{12}k_{21}}]/2$. The entries of the matrix, $\exp(\mathbf{A}t)$, are

$$A_{11} = \frac{(E_1 + k_2 + k_{21})e^{E_1 t} - (E_2 + k_2 + k_{21})e^{E_2 t}}{E_1 - E_2}$$

$$A_{22} = \frac{(E_1 + k_2 + k_{21})e^{E_2 t} - (E_2 + k_2 + k_{21})e^{E_1 t}}{E_1 - E_2}$$

$$A_{12} = \frac{k_{12}(e^{E_1 t} - e^{E_2 t})}{E_1 - E_2}$$

$$A_{21} = \frac{(E_1 + k_2 + k_{21})(E_2 + k_2 + k_{21})(e^{E_2 t} - e^{E_1 t})}{k_{12}(E_1 - E_2)}$$

Results such as these can be obtained from symbolic algebra computer programs or from standard texts on compartment models.

Laplace transforms If the rate equations describe a steady state, then we can use Laplace transforms as a 'black box' method. The operator, s, replaces the differential with respect to time in the equation of interest. This can then be solved and the result subjected to an inverse transformation to obtain the integrated rate. This inverse transformation can be found in a table of Laplace transforms.

Consider a system approaching equilibrium between two states with rates k_{12} and k_{21} in the two directions. Suppose that the system starts in state 1 with nonzero concentrations, $\mu_{1A}(0)$ and $\mu_{1B}(0)$ of two substances, but $\mu_2(0) = 0$

for the resulting substance. In order that mass balance be conserved, we must have $\mu_2(t) = \mu_{1A}(t) - \mu_{1A}(0)$. If we are interested in state 2, then we can write

$$\frac{\mathrm{d}\mu_2(t)}{\mathrm{d}t} = k_{12}\mu_{1B}(0)[\mu_{1A}(0) - \mu_2(t)] - k_{21}\mu_2(t) \tag{1.18}$$

Replacing the differential with the operator, s, we rewrite this as

$$s\mu_2(t) = k_{12}\mu_{1A}(0)\mu_{1B}(0) - \mu_2(t)[k_{21} + k_{12}\mu_{1B}(0)] \tag{1.19}$$

and solve to obtain

$$\mu_2(t) = \frac{k_{12}\mu_{1A}(0)\mu_{1B}(0)}{s + k_{21} + k_{12}\mu_{1B}(0)} \tag{1.20}$$

From a table of Laplace transforms, the inverse is

$$\mu_2(t) = \frac{k_{12}\mu_{1A}(0)\mu_{1B}(0)}{k_{21} + k_{12}\mu_{1B}(0)} e^{-[k_{21}+k_{12}\mu_{1B}(0)]t} \tag{1.21}$$

Now suppose instead that we were interested in substance A of state 1 in the same system. The differential equation is

$$\frac{\mathrm{d}\mu_{1A}(t)}{\mathrm{d}t} = -\mu_{1A}(t)[k_{12}\mu_{1B}(0) + k_{21}] + k_{21}\mu_{1A}(0) \tag{1.22}$$

Because $\mu_{1A}(0) \neq 0$, $s\mu_{1A}(0)$ has to be added to allow for the initial concentration, yielding

$$s\mu_{1A}(t) = -\mu_{1A}(t)[k_{12}\mu_{1B}(0) + k_{21}] + k_{21}\mu_{1A}(0) + s\mu_{1A}(0) \tag{1.23}$$

Solving this, we obtain

$$\frac{\mu_{1A}(t)}{\mu_{1A}(0)} = \frac{s + k_{21}}{s + k_{21} + k_{12}\mu_{1B}(0)} \tag{1.24}$$

From the table of transforms, the inverse is

$$\frac{\mu_{1A}(t)}{\mu_{1A}(0)} = \frac{k_{21} + k_{12}\mu_{1B}(0)e^{-[k_{21}+k_{12}\mu_{1B}(0)]t}}{k_{21} + k_{12}\mu_{1B}(0)} \tag{1.25}$$

Gutfreund (1995) provides further details on this use of Laplace transforms.

Further reading Box and Hunter (1962) provide an excellent introduction to model building.

Several books on generalized linear models are available: Aitkin et al. (1989), McCullagh and Nelder (1989), Dobson (1990), and Lindsey (1997).

Standard texts on nonlinear modelling, with a (multivariate) normal distribution, include Bates and Watts (1988), Davidian and Giltinan (1995), Ross (1990), Seber and Wild (1989), and Vonesh and Chinchilli (1997).

For the advanced theory of differential equations, see, for example, Braun (1983) or Dettman (1986), and for Laplace transforms, Guest (1991).

1.5 Exercises

(1) A three-period cross-over trial was performed to determine gastric half-emptying time in minutes. It involved 12 subjects, as shown in Table C.1. This is an analysis of variance type of design for duration data.

   (a) Find an appropriate model to determine if there are treatment effects.

   (b) Try several members of the generalized linear model family with various link functions.

   (c) Can you find a distribution outside of the exponential dispersion family that fits better?

(2) Patients with acute spinal cord injury and bacteriuria (bacteria in their urine) were randomly assigned to one of two groups and followed for up to 16 weeks. The first group (A) was treated for all episodes of urinary tract infection that occurred whereas the second group (B) was only treated if two specific symptoms appeared. All patients entered the study with bacteriuria so that the first observation is always positive. Having bacteriuria for a longer period does not necessarily mean that a patient is sicker. The resulting binary series for the 36 patients in each group having at least four weeks' observation are shown in Table C.2.

   (a) Develop an appropriate model to determine if there are differences between the two groups.

   (b) It appears that subjects in the first group systematically had bacteria removed whereas those in the second group would retain the infection for some time after acquiring it. What evidence do the data provide for this?

   (c) Have you appropriately taken into account dependence among observations on each subject?

2
Practical aspects

Nonlinear modelling is a complex area of statistics that requires a solid basis, especially for data manipulation, specifying models, and drawing conclusions. Some of these fundamental problems will be considered here.

2.1 Data

Data collected in medical studies can have very complex structures. For nonlinear models, unbalanced series of repeated measurements are often recorded on each subject. For example, these may be unequally spaced in time with different numbers of observations for each subject. Before even contemplating fitting any models, we must be able to manipulate the data easily and surely to ensure that we shall indeed really be fitting the models that we want. Nonstandard data structures are required.

Here, I shall describe the types of structures of data that may be encountered when nonlinear modelling is required. In Section A.1.1, I present one possible way of handling and storing such complex data, using the R software, that I have developed in an attempt to reflect closely the study design and to reduce the possibility of errors.

The classical rectangular data structure used in most software does not provide the means to distinguish between response, **y**, and covariates, **X**: they are grouped together in the same matrix. This may perhaps be justifiable in certain situations, such as for strictly multivariate data or for graphical models. However, in most contexts, these two classes of variables are fundamentally different; this should be reflected in the data objects containing them.

2.1.1 RESPONSE VARIABLES

A response variable carries the assumption of a (conditional) probability distribution within some given set of models (Section 1.1.2). This can entail a considerable amount of supplementary information. Let us first look at two examples.

- The usual longitudinal repeated measurements have times associated with them, as for example in Table 2.1. In contrast to much of classical time series, here the numbers of observations per individual are unequal and the time points are both unequally spaced and different for each individual. These data clearly do not have any natural rectangular structure; forcing

Table 2.1. An example of repeated response data for three selected individuals, from data analysed in Section 5.2. First line: times, measured from randomization (with negative times being pre-randomization baseline values). Second line: response measurement. (Lindsey, 1999a, p. 400)

−27	−13	28	56	84	168	259	331	427	504	672
561	334	157	374	191	465	125	212	232	177	98
771	834	945	1008	1092	1289	1306	1351			
207	127	202	143	174	216	245	237			
−14	−6	58	253	358	508	574	672	855	924	
429	587	446	269	131	50	145	634	273	144	
−14	−7	0	56	84	168	336	420	504	672	756
231	312	123	127	297	337	225	312	178	111	97
840	924	1000	1135	1260	1280	1337				
133	239	151	115	297	141	113				

it upon them would be difficult and uninformative, hiding the important distinction between observations on the same subject and those on different subjects—it could easily lead to errors.

- Times between events, as for example in Table 2.2, provide a different sort of complexity. If, in the previous example, the times might possibly have been fixed in advance, here this is impossible. It is the random times that are of direct interest. An additional complication is that observation of an individual may not terminate at an event, so that the last recorded time may be censored (Section B.6).

Thus, for each observation, we usually shall need to collect more than just a univariate response value or a set of multivariate responses. Even for simple independent observations, we may require, for each response,

(1) censor indicators (if durations);
(2) binomial denominators (if binary);
(3) unit of measurement (if continuous);
(4) calculated Jacobian of a transformation (if continuous); and/or
(5) weights.

In addition, for repeated measurements, at least one of the following must also be available:

(1) times (if longitudinal);
(2) nesting indicators (if clustered); and/or
(3) location coordinates (if spatial).

The first of these is required for individual time series as well.

Table 2.2. An example of repeated response data for six selected individuals. First line: times between recurrent events; second line: censor indicator. (Lindsey, 1999a, p. 436)

5	13				
1	0				
12	4	2			
1	1	0			
23					
0					
3	3	2	4	14	4
1	1	1	1	1	0
3	13	7			
1	1	1			
3	6	12	2		
1	1	1	0		

These last three types of information, related to repeated measurements, have a somewhat ambiguous status. They are required with the responses in order to define the dependencies among them. However, they may also be necessary, in some contexts, as covariates: times or locations for trends, nesting for fixed effects. I cover this point further in Section A.1.1.

All of the information described in this section will be necessary in order to construct statistical models based on probability distributions, even if no covariates are present. It should all be stored together, along with the corresponding response values, in one data object in a way such that mistakes cannot be made as to which information corresponds to what aspect of the response.

2.1.2 COVARIATES

For independent observations and for single time series, covariates generally have a simple structure, being in one-to-one correspondence with the response values. The same is not true for the repeated measurements so often used in nonlinear medical models. Some distinguish among the individuals (*inter-subject* or *time-constant*), staying identical for all responses on each individual, whereas others (*intra-subject* or *time-varying*) may change along with the responses on each subject.

Inter-subject covariates Many important covariates are either static characteristics of the subjects or are only measured once, at baseline. In the repeated mea-

Table 2.3. An example of repeated time-varying covariates for the three individuals in Table 2.1. First line: times, measured from randomization, but at different moments than the response. Second line: dose.

0	28	58	85	113	159	203	333	375	585
1.0	1.167	1.333	1.5	1.667	1.833	2.0	1.833	2.0	0.0
591	1306								
2.0	0.0								
0	218	312	352	403	406	973			
1.0	1.2	1.4	1.6	1.8	2.0	0.0			
0	29	57	87	119	164	203	241	287	818
1.0	1.2	1.4	1.6	1.8	2.0	2.2	2.4	2.6	0.0
835	1280								
2.4	0.0								

surements context, the rectangular data matrix paradigm forces the user to replicate such inter-subject covariates as many times as there are repeated responses. Not only is this wasteful of storage space (and copying time in certain statistical software) and subject to error, but often statistical algorithms can be designed more logically, and perhaps more efficiently, if each such covariate has only one value per subject.

Intra-subject covariates Other covariates vary among individuals in a cluster or change over time for each subject. Consider again the example responses above in Table 2.1; the time-varying covariate, dose, is also available. The dose level changes over time for each patient. These values are presented in Table 2.3. Here, not only is the covariate recorded at unequally spaced times, different for each individual, but the times are different from those for the responses. Thus, some kind of matching may be required in order to know, in the model, what covariate value is in effect at the time a given response value is measured.

When the observation times for the response(s) and a time-varying covariate differ, we must consider what value of the covariate is most appropriate to use at the time the response was recorded. Often, we can use the most recently recorded value as the best information currently available. However, care must be taken with ties in the times when the response(s) and the covariate are recorded. Can we assume that the covariate takes effect instantaneously? For example, if the covariate is, say, blood pressure, the current value should be used, but if it is the new level of dose of medication, the change will not usually have had time to take effect, and the previous dose level should generally be used.

Thus, an intra-subject covariate requires one value per response value, in contrast to an inter-subject covariate that needs only one value per individual. And it may require manipulation before storage and use.

2.2 Specifying models

Once the data are available in a suitable form, the next requirement is to be able to communicate the desired models easily to your chosen software.

2.2.1 SOFTWARE

Some general criteria for choosing among the available statistical software packages include whether or not they have the following features:
- clear documentation;
- flexibility for reading data from files;
- data management, such as editing;
- a reasonable maximum amount of data accepted;
- user friendliness and interactivity;
- accuracy, precision, and speed;
- a wide choice of appropriate statistical methods appropriate for the problems at hand;
- clear and easy ways of specifying the structure of nonlinear models;
- choice of stochastic dependencies among responses;
- treatment of missing values;
- clear, self-explanatory output;
- a variety of high-resolution graphics;
- good reputation and reasonable cost;
- good error handling

(adapted from Altman, 1991, p. 110).

Once data are available in an appropriate form (Sections 2.1 and A.1.1) and some model has been chosen, the major role of the statistical software is to fit the model by likelihood methods and then to provide any required information about the results. Various criteria can be specified for such a process. Among others, these include
- correct model formulation, given the specification provided by the user;
- speed: wherever possible, fitting in real time;
- ease of model specification;
- default information which, when displayed, should not be erroneous or misleading in any context.

Readers will have varying orders of preference for these criteria and will certainly add others.

2.2.2 MODEL COMPONENTS

As we have seen, statistical models generally have two basically distinct parts, the probability distribution (Sections 1.1.2 and 1.1.3) and the regression function(s) (Section 1.1.4), although the latter is not always present. These are reflected in the data objects described above and in Section A.1.1.

When a selection of probability distributions is available, the user can generally choose among them from a list of possibilities, as in implementations of generalized linear models. In the future, one might expect that software may even be able to optimize over some set of pre-specified model functions in the same way as over a set of parameter values; from a likelihood point of view, the two are logically equivalent. However, stepwise and all subsets regression illustrate the misuse of such automatic optimization procedures.

Regression functions describe the ways in which the various parameters (location, dispersion, shape) of a distribution depend on covariates. For linear (parts of) regression functions for the mean, the standard way in most statistical software is now by a Wilkinson and Rogers (1973) formula set up by the user (in SAS and SPSS, there is no standard way, the procedure varying with the type of model fitted).

Probability distribution The first criterion for probability distributions is to have a wide choice available. The five generalized linear models usually provided (even the Weibull distribution is excluded!) by statistical software are entirely insufficient (Section 1.2.2). This current restriction is essentially a technical one: the linear parameters of all generalized linear models can easily be estimated by the iterated weighted least squares (IWLS) algorithm without requiring the user to supply initial values (Section 1.2.1).

For repeated measurements, the stochastic dependence relationships among the responses of an individual must also be specified (Section 1.2.4 and Appendix B). These include longitudinal serial and/or clustering dependencies. Except in special cases, calculations for the former will require recursive updating. The latter are generally handled by random effects, but this requires either some form of efficient multidimensional integration or recursive updating. For speed, recursive likelihoods (such as Kalman filtering; see Section B.4) must be calculated in a lower level language such as C or Fortran, dynamically loaded into an interpreted language like R. Only vectorized operations are sufficiently fast for repetitive everyday use in likelihood construction directly in a high-level language such as R, and such recursion cannot be vectorized.

Regression formulæ Models involve mathematical formulæ; these must be communicated in some way to the software. Here, a first criterion is a user-friendly way of specifying nonlinear functions (Section A.2.3). For models containing nonlinear regression functions, the Wilkinson and Rogers (1973) notation is not adequate. No standard approach is available in various software packages. One must be able to write down the regression formula, including both covariates and unknown coefficients, in an intuitive way, but such that the software can interpret it. Thus, an interpreter, such as those available in symbolic algebra packages, is necessary. One possible implementation, in R, of the specification of formulæ with unknowns is described in Section A.2; I have used it to analyse the examples in this book.

A second criterion is that any parameter of the probability distribution, not just the mean, be allowed to depend on covariates (Section 1.1.4). For example, models involving a normal distribution with heteroscedastic variance are now fairly widely known. However, models based on any probability distribution should be allowed to have nonconstant dispersion and shape parameters, depending on covariates or on the location parameter in some arbitrary way. Again, the fixed relationship between the mean and the dispersion in generalized linear models is insufficiently flexible (Section 1.2). As well, when a model contains regression functions for several parameters, these may need to have certain parameters in common.

2.3 Calculating the likelihood

Once the functional form of a model has been decided upon, the likelihood function can be set up (Section A.3), generally in some fairly automated way.

2.3.1 NONLINEAR OPTIMIZATION

The basic procedure for obtaining maximum likelihood estimates of the unknown parameters in the likelihood function is to solve the score equations obtained by setting the first derivative of the log likelihood function, with respect to these parameters, equal to zero. As discussed in Section 1.3, except for the linear normal case, these equations to solve will be nonlinear. The most common iterative procedure to solve them is some variation of Newton–Raphson which requires the second derivatives of the log likelihood function. That used in this book (contained in R; see Dennis and Schnabel, 1983) calculates both sets of derivatives numerically so that only the (negative) log likelihood need be supplied.

Thus, one of the most valuable things with which the applied statistician can arm him- or herself is a good nonlinear optimization routine. For simple examples of ways of setting up the specification of a likelihood for such an optimizer, see Section A.3.

Note that, if certain derivatives do not exist, special care must be taken (Sections 1.3, 3.3.3, and 4.4) as Newton–Raphson procedures will not work. In such cases, a grid search over values of the problematic parameter may be sufficient.

Multimodal likelihood functions In much of classical statistics, including most of the generalized linear model family, the likelihood function is usually well behaved. It has one unique mode and hence a unique maximum likelihood estimate. Such a situation is not always true for nonlinear problems. Depending on the number of observations and on the parametrization, the log likelihood may be far from a quadratic shape and may have local maxima.

In certain situations, if the various maxima yield fairly similar or even identical likelihood values, this is not of concern. It simply means that models with several distinct sets of parameter values predict the observed data about equally well. Often, only one set is biologically meaningful (see, for example, Section

3.2.1); if not, further data may be required to distinguish among the competing models. However, in most situations, local maxima are far from optimal and pains must be taken to find the global maximum, if it exists.

In summary, because most optimization routines use quadratic approximations, great care must be taken with parametrization and checking convergence if the log likelihood surface is far from quadratic.

2.3.2 PARAMETRIZATIONS

Parameter transformations do not affect the assumptions of a model, neither its systematic nor its stochastic parts; they may, however, make interpretation more or less easy. In contrast, transformation of the response modifies the stochastic part and, even if the regression function for the location parameter is also so transformed, does not result in a regression function for that parameter on the original scale (Sections 1.2.5 and 1.3.3).

Parameter constraints Often parameters in a mechanistic model involve constraints. For example, rates must be positive. It is generally dangerous to attempt optimization without these constraints because wild oscillations or numerical overflow may occur. Constrained optimization algorithms are available but they are often not as efficient as the standard ones. Usually, the constraints can be handled by some simple transformation. For example, if a parameter, θ, must be positive, apply a log transformation to it:

$$\theta = e^{\kappa} \tag{2.1}$$

if it must lie between zero and one, apply a logit transformation:

$$\theta = \frac{1}{1 + e^{-\kappa}} \tag{2.2}$$

and then optimize the new parameter, κ, that can take values on the whole real line.

Shape of the likelihood Parameter transformation to make contours of the likelihood surface more like symmetrical ellipsoids will generally facilitate numerical optimization. One should look for

- an interpretable relationship between parameters and data, helping to obtain reasonable initial estimates;
- rapid convergence (few iterations) of the nonlinear optimization algorithm;
- numerical accuracy at well-determined maxima;
- successful convergence for different starting values.

(See Ross, 1990, pp. 16–17.) These goals can often be aided by centring and/or scaling the data.

One indication that reparametrization has been successful is that the correlation among the parameter estimates is reduced. These correlations, printed out by the software, should be examined to see if this has been accomplished. Parameter estimates that have low correlation, with the log likelihood function approximately quadratic, are said to be *stable* because small changes in one parameter have little effect on the others. See Section 1.3 for other details.

Simple linear example Consider possible reparametrizations of a polynomial function of some covariate, such as the quadratic function

$$\mu_i = \beta_0 + \beta_1 x_i + \beta_2 x_i^2 \tag{2.3}$$

The parameters may be more easily interpretable if we write this as

$$\mu_i = \alpha_1 - \alpha_3(x_i - \alpha_2)^2 \tag{2.4}$$

where α_1 is the maximum of μ_i corresponding to $x_i = \alpha_2$. However, this is no longer a linear function of the unknown parameter vector, $\boldsymbol{\alpha}$. On the other hand, for numerical stability in calculations, orthogonal polynomials are preferable:

$$\mu_i = \psi_0 + \psi_1(x_i - \bar{x}_\bullet) + \psi_2[(x_i - \bar{x}_\bullet)^2 - \overline{(x_i - \bar{x}_\bullet)^2}] \tag{2.5}$$

where the bars over variables indicate means. One would hope to obtain the same final results, after the appropriate back transformations, from all three of these formulations (Ross, 1990, p. 12).

Nonlinear growth curve example Consider a logistic growth curve regression function (Section 3.1.3). This is often written

$$\mu(t) = \frac{\alpha}{1 + e^{-(\beta_0 + \beta_1 \gamma t)}} \tag{2.6}$$

with asymptote, α. However, the form

$$\mu(t) = \frac{\alpha}{1 + e^{-(t - \psi_1)/\psi_2}} \tag{2.7}$$

may sometimes be more meaningful. Here, α is still the asymptote, ψ_1 is the time at which μ is one-half the asymptote, and ψ_2 is a scale parameter.

2.3.3 INITIAL ESTIMATES

In the special case of generalized linear models, initial estimates are not necessary; they can be obtained automatically from the data by the software (Section 1.2.1). In other cases, they must be supplied. If these initial estimates are far from the maximum likelihood estimates, there is a good chance that the optimization may converge to a local maximum, if one exists. Thus, their choice can have a critical impact on the resulting solution so that several distinct sets of values should be tried. In this way, checks can be made as to whether one has found a local, or the global, maximum of the likelihood function.

Thus, for any nonlinear optimization procedure, good starting values are essential. Bates and Watts (1988, pp. 72–76) suggest several possible procedures for choosing them:

- interpret the behaviour of the regression function analytically or graphically;
- do this with its derivatives, if relevant;
- transform the regression function to a simpler, preferably linear, form (see Section 1.3);
- fix some of the parameters at reasonable values and optimize over the others.

In a mechanistic model, the parameters will usually have physical meaning. Scientists may have possible reasonable values available, perhaps from related studies. Certain values may be deducible from behaviour near the (time) origin. Sometimes, this can be most easily done in terms of the derivatives, when they are available.

Sums of exponentials When the regression function is a sum of exponentials (Section 3.2), the process of *peeling* can be used. Consider, for example,

$$\mu(t) = \theta_1 e^{-\theta_2 t} + \theta_3 e^{-\theta_4 t} \tag{2.8}$$

with all parameters constrained to have positive values. For large t, we have $\log[\mu(t)] \doteq \log(\theta_3) - \theta_4 t$ if $\theta_2 > \theta_4$ from which initial values for θ_3 and θ_4 can be obtained (replacing $\mu(t)$ by the appropriate response values). Using the parameter values so obtained, we can calculate those for θ_1 and θ_2 from $\log[\mu(t) - \theta_3 e^{-\theta_4 t}] \doteq \log(\theta_1) - \theta_2 t$ in a similar way.

Alternatively, we may study the derivatives of this same equation. For large t, $\mu(t) \doteq \theta_3 e^{-\theta_4 t}$ so that the rate of change here provides an estimate of θ_4. For small t, $\mu(t) \doteq \theta_1 e^{-\theta_2 t} + \theta_3$ so that the rate of change provides an estimate of θ_2.

Growth curves Initial parameter estimates are most easily obtained when an interpretable parametrization is used, such as in Equation (2.7).

To obtain initial estimates, calculate the average response value at each time point. An initial estimate of α is the maximum response. That of θ_1 is the time corresponding to when the average response is about one-half the maximum. The scale, θ_2, can be estimated by the difference in time between a mean response at one-half the maximum and at three-quarters the maximum.

2.3.4 CHECKING CONVERGENCE

Because the log likelihood functions to be optimized in nonlinear modelling are often multimodal, reaching convergence can be difficult. If reasonable initial values have been used and the model is suitable for the data, generally there should not be too much of a problem. If these conditions are fulfilled and there are still problems, the first thing to check is that the model has indeed been correctly specified to the software.

Where possible, a good procedure is to start with the simplest possible model so that few parameters need to be estimated. Then, the model can be built up as necessary using, as initial values of those parameters present at previous stages, their previous estimates. As well, starting with a simple model is good scientific practice.

On the other hand, if a model has too many parameters, so that not all can be estimated, convergence will be very slow or impossible. This is called the problem of *identifiability*. It occurs if the regression function, say $\mu(\theta)$, here written as a function of the parameters, is such that, for at least two sets of parameter values, $\mu(\theta_1) = \mu(\theta_2)$ for all covariate values. Careful inspection of the regression function will usually reveal this.

Identifiability of a model holds for all possible covariate values. Sometimes, the observed configuration of covariate values does not yield sufficient information to obtain estimates of all of the desired parameters. The data are not adequate for the model of interest. This is called *ill conditioning*. The only solutions are either to accept that only a simpler model can be fitted given the available information or to obtain supplementary observations with the required covariate values. This also has the implication that very accurate data can yield very imprecise parameter estimates if the covariate values are not appropriately spaced.

Nonlinear regression functions of quite different form can sometimes give rise to almost identical curves. This is especially true of sums of exponentials, as in compartment models (Section 3.2.1). If one of the functions contains more parameters than the other, this is called *parameter redundancy*. In some cases, this can cause convergence problems.

Once convergence has been obtained, the first things to do are to check that the parameter values are reasonable and to plot the mean regression function with the data to make sure that they agree. Next, different starting values should be tried to see if convergence was to a local optimum. This may only be important if the height of the global optimum is much different than that of the local one. If not, then several different sets of parameter values are indicated as about equally plausible. Either all sets may be retained, or only those that make scientific sense.

A more computationally intensive, but also more informative, method is to plot profile likelihood curves for parameters (Section 2.4.2). This will often allow one to detect any nonconvergence by the stepping through values of parameters.

2.4 Inference

To conclude this chapter, it is appropriate to explain briefly the methods of inference to be used here.

2.4.1 MODEL SELECTION

This book is about the construction and analysis of nonlinear models. In modern statistics, with several competing approaches to making inferences, the lowest common denominator is the (log) likelihood ratio comparing competing models; this will be used here for drawing the required inferences. Thus, the basic assumption underlying this approach is the Fisherian one that a model is more plausible or likely if it makes the observed data more probable, that is, if it better predicts the available data. Notice that this is a *relative* criterion for *comparing* models; it says nothing about the absolute goodness of fit of a model to the data.

A set of probability-based models, that one is entertaining as adequately describing the possible data-generating mechanism for the observed data, defines the likelihood function. If this function is so complex as to be intractable, then there is a good chance that it cannot provide useful and interpretable information about the data-generating mechanism.

However, a likelihood value, by itself, does not take into account the complexity of the model, as usually measured by the degrees of freedom. It is not clear that these incommensurable quantities (fit measured by the likelihood and complexity measured by the number of estimated parameters) can be sensibly compared statistically, as opposed to scientifically. The common approach is to calibrate the deviance, at least approximately, by the appropriate value from a chi-squared distribution. This will not be used here. Instead, the negative log likelihood (not multiplied by two) will be penalized by adding to it the number of parameters estimated, a form of the Akaike (1973) information criterion (AIC). Smaller values will indicate models fitting relatively better to the data, given the constraint on the degree of complexity.

Innumerable new models are enthusiastically promoted in the statistical literature, illustrated by data that are, in fact, often entirely inappropriate. The authors generally provide only point estimates and standard errors, so that the reader has no means of judging the validity of the analysis. Provision of values of the (full) likelihood function to allow objective comparisons can yield many surprises.

2.4.2 LIKELIHOOD REGIONS

Once one or more appropriate models have been selected, one will wish to study the precision of the parameter estimates. In multiparameter models, the complex likelihood surface cannot be graphed in any simple way. The standard errors will provide some rough idea of the precision of each parameter, but this should be checked by removing each parameter in turn (where possible) from the model to see the change in log likelihood.

A next step is to produce profile likelihood graphs of each parameter of special interest. This is done by fixing that parameter at a series of successive values around the maximum likelihood estimate and optimizing over the others in the model. (Use the values of these latter parameters obtained at each step as the new initial estimates at the next step.) These will provide more reliable precision intervals than the standard errors which rely on a quadratic approximation.

Unfortunately, in nonlinear models, the parameters may be inter-related in complex ways so that the profile likelihoods for single parameters can hide a great deal. The correlations among them do not tell the whole story either. It is wise to produce bivariate profile likelihood plots of important pairs of parameters to see what happens with one when the other is changed. This can be accomplished by fixing both parameters over a grid of reasonable values and optimizing over the remaining parameters for each point on the grid. Then, the resulting likelihood surface can be plotted using either a contour or a 3-D function, or preferably both. Obviously, this step can be very time consuming.

If the chosen parametrization for optimization is stable (Section 2.3.2), the contours should be reasonably elliptical. The contours should also be plotted in the parametrization that is most interpretable scientifically. In nonlinear models, these can sometimes be extremely 'banana' shaped or have other strange forms.

One advantage of these profile likelihood plots is that they allow precision regions for parameters easily to be reported on the scale that is most scientifically meaningful. For example, they can be given for rates instead of log rates, although the latter are used in the optimization to ensure the positivity constraint (Section 2.3.2).

An alternative possibility that may be useful in certain cases is to produce cross-sectional contour plots of the likelihood surface for a pair of parameters for fixed values of all other parameters, instead of optimizing over the latter.

2.4.3 GOODNESS OF FIT

When the distribution is not normal, the variance is not constant, the regression function is nonlinear, and responses on each subject are interdependent (Appendix B), evaluating goodness of fit can be difficult. Differences between fitted values and response values (fitted value residuals) may be impossible to interpret, even when standardized in some seemingly appropriate way. (Even for the normal distribution, if there is considerable intrinsic nonlinearity, care must be taken; see Seber and Wild, 1989, pp. 174–181.) There will usually be no useful saturated model, as for generalized linear models, upon which deviance residuals can be based.

The most reliable single criterion will be choice of the best model among those being entertained, as indicated by the AIC, ascertaining that no parameters can be eliminated. In certain situations, a more general model may exist, containing, as special cases, several of the competing models of special interest, perhaps distinguished by the values of one of the parameters (see, for example, Section 7.2.5). Fitting this model will then provide additional information about which of the competing models has the best fit.

Plots of underlying and individual profile curves against the corresponding observations are very important. If they show inadequacy, the model should be modified in a scientifically sensible way. Certain departures relate to stochastic properties of the model. For example, if the observations wobble around the

Table 2.4. Twenty observations believed to have a Cauchy distribution.

9.57	−4.34	0.01	−1.84	1.82
−0.01	0.36	−2.47	0.54	2.19
−4.61	0.47	1.95	−0.44	2.48
0.39	9.79	0.61	2.64	1.25

corresponding individual profile over time, consistently on one side for several time points, then the other, some form of autoregression (Section B.2) is indicated.

Subgroups should be examined for unexpected differences: demographic, time, geographic differences. Outlying observations should be rechecked (the data were properly cleaned, were they not?) for contamination. If everything is in order, a distribution with heavier tails may provide a better (more 'robust') fit (Section 1.2.5).

Further reading For a more complete presentation of the inference approach used here, see Lindsey (1996, 1999c).

2.5 Exercises

(1) Give the steps, using R functions, to set up the data sets of the exercises in the previous chapter as the data objects described in Sections 2.1 and A.1.1.

(2) Using the procedures outlined in Sections 2.3.1, A.2, and A.3:
   (a) Write, from first principles, a log likelihood function for the beta binomial distribution that will handle regression functions for the two parameters.
   (b) Repeat, using a density function for this distribution available in the software.

(3) The data in Table 2.4 are believed to have arisen from a Cauchy distribution.
   (a) Plot the profile likelihood functions for each of the two parameters and the joint likelihood of the two parameters.
   (b) How well are they approximated by a normal distribution?

3
Families of nonlinear regression functions

In this chapter, I shall review briefly some of the basic classes of nonlinear regression functions that are important in medical research.

3.1 Growth curves

One of the most common types of studies where nonlinear regression functions are usually necessary involves the analysis of growth curves. As the name indicates, they are usually associated with studies over time. As compared to other types of longitudinal data, these curves have a number of special characteristics, only some of which they share with other series of observations over time:

- the growth profile will generally be a nonlinear function of time, often reaching an asymptote;
- random variability will generally increase with size, so that the dispersion is not constant (Section 1.1.4);
- the successive responses are measured on the same subject so that they will generally not be independent (Appendix B);
- different individuals may have different growth rates or profiles, either inherently or due to environmental effects (Section B.1);
- by definition, growth is not stationary; occasionally, the increments, or innovations, may be (Sections B.2 and B.4).

A wide class of different functions is available for studying such phenomena.

3.1.1 POLYNOMIALS

Classically (Box, 1950; Potthoff and Roy, 1964; Laird and Ware, 1982), growth curves have often been handled by simple polynomials in time. When such polynomials are used, they may be thought of as a Taylor or Maclaurin series approximation

$$g(\mu) = c(0) + \frac{\partial c(0)}{\partial t} t + \frac{\partial^2 c(0)}{\partial t^2} \frac{t^2}{2} + \cdots$$
$$= \beta_0 + \beta_1 t + \beta_2 t^2 + \cdots \quad (3.1)$$

to some unknown nonlinear functional form, $c(t)$, of the time, t.

Voit and Knapp (1997) provide examples of theoretical derivation of such approximations. However, this approach should only be considered when the regression function is unknown theoretically, generally when there is no asymptote or when all responses are far from the asymptote. And care should be taken not to use polynomials of too high an order, usually not more than quadratic, because otherwise the model will be inherently unstable in replications of the data (Lindsey, 2001).

Sandland and McGilchrist (1979) provide several reasons why such polynomials are unattractive for growth functions:

(1) Growth processes can undergo changes of phase that cannot be accommodated by polynomials.
(2) The stochastic structure of the model will be distorted if the polynomial is inappropriate.
(3) Polynomials cannot easily represent the asymptotic behaviour of a growth curve.

They also emphasize that growth curve data are usually nonstationary and that polynomials do not represent biological mechanisms of growth.

Fortunately, a number of more realistic general functions are available. One simple possibility is to use inverse polynomials (Nelder, 1966). The reciprocals of time are used in the polynomial; this allows an asymptote to be reached. A simple example is provided by the reparametrization of the Michaëlis–Menten function given in Equation (1.8). However, such a procedure generally still does not provide a mechanistic explanation of the process.

3.1.2 EXPONENTIAL FORMS

Exponential growth Suppose that the rate of growth is proportional to the size already attained:

$$\frac{dy_t}{dt} = \gamma y_t \qquad (3.2)$$

Solving this (Section 1.4.2) yields one of the simplest curves for growth, the *exponential* curve:

$$y_t = \iota e^{\gamma t} \qquad (3.3)$$

where $\iota = y_0$ is size at time zero. Usually, such a function will only be realistic in the early stages of growth; nothing can continue growing exponentially forever. On the other hand, with $\gamma < 0$, it may be a reasonable model of exponential decline.

As it stands, Equation (3.3) describes a deterministic relationship between response and time. A stochastic element can be introduced in at least two ways. The response may have some distribution, say in a normal or gamma distribution, with a log link such that the linear predictor is

$$\log[\mu_y(t)] = \log(\iota) + \gamma t \qquad (3.4)$$

or

$$\mu_y(t) = \iota e^{\gamma t} \qquad (3.5)$$

Another possibility is to assume that the log response has some distribution, such as the normal or gamma, yielding a log normal or log gamma distribution, with the identity link and linear predictor,

$$\mu_{\log(y)}(t) = \log(\iota) + \gamma t \qquad (3.6)$$

The resulting curves can differ rather significantly, both in their fit to observed data and in the predictions they yield. In the first model, the curve goes through the arithmetic mean of the data, whereas, in the second, it goes through the geometric mean (see Section 1.3.3).

The stochastic variability modelled by the two equations is also quite different. For example, for the first model, with a normal distribution, the variance of the log response is constant, implying that the variance of the response is increasing with size. In the second, again with a normal distribution, the variance of the response is constant. If Equation (3.4) is used with a gamma distribution, the ratio of standard deviation to mean, the coefficient of variation, is assumed constant. Other distributions will carry still other assumptions about how the variability is changing with mean response, that is, over time.

Monomolecular growth With the exponential growth curve, the response continues to increase indefinitely. For many phenomena, this is not reasonable, except over short periods. One of the simplest assumptions leading to an asymptote, say α, is that the growth rate is proportional to the remaining size:

$$\frac{d\mu(t)}{dt} = \gamma[\alpha - \mu(t)] \qquad \gamma > 0 \qquad (3.7)$$

yielding

$$\begin{aligned}\mu(t) &= \alpha - (\alpha - \iota)e^{-\gamma t} \\ &= \alpha - \zeta e^{-\gamma t}\end{aligned} \qquad (3.8)$$

where $\iota = \alpha - \zeta$ is the mean initial size. Growth occurs if $\alpha > \iota > 0$. This is called the *monomolecular* growth function.

When $\alpha = \zeta$ so that initial size is zero, this is called the von Bertalanffy growth curve, used in ecology to describe animal growth.

3.1.3 SIGMOIDAL CURVES

We can combine the assumptions of the two previous models. Thus, suppose now that the growth *rate* increases to a maximum before steadily declining to zero. This can be accomplished by having this rate proportional to a product of functions of the current and remaining sizes:

$$\frac{d\mu(t)}{dt} = g_1[\mu(t)]\{\alpha - g_2[\mu(t)]\} \qquad (3.9)$$

These will yield sigmoidal behaviour for the growth curve.

Logistic growth One possibility, perhaps the simplest, is that the rate is directly proportional to the two sizes:

$$\frac{d\mu(t)}{dt} = \frac{\gamma}{\alpha}\mu(t)[\alpha - \mu(t)] \qquad (3.10)$$

yielding the symmetric S-shaped *logistic* curve that has the form

$$\mu(t) = \frac{\alpha}{1 + \zeta e^{-\gamma t}} \qquad (3.11)$$

where α is the asymptotic maximum value of the response. For other parametrizations, including a more interpretable one, see Section 2.3.2.

We can transform this to a linear structure by using a logit link:

$$\log\left[\frac{\mu(t)}{\alpha - \mu(t)}\right] = -\log(\zeta) + \gamma t \qquad (3.12)$$

If α were known, this could be fitted as a generalized linear model.

A handicap of this function as a growth curve is that it is symmetric. Often, there is no biological reason why the shape of the curve of increasing early growth should be identical to that of decreasing late growth.

Gompertz growth A second commonly used growth curve with an asymptote has growth rate defined by

$$\frac{d\mu(t)}{dt} = \gamma\mu(t)\{\log(\alpha) - \log[\mu(t)]\} \qquad (3.13)$$

The solution to this is called the *Gompertz* curve,

$$\mu(t) = \alpha e^{-\zeta e^{-\gamma t}} \qquad (3.14)$$

where, again, α is the unknown asymptotic maximum value. This curve is not symmetric about its point of inflection. Again, we can obtain a linear structure, this time by means of a log log link:

$$\log\left[-\log\left(\frac{\mu(t)}{\alpha}\right)\right] = \log(\zeta) - \gamma t \qquad (3.15)$$

If we invert the asymmetry, we have

3.1. GROWTH CURVES

$$\mu(t) = \alpha \left(1 - e^{-\zeta e^{-\gamma t}}\right) \tag{3.16}$$

with linear structure given by a complementary log log link:

$$\log\left[-\log\left(1 - \frac{\mu(t)}{\alpha}\right)\right] = \log(\zeta) - \gamma t \tag{3.17}$$

Richards growth The growth rate of a living being is the difference between the metabolic forces of anabolism and catabolism, the synthesis of new body matter and its loss. Catabolism can be taken proportional to weight whereas anabolism can be assumed to have an allometric relationship (see Section 3.3.1) to weight:

$$\frac{d\mu(t)}{dt} = \gamma[\mu(t)]^{\kappa+1} - \alpha\mu(t) \tag{3.18}$$

This, and the previous functions, can be generalized to

$$\frac{d\mu(t)}{dt} = -\frac{\gamma}{\kappa}\mu(t)\left[\left(\frac{\mu(t)}{\alpha}\right)^{\kappa} - 1\right] \tag{3.19}$$

with solution

$$\mu(t) = \alpha\left(1 + \kappa e^{-\gamma(t-\zeta)}\right)^{-1/\kappa} \qquad \kappa \neq 0 \tag{3.20}$$

called the *Richards* curve. When $\kappa = -1$, this is the von Bertalanffy special case of the monomolecular function, when $\kappa = 1$, the logistic function, and when $\kappa \to 0$, the Gompertz function.

This curve can be thought of as describing initial exponential growth that is increasingly damped as the size increases until it eventually stops. For another derivation, in a different context, see Section 4.2.1.

Generalized logistic curve Nelder (1961, 1962) has called a closely related parametrization of the Richards function the generalized logistic growth curve; this may have an easier interpretation in certain contexts. Suppose that the change in mean response obeys the following differential equation:

$$\frac{d\mu(t)}{dt} = \gamma\mu(t)\{d(\alpha,\kappa) - d[\mu(t),\kappa]\} \tag{3.21}$$

where

$$d(\mu,\kappa) = \begin{cases} \frac{\mu^{\kappa}-1}{\kappa} & \kappa \neq 0 \\ \log(\mu) & \kappa = 0 \end{cases}$$

with initial condition $\mu(0) = \iota$ at $t = 0$. The solution is

$$\mu(t) = \begin{cases} \alpha\left[1 + \left(\left[\frac{\alpha}{\iota}\right]^\kappa - 1\right)e^{-\gamma(t-t_0)\alpha^\kappa}\right]^{-1/\kappa} & \kappa \neq 0 \\ \alpha\left(\frac{\iota}{\alpha}\right)e^{-\gamma(t-t_0)} & \kappa = 0 \end{cases} \qquad (3.22)$$

Then, $\alpha = \lim_{t \to \infty} \mu(t)$ is the asymptote. The parameters γ and κ control the rate of growth. If $\gamma < 0$ and $\alpha > \iota$ or $\gamma > 0$ and $\alpha < \iota$, we have negative growth or decay. The parameter κ determines the type of the curve, varying from the Mitscherlich ($\kappa = -1$) through the Gompertz ($\kappa = 0$), and the logistic ($\kappa = 1$) to the exponential ($\kappa \to \infty$ and $d(\alpha, \kappa) \to$ constant). Heitjan (1991a, 1991b) has applied this function to clinical trial data, including autocorrelation and random effects, as we shall see in Section 5.2.

3.2 Sums of exponentials

As we saw in Section 1.4.2, the solution of linear differential equations involves exponential functions. Thus, regression functions based on rates will often have the form of sums of exponentials.

3.2.1 COMPARTMENT MODELS

One way to construct a mechanistic model for a process is to divide the system into *compartments* and to assume that the rate of flow of the substances between these obeys first-order kinetics. In other words, the rate of transfer to a receiving or sink compartment is proportional to the concentration in the supply or source compartment, so that the differential equations are linear. These are called the *mass balance equations*. We saw in Section 1.4 how to solve such equations. There may be inputs (ingestion, injection, infusion, and so on) into and outputs (excretion) from one or more compartments.

For example, in a study of the body, a three-compartment model might correspond to blood, soft tissue, and muscle, plus the outside environment from which the substance comes and to which it is eliminated. An important assumption in such models is that the substance under study is well mixed in all compartments. It is also assumed to have identical kinetic behaviour within each one.

Such compartment models have wide application in medicine. Perhaps, the most important area is pharmacokinetics (Chapter 7), but they are also used in radioactive tracer studies in physiology and to describe how individuals pass through a series of healthy and diseased states (Sections 4.5.1 and 6.1.2), called event history analysis. To keep the description concrete, let us only consider here the application of compartment models to the movement of a substance through the body.

Basic models A substance may enter the body in various ways, such as ingestion, infusion, or injection. Difference models will be required in each case.

3.2. SUMS OF EXPONENTIALS

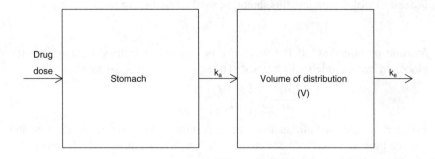

Fig. 3.1. Graphical presentation of an open, first-order, one-compartment model.

Ingestion When a substance is ingested, one commonly used nonlinear regression function is called the open, first-order, one-compartment model. The process that it models is illustrated in Figure 3.1 (although often the first source compartment is not drawn). It corresponds to the differential equations

$$\frac{d\mu(t)}{dt} = k_a \mu_a(t) - k_e \mu(t)$$
$$\frac{d\mu_a(t)}{dt} = -k_a \mu_a(t) \tag{3.23}$$

from which the regression function can be derived, where μ is the concentration of the substance in the body, usually measured in the blood, μ_a the amount at the absorption site (often the stomach), k_a is the absorption rate, and k_e the elimination rate. Generally, direct information is only available about $\mu(t)$. Indirect information about $\mu_a(t)$ comes from the dose administered.

The resulting nonlinear function is

$$\mu(t) = \frac{xk_a}{V(k_a - k_e)} \left(e^{-k_e t} - e^{-k_a t} \right) \tag{3.24}$$

where x is usually the dose of the substance given, t is the time after administration, and V the 'apparent volume of distribution'. This is sometimes called the Bateman equation (Gutfreund, 1995, p. 111). The parameters to be estimated are k_a, k_e, and V (exceptionally, I do not use Greek letters, in order to conform to standard usage in pharmacokinetics).

Notice that the two rate parameters may be interchanged in Equation (3.24) without fundamentally changing the model. Only a simple transformation of V is required. Thus, the likelihood will have two symmetric maxima of equal height. In most situations, the solution with $k_a > k_e$ is the meaningful one.

If the absorption and elimination rates are identical, Equation (3.24) simplifies to

$$\mu(t) = \frac{xkte^{-kt}}{V} \tag{3.25}$$

For stability of estimation, this should be used when the two rates are very similar.

Infusion or injection If the substance is injected or infused directly into the blood, different models will be used. The simplest differential equations are

$$\frac{d\mu(t)}{dt} = \begin{cases} x - k_e\mu(t) & t \leq c \\ -k_e\mu(t) & t > c \end{cases} \quad (3.26)$$

where k_e is again the elimination rate, x is now the known rate of infusion, and c is the time at which infusion stops, which is zero for injection. A zero-order, one-compartment model can then be derived:

$$\mu(t) = \begin{cases} \frac{x}{Vk_e}\left(1 - e^{-k_e t}\right) & t \leq c \\ \frac{x}{Vk_e}\left(1 - e^{-k_e c}\right)e^{-k_e(t-c)} & t > c \end{cases} \quad (3.27)$$

Other, more complex functions may be required depending on the specific characteristics of the process under study (see, for example, Section 7.1.2).

3.2.2 DIFFUSION MODELS

Diffusion processes were originally primarily used in physics to describe various processes such as heat conduction, Brownian motion of pollen particles, and turbulent flow of fluids. The basic equation for spread in two dimensions is

$$\frac{\partial \mu(t,x,y)}{\partial t} = \delta \left(\frac{\partial^2 \mu(t,x,y)}{\partial x^2} + \frac{\partial^2 \mu(t,x,y)}{\partial y^2} \right) \quad (3.28)$$

where δ is the diffusion coefficient determining how rapidly the spread occurs. This equation can be derived in many ways, for example as a random walk or from Fick's law (Section 9.5.2; see Murray, 1993, pp. 234–235).

If initial conditions are such that the mean is $\mu(0,0,0) = \mu_0$ at the origin and zero elsewhere, the solution is

$$\mu(t,x,y) = \frac{\mu_0}{4\pi\delta t} \exp\left(-\frac{x^2 + y^2}{4\delta t}\right) \quad (3.29)$$

the form of a bivariate normal density. The characteristics of this distribution can be used to describe the process of diffusion. Notice that, as it stands, it is symmetric in all directions.

Local growth If, in addition to diffusion, there is local population growth, Equation (3.28) can be generalized, for example to

$$\frac{\partial \mu(t,x,y)}{\partial t} = \delta \left(\frac{\partial^2 \mu(t,x,y)}{\partial x^2} + \frac{\partial^2 \mu(t,x,y)}{\partial y^2} \right)$$
$$+ \frac{\gamma}{\alpha}[\alpha - \mu(t,x,y)]\mu(t,x,y) \quad (3.30)$$

where logistic growth has been chosen, using Equation (3.10). This model was originally proposed by Fisher (1937) for the one-dimensional case.

This equation does not have an explicit solution but must be solved numerically. Skellam (1951) used a simplified special case of this equation, based on exponential growth described by Equation (3.2), that does have an explicit solution. However, it has the unfortunate property that the mean eventually becomes infinite.

Drift If there is drift, say in the x direction, Equation (3.28) generalizes to

$$\frac{\partial \mu(t,x,y)}{\partial t} = \delta \left[\frac{\partial^2 \mu(t,x,y)}{\partial x^2} + \frac{\partial^2 \mu(t,x,y)}{\partial y^2} \right] - \gamma \frac{\partial \mu(t,x,y)}{\partial x} \quad (3.31)$$

with solution

$$\mu(t,x,y) = \frac{\mu_0}{4\pi\delta t} \exp\left[-\frac{(x-\gamma t)^2 + y^2}{4\delta t}\right] \quad (3.32)$$

where γ is the speed of drift.

3.3 Other nonlinear functions

Specific functions often have to be developed for a particular problem. A few general families are given below, using only simple examples as illustrations.

3.3.1 POWER FUNCTIONS

Power functions often appear in the description of body size, for example in allometry. In its simplest form, we have

$$\frac{d\mu(t)}{dt} = \kappa [\mu(t)]^\delta \quad (3.33)$$

with solution

$$[\mu(t)]^{1-\delta} = [\mu(0)]^{1-\delta} + (1-\delta)\kappa t \quad (3.34)$$

If this is used as a description of body weight, δ is often about 0.75.

Some other power functions are developed as diffusion models in Section 9.5.2.

3.3.2 CYCLIC FUNCTIONS

A major problem with the sigmoidal growth curves derived from Equation (3.9) is that the effects are assumed to be instantaneous; the change in $\mu(t)$ depends only on its present size. Consider, for example, the logistic growth curve derived from Equation (3.10). If the remaining size has a delayed effect, we can write

$$\frac{d\mu(t)}{dt} = \frac{\gamma}{\kappa} \mu(t)[\kappa - \mu(t-\delta)] \quad (3.35)$$

where $\delta > 0$ is the delay parameter. However, in this model, we assume that the delay effect only occurs at one specific moment in the past. A more general model involves an average over past time yielding an integro-differential equation:

$$\frac{d\mu(t)}{dt} = \frac{\gamma}{\kappa}\mu(t)\left[\kappa - \int_{-\infty}^{t} w(t-u)\mu(u)du\right] \tag{3.36}$$

where $w(\cdot)$ is an appropriate weight function. These equations can only be solved numerically and generally yield periodic equations.

As a very simple example, consider

$$\frac{d\mu(t)}{dt} = -\frac{\pi}{2\delta}\mu(t-\delta) \tag{3.37}$$

which can be solved, yielding

$$\mu(t) = \kappa \cos\left(\frac{\pi t}{2\delta}\right) \tag{3.38}$$

The solutions to Equations (3.35) and (3.36) may or may not yield stable limit cycles (Murray, 1993, pp. 8–9).

For an application of cyclic functions, arising from compartment models, to epidemics, see Section 4.5.

3.3.3 CHANGE-POINT MODELS

A further important class of nonlinear regression functions in medical research involves abrupt changes over time. When individuals are followed over time, they may change state at some point in time. This means that the distribution of the response is altered at this time point. The response variable, Y_t, at time t may be modelled as

$$\begin{array}{ll} f(y_t;\boldsymbol{\phi}_1) & t < \tau \\ f(y_t;\boldsymbol{\phi}_2) & t \geq \tau \end{array} \tag{3.39}$$

where $f(\cdot)$ is some given distribution and τ is an unknown parameter giving the change-point time. Some or all of the elements of the vector of parameters, $\boldsymbol{\phi}$, in the distribution may change. Time may be either discrete and equally spaced or continuous. Notice that the derivative of ϕ does not exist at $t = \tau$ so that care must be taken in the estimation of this parameter. In a more complex situation, the distribution function itself might change.

This problem may be approached in at least two ways. The probability model may be set up as just stated and τ estimated, along with the other parameters (as will be done in Section 4.4). Or a hidden Markov model (Section B.5.2) with two hidden states may be used.

Further reading A fundamental book on nonlinear models in biology is Murray (1993).

Seber and Wild (1989, pp. 327–342) provide a presentation of a variety of growth curves. For sums of exponentials functions, see the references at the end of Chapter 7. Bunke and Bunke (1989, pp. 73–105) give a very technical discussion of change-point models.

3.4 Exercises

(1) Many growth curve functions have forms similar to cumulative distribution functions.
   (a) Suggest some such cumulative distributions that might be used as regression functions and that are not described in this chapter.
   (b) Do these have any mechanistic interpretations?
(2) Many sums of exponentials functions have forms similar to some probability density function.
   (a) Suggest some such densities that might be used as regression functions.
   (b) Do these have any mechanistic interpretations?

4
Epidemiology

As its name suggests, the field of epidemiology arose from the study of epidemics. However, this discipline now has a much wider coverage, looking at public health in all its aspects, not just those involving infectious diseases. It uses a number of special techniques and some rather specific terminology.

4.1 Studying natural populations

Epidemiological research aims to study phenomena related to health in natural populations. It attempts to detect nonstandard events and to determine the reasons, called *risk factors*, behind them.

Many of the techniques are observational so that great care must be made in drawing causal conclusions. The public is often concerned with apparent clustering of disease events, whether in space or in time. This can make reasonably objective analysis of the situation difficult, especially if the problem is widely publicized in the news media. On the other hand, many new relationships between human health and *exposure* to various environmental or genetic factors have first been detected by epidemiological means, later to be confirmed by more controlled clinical techniques.

4.1.1 GOALS

To judge if something exceptional is occurring requires a point of comparison. Thus, standardized models for ordinary healthy populations are necessary, such as growth curves for children or pregnant women and death rates in large populations of standard composition. In the first case, the progress of individuals can be compared to the standard curve; in the second case, subgroups can be monitored for abnormal risks.

A vast array of models for epidemics and the spread of disease is also available; see, for example, Section 3.2.2. However, sufficient data are usually not available to allow statistical model fitting to be applied. In this chapter, I shall only consider two simple aspects of the study of epidemics.

The principal statistical techniques commonly used in epidemiology are logistic regression for probability of contracting a disease, log linear Poisson regression for rates, and survival models (Section B.6). In most cases, these do not involve nonlinearity in the regression functions.

Incidence studies are similar to survival studies (Section B.6), except that the duration is measured from birth instead of from diagnosis or start of treatment; it is a rate of occurrence, obtained by longitudinal follow-up. In contrast, *prevalence* is the frequency of a disease in a population at a given time point. Naively, in a population of fixed size, prevalence = incidence × duration. Survival and incidence are modelled by an intensity, whereas prevalence is a probability.

Because of the observational nature of much of epidemiology, the danger is always present that some unmeasured *confounding* variable is present that has an influence on the outcome of interest. Thus, differences apparently due to observed exposure may, in fact, result from these confounding variables.

4.1.2 DESIGNS

Epidemiology has a number of study designs that are typical of this discipline. In a *cohort design*, a group of individuals is followed over time and new cases of the disease are recorded. These are related to covariates that may measure differential exposure to the disease. In simple cases, a dose–response model may be used.

When a disease to be studied is rare, a very large random sample from the population would be required in order to obtain sufficient cases. Thus, instead, a retrospective *case–control design* is used. Here, cases are available, but in a nonrandom way. Subjects with the condition of interest are identified, as well as a group of controls without the condition. The latter are matched as closely as possible to the cases. They can then be compared as to their *previous* exposure to any risk factors of interest. The main advantages of such a design are practicality, simplicity, speed, and low cost. However, the disadvantages are many, especially the nonrandom selection of the cases. The analysis involves use of logistic regression models.

More experimental methods are also used in clinical epidemiology.

4.1.3 ECOLOGICAL REGRESSION

Ecological regression involves fitting models to aggregates, such as averages or proportions from geographic regions, and attempting to interpret the results at the individual level. In certain situations, no other information is available and this is the only approach possible. However, it involves making assumptions that cannot be checked at the aggregate level. I shall not provide examples in this text, but a few words of caution are necessary for cases when nonlinear regression functions are required.

Consider first the case of simple linear regression:

$$E(Y_{ij}) = \beta_{0j} + \beta_{1j} x_{ij} \qquad (4.1)$$

where i indexes the individuals in region j. If only aggregate data, $(\bar{y}_j, \bar{x}_j)$, from the regions are available, the corresponding function,

$$E(\bar{Y}_j) = \beta_{0j} + \beta_{1j} \bar{x}_j \qquad (4.2)$$

can be derived by averaging. However, if the regression function is nonlinear, this no longer works.

Consider the simple case of a log linear regression function, that is, using a log link (Section 1.2.1),

$$E(Y_{ij}) = e^{\beta_{0j} + \beta_{1j} x_{ij}} \tag{4.3}$$

Here, the aggregate level function for region j with n_j individuals is

$$E(\bar{Y}_j) = \frac{1}{n} \sum_{i=1}^{n_j} e^{\beta_{0j} + \beta_{1j} x_{ij}} \tag{4.4}$$

Thus, the individual observations are required. The same problem arises for any nonlinear function. Various solutions have been suggested when only aggregate data are available, but none is really satisfactory.

4.2 Growth curves

It is important, in many situations, to estimate curves over time for individuals undergoing some rapid change, as for example the growth of young children. Such curves can then be used to determine the deviation of a given individual from the mean or to compare different groups of individuals. The latter is important in epidemiology to aid in detecting changes in subpopulations that may indicate health problems.

One of the most important classes of such curves are the growth curves (Section 3.1). Here, I need only look at a special derivation of one of them.

4.2.1 RICHARDS CURVE

The sigmoid shape of growth curve data suggests that two processes are in competition (Day, 1966): a growth process, say

$$\frac{d\mu(t)}{dt} = \mu(t)^{\kappa+1} [c - \nu(t)]^{\gamma_1} \tag{4.5}$$

and an aging process

$$\frac{d\nu(t)}{dt} = \gamma_2 [c - \nu(t)] \tag{4.6}$$

inhibiting growth. Equation (4.6) can be solved; see Equation (3.7). This can be used to eliminate $\nu(t)$ from Equation (4.5), yielding

$$\mu(t) \frac{d^2 \mu(t)}{dt^2} - (\kappa + 1) \left(\frac{d\mu(t)}{dt} \right)^2 + \gamma \mu(t) \frac{d\mu(t)}{dt} = 0 \tag{4.7}$$

where $\gamma = \gamma_1 \gamma_2$. The solution to this equation is the Richards growth curve of Equation (3.20):

Table 4.1. AICs for various logistic growth curve models for weight gains of pregnant women.

	Normal	Log normal
Same intercept	473.2	470.0
AR(1)	247.0	241.6
Different intercept	307.9	305.8
AR(1)	240.0	236.6
Random intercept	331.9	317.8
AR(1)	248.0	242.6

$$\mu(t) = \alpha \left(1 + \kappa e^{-\gamma(t-\varsigma)}\right)^{-1/\kappa}$$

Generally, one would expect the parameter defining the family, κ, to be identical for all individuals following the same process.

I looked at this model in more detail in Section 3.1; other special cases were also described there.

4.2.2 WEIGHT GAINS OF PREGNANT WOMEN

One phenomenon of life that is generally closely followed is pregnancy. Thus, a series of weights is usually recorded for pregnant women. Standard curves allow doctors to detect deviations from what would be expected. In one study (Day, 1966), ten clinically normal women were weighed at irregular time intervals during their pregnancies.

Because weight gain during pregnancy does not start at zero, we must modify Equation (3.20) by adding an intercept:

$$\mu(t) = y_0 + \alpha(1 + \kappa e^{-\gamma(t-\iota)})^{-1/\kappa} \tag{4.8}$$

where y_0 is the normal weight when not pregnant. Unfortunately, for these data, this information is not available so that I must replace it by an unknown parameter that may be expected to vary among women:

$$\mu(t) = \alpha_0 + \alpha(1 + \kappa e^{-\gamma(t-\iota)})^{-1/\kappa} \tag{4.9}$$

When I fit this model to these data, I discover that the likelihood function is very flat in the direction of κ, with $\kappa = 1$, the logistic growth curve, providing a reasonable model.

In contrast to height data, weight data are known generally to be skewed. Hence, it is not surprising that the log normal distribution fits better than the normal distribution, as can be seen in the first line of Table 4.1. Here, the log weight has mean described by the logarithm of Equation (4.9). So far in these models, I have not looked at the variability among the women, nor at the dependence among observations on each woman.

4.2.3 DIFFERENCES AMONG WOMEN

Different intercepts Women start pregnancy at greatly varying weights. When this weight is available, it can be used directly in the model for prediction. Here, if I introduce a different (estimated) intercept for each woman, a fixed-effects model, the fit is greatly improved (third line of Table 4.1).

Random intercepts Care must be taken in introducing random intercepts into a nonlinear model. For the normal distribution, Equation (4.9) can be modified as follows:

$$\mu(t) = \alpha_0 + u_i + \alpha(1 + \kappa e^{-\gamma(t-\iota)})^{-1/\kappa} \tag{4.10}$$

where u_i is the random difference from the mean, α_0 for the ith women. However, for the log normal distribution, it is not appropriate to take the logarithm of this equation; the weights are so variable that Equation (4.10) yields negative values and the logarithm cannot be calculated. In any case, the standard random intercepts model for the log normal distribution (when fitted by taking logarithms of the response variable and using the normal distribution) has

$$\mu(t) = \log\left[\alpha_0 + \alpha(1 + \kappa e^{-\gamma(t-\iota)})^{-1/\kappa}\right] + u_i \tag{4.11}$$

This model, with normally distributed random effects, fits less well than the fixed-effects one, as can be seen in the fifth line of Table 4.1.

Because of the great variability among women, one might be led to the conclusion that the normal mixing distribution is not appropriate. However, the longer tailed Cauchy distribution, still with a log normal distribution, provides an even poorer fit: the AIC is 320.4.

Another possibility is to use a multiplicative random effect with mean 1 instead of 0,

$$\mu(t) = \log\left[\alpha_0 u_i + \alpha(1 + \kappa e^{-\gamma(t-\iota)})^{-1/\kappa}\right] \tag{4.12}$$

say with a gamma mixing distribution. However, this is even worse (AIC 329.9).

Autoregression There is considerable variability about the mean growth curve so that an autoregression effect might be expected. When this is added to each of the previous models, the fit is always much improved (Table 4.1). The best model has a different intercept for each woman and an AR(1) to allow for this dependence among observations.

The underlying (marginal) growth curves and the individual curves for the first nine women are plotted in Figure 4.1. Most of the women follow the underlying curve rather closely. Individuals 1 and 8 appear to have a larger slope and individuals 6 and 10 (not shown) a smaller one, but these variations are handled fairly well by the AR(1).

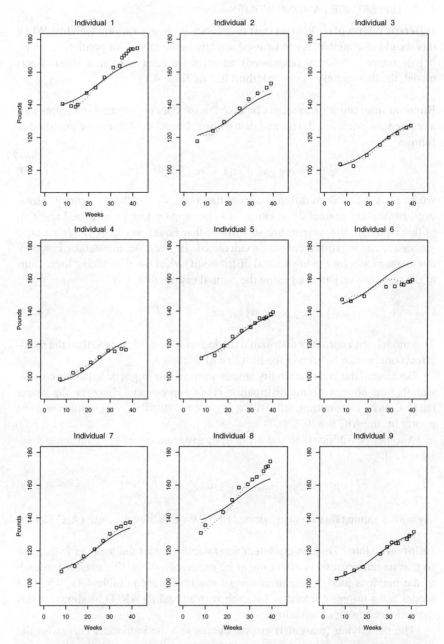

Fig. 4.1. Weights of nine clinically normal women during pregnancy, with the fitted log normal AR(1) model with different intercepts (solid: underlying profile; dotted: individual profile, both as geometric means).

Thus, perhaps surprisingly, it is not possible to replace the ten different intercepts by a random intercept. The dependence among observations is due primarily to fluctuations from the growth curve over time, not to static differences among the women. In fact, this is an advantage for using the model because the initial weight of a woman will be available and her individual curve can be updated at each measurement using the AR(1) model.

4.3 Death rates

One of the most important indicators studied in epidemiology is death rates. Differential rates among subpopulations or over time can point to significant health problems.

4.3.1 LOG LINEAR MODELS

In standard analyses, Poisson log linear regression is used for the number of events with the logarithm of the size of the population as an offset. In this way, the ratio of events to population size, the rate, is, in fact, being modelled. Here, I shall look at a case were the log linear assumption is questionable and a more nonlinear model is required.

4.3.2 MALIGNANT NEOPLASMS

In the 1970s, there was concern that fluoridation of water supplies could possibly be associated with cancer. A study was conducted to compare cancer mortality in the ten largest USA cities that were fluoridated between 1951 and 1956 (San Francisco, Washington, DC, Chicago, Baltimore, St Louis, Buffalo, Cleveland, Philadelphia, Pittsburgh, and Milwaukee) with the ten that were not before 1969 (Los Angeles, Atlanta, New Orleans, Boston, Kansas City, Newark, Cincinnati, Columbus, Portland, and Seattle). Population totals were available for these cities in 1950, before fluoridation, but only national death rates (Table 4.2). The idea was to compare the situation then with that in 1970, after fluoridation.

The cancer rates in the ten fluoridated cities in 1950 were 180.76 per 100 000 and, in the unfluoridated cities, 178.96. In 1970, these were respectively 217.38 and 197.16, seeming to indicate a link between the rate and fluoridation. However, because cancer mortality rates differ with age, sex, and race, among other factors, differential changes in these demographic variables could possibly explain the differences in rates between the two groups of cities in 1970.

Here, I shall study this differential mortality in 1950, as it may depend on sex, race, and age. The death rates are plotted in Figure 4.2, showing a somewhat sigmoidal form. Although there is no mechanistic reason for this, a growth curve may prove adequate. Notice that a log linear model corresponds to an exponential growth curve. In fitting the counts of deaths, the growth function must be multiplied by the appropriate totals (the sum of fluoridated and unfluoridated populations for a given age, sex, and race). Because of the variability, an overdispersed distribution will probably be necessary.

Table 4.2. Population totals from ten fluoridated and ten unfluoridated cities in the USA in 1950 and national deaths from malignant neoplasms standardized to these population totals (both rounded from rates). (Oldham and Newell, 1977)

Age	White				Black			
	Male		Female		Male		Female	
	National deaths							
0–5	86		71		13		11	
5–15	72		59		11		8	
15–25	99		81		14		19	
25–35	222		278		44		96	
35–45	503		912		124		285	
45–55	1500		1955		353		446	
55–65	3312		3068		437		410	
65–75	3577		3311		291		245	
75–85	2005		2202		103		88	
85+	370		524		18		25	
	Population totals for fluoridation							
	Yes	No	Yes	No	Yes	No	Yes	No
0–5	403749	290382	387599	279948	94854	54520	94316	53712
5–15	561480	389429	549206	381273	128661	72522	131461	73698
15–25	590657	409047	631786	446667	117895	66864	144273	81413
25–35	740852	513752	785426	543290	157946	88687	184002	101839
35–45	669039	462392	721580	502216	141151	81119	151164	87364
45–55	589796	404932	617789	434470	110035	60251	103037	60178
55–65	489559	319479	495588	350706	57171	32991	52864	32330
65–75	259476	188322	298774	238360	27347	18590	30577	20794
75–85	81180	65395	115418	99047	7214	4996	9152	6025
85+	11305	10066	20457	18443	1184	808	2046	1470

4.3.3 OVERDISPERSION

For a negative binomial distribution, the AICs are 242.6 for an exponential curve (1310.5 for the Poisson distribution), 297.0 for the logistic curve, and 240.3 for the Gompertz curve. There is no indication of a difference in parameter values with sex or race. However, from Figure 4.2, it appears that the form of the curves for Blacks changes at about age 60. If I allow for a different asymptote for them after this age, the AIC reduces slightly, to 239.7, giving some indication of a possible change; allowing a different slope does not improve the model. The three curves are plotted in Figure 4.2.

From these models, I can find no differences among sex or race that cannot be ascribed to random variation. However, they are not mechanistic models and even the third one does not seem to follow the data very closely.

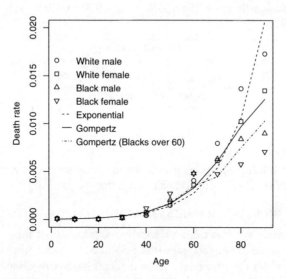

Fig. 4.2. Observed rates of malignant neoplasms in four subpopulations with three fitted growth curves.

4.4 Change points

A common problem in epidemiology is to determine if the incidence of a disease is changing over time. If the change is relatively abrupt at some point in time, determination of that time point is called the change-point problem (see Section 3.3.3).

4.4.1 POISSON PROCESS

Because we are interested in counts of the disease over time, a simple model is the Poisson process (Section B.6.2). When such a process is in operation, the rate of occurrence of new cases of the disease remains constant over time, the counts following a Poisson distribution within small intervals of time. If there is a change point, the mean of the Poisson distribution has changed at that point in time. Thus, we shall have a special case of Equation (3.39):

$$Y_t \sim \begin{cases} f(\mu_1) & t = 1, \ldots, \tau \\ f(\mu_2) & t = \tau+1, \ldots, T \end{cases} \quad (4.13)$$

where $f(\cdot)$ is a Poisson distribution and τ is an unknown parameter giving the change-point time. Hence, for a single series, there will be three parameters to estimate, the two means, before and after, and the change point.

Unfortunately, for such models, the likelihood function can be very irregular, with local maxima; standard optimization algorithms, especially those using derivatives, will have trouble finding the maximum. A simple approach is to fix a

Table 4.3. Annual numbers of cases of hæmolytic uræmic syndrome in Birmingham and Newcastle-upon-Tyne, UK, from 1970 to 1989. (Henderson and Matthews, 1993)

Birmingham									
1	5	3	2	2	1	0	0	2	1
1	7	11	4	7	10	16	16	9	15
Newcastle-upon-Tyne									
6	1	0	0	2	0	1	8	4	1
4	0	4	3	3	13	14	8	9	19

grid of values of the change-point parameter and optimize over the other parameters. The resulting set of likelihood values can then be plotted.

4.4.2 THE HÆMOLYTIC URÆMIC SYNDROME STUDY

Hæmolytic uræmic syndrome is a severe illness, primarily of infants and young children, that can be life threatening. It is associated with diarrhoea but its ætiology is unknown. Various bacterial and viral agents have been suspected, particularly an association with the level of *E. coli* in the environment. Health authorities in the UK were concerned that this illness may have increased in the 1980s.

Annual numbers of cases were available from two specialist centres, in Birmingham and Newcastle-upon-Tyne, from 1970 to 1989, as shown in Table 4.3. If we plot the cumulative numbers of cases separately for the two centres, as in Figure 4.3, we see that the slope appears to increase most sharply in about 1980 for Birmingham and in about 1984 for Newcastle-upon-Tyne.

4.4.3 DETECTING A CHANGE POINT

If I fit a common Poisson distribution to all times at both centres, the AIC is 162.8, whereas it is 163.4 when each centre is allowed to have a different mean. Thus, over the 20 years, the average number of cases per year is about the same in the two centres. This appears to be quite accidental because these are not rates and the sizes of the catchment areas of the two centres could be very different.

If I fit a log linear model where the mean depends on time, the AIC reduces to 105.3 with the same curve for both centres. There is no indication that a different intercept or slope is necessary for the two centres. Clearly, the mean number of cases is changing over time.

When I allow for a change in mean at some unknown point in time, the same for both centres, the AIC reduces to 104.7 if the means, before and after, are the same for both centres, and increases to 106.0 if the (four) means are different. Again, I find no difference between the centres. The log likelihood for the first of these two models is plotted in Figure 4.4. (That for the second model is very similar.) We can see how irregular it is, with a double mode. The change point is estimated to be between 1984 and 1985. (The second mode is 4.4 lower, a much poorer model.)

4.4. CHANGE POINTS

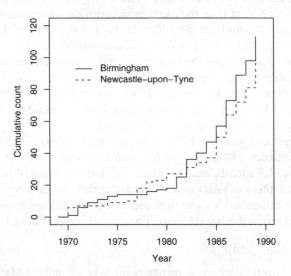

Fig. 4.3. Cumulative counts of hæmolytic uræmic syndrome in Newcastle-upon-Tyne and Birmingham, 1970–1989.

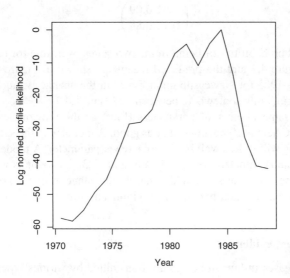

Fig. 4.4. Log normed profile likelihood function for the date of change being the same in Newcastle-upon-Tyne and Birmingham, with common means for the two centres.

Up until now, I have assumed that the change point occurred at the same time for both centres. Let us now look more closely at this assumption. If I fit a different change-point time for each centre, with the same means before for both centres and after for both, the AIC is further reduced to 97.9. With different means, it is 98.2. Again, there is no indication of difference in mean between centres, either before or after the change, but the change occurred in a different year at each centre. The joint log likelihood surface for the two change points is plotted in Figure 4.5. This surface is also very irregular, with several local maxima. Notice the difference in impression of what are plausible values that are given by the plots of likelihood and log likelihood.

The change-point times are estimated to be between 1980 and 1981 for Birmingham and between 1984 and 1985 for Newcastle-upon-Tyne. The means are 2.1 before and 11.3 after the change. These are plotted in Figure 4.6.

Note that, in this analysis, I have assumed that there is only one change point. There is some evidence that more than one change might have occurred but, for only two short series, that would seem to be a rather complex model.

4.4.4 A DYNAMIC MODEL

Another approach to detecting a change point is to use hidden Markov models (Sections 3.3.3 and B.5.2). I shall use a model with two hidden states and the same Poisson mean for the two cities in a given state. The means in the two states are estimated to be 1.9 and 11.1 and the matrix of hidden transition probabilities to be

$$\begin{pmatrix} 0.91 & 0.09 \\ 0.12 & 0.88 \end{pmatrix}$$

The predicted probabilities of being in the two states over time for each city are plotted in Figure 4.7 and the predicted means are shown in Figure 4.8. These point to 1984–1985 for Newcastle-upon-Tyne but the change is much less clear for Birmingham, lying somewhere between 1980 and 1984.

With the same number of parameters (four) as the previous change-point model, the AIC here is 106.3, not nearly as good. A model with the second hidden state absorbing will fit less well but has one fewer parameter. A model with three hidden states and estimated means, 1.0, 4.6, and 12.3, fits about as well: AIC of 106.6 with nine parameters. An additional disadvantage of this approach is that it does not have an explicit parameter providing an estimate of when the change took place.

4.5 Recurrent epidemics

Infectious diseases in human beings are transmitted by various types of microorganisms, primarily bacteria and viruses. Many approaches to the study of the development and spread of epidemics involve compartment models (Section 3.2.1). In this section, I shall look at one of the best known of these models and

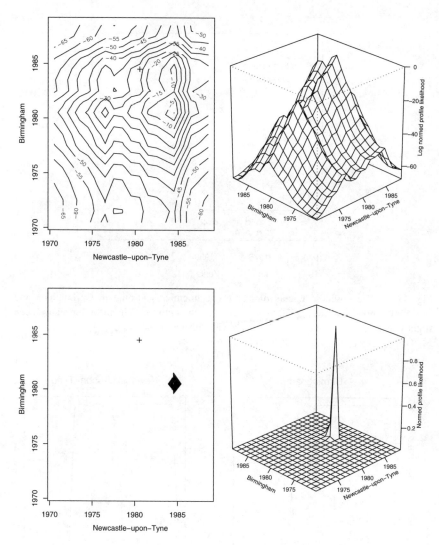

Fig. 4.5. Likelihood surface for the date of change being different in Newcastle-upon-Tyne and Birmingham, with common means for the two centres. Top panel: log normed profile likelihood. Bottom panel: normed profile likelihood (contours from 0.1 to 0.9 in steps of 0.1).

show how it can be adapted to the situation where a disease recurs at frequent intervals.

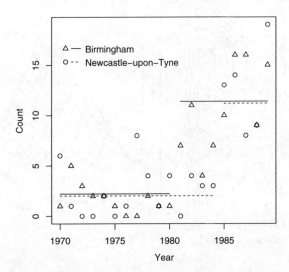

Fig. 4.6. The observed counts of hæmolytic uræmic syndrome in Birmingham and Newcastle-upon-Tyne from 1970 to 1989 and the fitted model. (The mean lines have been slightly displaced vertically so that both are visible.)

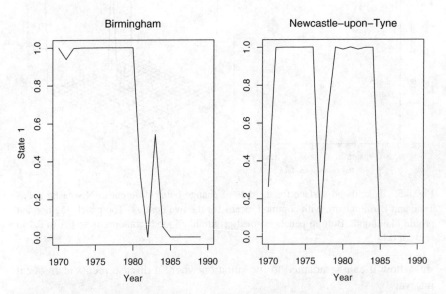

Fig. 4.7. The probability of being in the first state of the hidden Markov model for the hæmolytic uræmic syndrome in Birmingham and Newcastle-upon-Tyne from 1970 to 1989.

4.5. RECURRENT EPIDEMICS

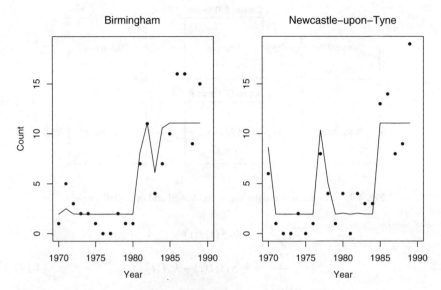

Fig. 4.8. The predicted individual mean profiles from the hidden Markov model for the hæmolytic uræmic syndrome in Birmingham and Newcastle-upon-Tyne from 1970 to 1989.

4.5.1 EPIDEMIC MODELS

SIR model Suppose that a nonfatal infectious disease confers immunity upon recovery. We can then divide a given population into three distinct categories:

(1) susceptibles (S) who can catch the disease;
(2) infectives (I) who have the disease and are contagious so that they can transmit it;
(3) recovered (R), who have had the disease and are now immune.

The stages can then be described by a compartment model, as shown in the top panel of Figure 4.9. This is called the (closed) SIR model and is an example of an event history model (Section 6.1.2).

Let us assume that

- the rate (k_2) of exit from the susceptible category and entry to the infective category is proportional to the present numbers of infectives and susceptibles;
- the rate (k_3) of exit from the infective category and entry to the recovered category is proportional to the present number of infectives;
- each category of people is uniformly mixed so that every pair of individuals has the same probability of meeting; and
- the population is of constant size.

Then, the model can be defined by the differential equations

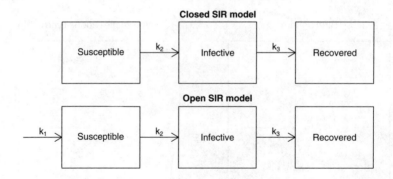

Fig. 4.9. Graphical presentation of the closed and open SIR models.

$$\frac{dS(t)}{dt} = -k_2 S(t) I(t)$$
$$\frac{dI(t)}{dt} = k_2 S(t) I(t) - k_3 I(t) \quad (4.14)$$
$$\frac{dR(t)}{dt} = k_3 I(t)$$

with initial conditions $S(0) = S_0 > 0$, $I(0) = I_0 > 0$, and $R(0) = 0$. If $S_0 < k_3/k_2$, the infection eventually dies out and no epidemic occurs.

If the population is not closed so that susceptibles are born or can immigrate at the constant rate k_1, the stages are now given by the compartment model in the bottom panel of Figure 4.9 and the first equation becomes

$$\frac{dS(t)}{dt} = k_1 - k_2 S(t) I(t) \quad (4.15)$$

This is an open SIR model. The system will reach an endemic level or equilibrium at $S_\infty = k_3/k_2$ and $I_\infty = k_1/k_3$, obtained by setting the above equations equal to zero.

Oscillations However, with stochastic variability, there will be damped oscillations around the equilibrium starting after each disturbance. If the deviations from the equilibrium values are small, the appropriate functions can be derived. Generally, information is only available on infectives, so that I shall concentrate on this. The resulting function will be

$$I(t) = I_\infty \left[1 + \kappa e^{-t/(2\sigma)} \cos(\xi t) \right] \quad (4.16)$$

where $\sigma = \frac{k_3}{k_2 k_1}$ and $\xi = \sqrt{\frac{k_2}{\sigma} - \frac{1}{4\sigma^2}}$ (Bartlett, 1960, pp. 62–63). The maximum magnitude of the oscillations from the equilibrium value is given by κ and the period by $2\pi/\xi$. Notice that oscillations are symmetric about I_∞.

4.5. RECURRENT EPIDEMICS

Table 4.4. Monthly numbers of cases of measles and chicken pox in Philadelphia, USA, from January 1941 to December 1943. (Bartlett, 1960, p. 73)

	Measles			Chicken pox		
Month	1941	1942	1943	1941	1942	1943
Jan	2906	62	4923	705	1021	556
Feb	4770	93	4759	555	991	439
Mar	6991	132	3583	720	1167	461
Apr	5457	222	1428	827	1144	432
May	2203	194	1198	582	974	550
Jun	527	135	821	739	531	548
Jul	77	70	235	79	92	214
Aug	8	38	10	25	16	80
Sep	7	44	14	22	18	32
Oct	10	275	22	87	124	160
Nov	19	1122	23	360	227	345
Dec	16	2770	22	730	387	585

If the stochastic disturbances occur frequently enough, damping will not have had time to take effect and we have

$$I(t) = I_\infty \left[1 + \kappa \cos(\xi t)\right] \qquad (4.17)$$

Notice that, from this function, we can no longer obtain estimates of all three rate constants because they now only relate to two parameters, I_∞ and ξ.

4.5.2 CHILDHOOD INFECTIONS

Measles and chicken pox are well-known childhood diseases; they have been closely studied in epidemiology. They have immunizing characteristics that make the susceptible population and the new recruits well defined. However, measles tends to have periodic epidemics about once every two years in large enough populations, at least if vaccination is not widely available, whereas chicken pox has a more stable seasonal variability. This can be seen in the data from Philadelphia, USA, for the early 1940s, given in Table 4.4.

Chicken pox Let us consider first the chicken pox infections. Because the cosine function has a maximum at 0, I set time to be zero for March 1941. For the regression function in Equation (4.16), the Poisson distribution gives an AIC of 1206.8. However, there is a great deal of overdispersion so that the negative binomial distribution has 227.6. I obtain $\hat{\sigma} = 411.8$ indicating that damping is not in effect. Thus, Equation (4.17) has an AIC of 227.1. The period is estimated to be 11.9 months, the equilibrium value is $\widehat{I_\infty} = 462.1$, and $\hat{\kappa} = 0.96$ so that the maximum is almost double the equilibrium value. The fitted curves for the Poisson and negative binomial distributions are plotted in the top graph of Figure

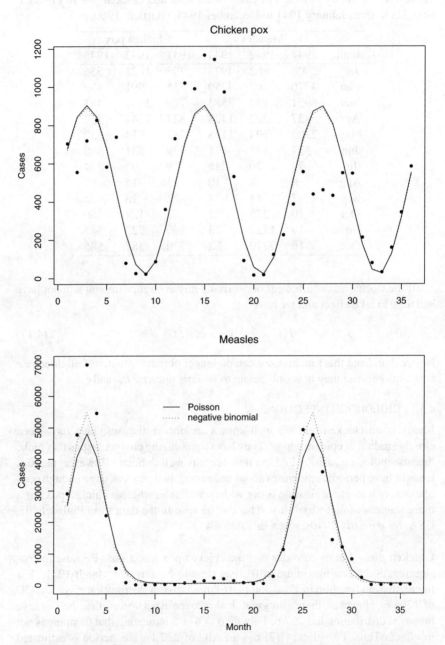

Fig. 4.10. Observed cases of measles and chicken pox in Philadelphia, USA, from January 1941 to December 1943, with the fitted Poisson and negative binomial models.

4.10. These curves are very similar but, of course, the variation about the curves is very different in the two cases.

Measles Let us now look at measles. For the Poisson and negative binomial distributions, Equation (4.16) gives, respectively, 20 705.1 and 265.0. Here, I have $\hat{\sigma} \to \infty$ and Equation (4.17) with the negative binomial distribution gives 264.2. The equilibrium value is estimated to be $\widehat{I_\infty} = 839.3$, whereas the maximum observed number of cases is 6991. Thus, the oscillations cannot be symmetric about I_∞, reach near the peak, and still always remain positive.

Two possible ways to obtain an asymmetric function by modifying Equation (4.17) are

$$I(t) = I_\infty e^{1+\kappa \cos(\xi t)} \tag{4.18}$$

and

$$I(t) = I_\infty \left[1 + e^{\kappa \cos(\xi t)}\right] \tag{4.19}$$

These yield, respectively, AICs of 255.7 and 246.9 for the negative binomial distribution. For the latter curve, the period is estimated to be 23.0 months and the equilibrium value is now $\widehat{I_\infty} = 53.2$. This model is plotted in the bottom graph of Figure 4.10 for the Poisson and negative binomial distributions. Here, there is somewhat more difference between the two curves than for chicken pox.

4.6 Infectious disease outbreaks

One important goal of epidemiology is to understand the mechanisms of transmission of a given disease, generally through the study of observed cases. When an outbreak occurs, this knowledge can aid in controlling further transmission.

4.6.1 MICRO-ORGANISM SUBTYPING

For many infectious diseases, the micro-organisms' genetic characteristics remain constant during the cycle within the host and during transmission. (A major exception is HIV, the cause of AIDS.) Molecular biology provides useful tools in this investigation. It can be used to identify *subtypes* of the micro-organism involved in a cluster of cases of the disease (of size N, say). This information can be used, along with that concerning personal contacts among the people in the cluster, to study possible mechanisms of transmission.

The first identified case of the disease in a cluster is called the *index case*. Blood samples are obtained from the case and from as many others in the cluster as feasible. These are cultured for the micro-organism to identify subtypes. Cases having the same subtype of micro-organism may possibly be related by direct transmission whereas transmission among those within different subtypes may be excluded if the genetic characteristics have remained constant.

One possible problem is that the subtype localized is, in fact, widely spread in the population, in which case this procedure provides little support for direct transmission. To check this, the typing procedure should be carried out on a control or reference group of subjects (of size M, say) having the same infectious disease, but unrelated to the cluster of interest *and to each other*. If the subtype in the cluster is rare or nonexistent in this reference group, then there is a much higher chance that the cases in the cluster are related by direct transmission.

4.6.2 TYPING MODEL

The comparison of the cluster and the reference groups involves the difference in the proportion of subjects with the given subtype of micro-organism in each group: n out of N and m out of M, respectively, have the same subtype as the index case. To study this difference, we require a statistical model (Mellen, 1999).

Let π_p be the probability of the subtype in the population and π_c that in the cluster. Note that we assume that the subjects in the cluster are interdependent. However, because the subjects in the reference group are unrelated among themselves and not related to the cluster, these observations can be assumed to have a binomial distribution

$$\Pr(m|M;\pi_p) = \binom{M}{m} \pi_p^m (1-\pi_p)^{M-m} \quad (4.20)$$

Now, let $\delta = 1$ if transmission occurred from the index case to the cluster and $\delta = 0$ otherwise. If $\delta = 0$, the index case is related neither to the cluster nor to the reference group and has the same probability as those in the latter group so that it can be included in the latter:

$$\Pr(m+1|M+1;\pi) = \binom{M+1}{m+1} \pi_p^{m+1} (1-\pi_p)^{M-m+1} \quad (4.21)$$

On the other hand, if the index case is related to the cluster, its probability is π_c so that the combined probability is

$$\Pr(m|M;\pi_p,\pi_c) = \pi_c \binom{M}{m} \pi_p^m (1-\pi_p)^{M-m} \quad (4.22)$$

From this development, the likelihood can be written as

$$L(\delta,\pi_p,\pi_c) = [\delta\pi_c + (1-\delta)\pi_p] \binom{M}{m} \pi_p^m (1-\pi_p)^{M-m}$$
$$\times \Pr(n|N;\pi_c) \quad (4.23)$$

where $\Pr(n|N;\pi_c)$ is the probability for the cluster. This will not be binomial because of the dependence through transmission, although we can nevertheless estimate $\hat{\pi}_c = n/N$. However, the probability of the cluster does not depend on δ or π_p so that the profile likelihood is

$$L(\delta, \pi_p, \pi_c = n/N) \propto \left[\delta\frac{n}{N} + (1-\delta)\pi_p\right] \pi_p^m (1-\pi_p)^{M-m} \quad (4.24)$$

With this profile likelihood, we can make inferences about whether or not transmission occurred from the index case to the cluster (δ). However, if we want to study plausible values of π_c, we must specify some dependency model for $\Pr(n|N;\pi_c)$.

4.6.3 THE MAINE TUBERCULOSIS OUTBREAK

From 1989 to 1992, an outbreak of tuberculosis occurred in a small town in Maine, USA (Mellen, 1999). One patient was diagnosed with active tuberculosis and was able to identify his or her contacts. Of the patients isolated, 21 had active tuberculosis. The first patient turned out to be the index case.

Mycobacterium tuberculosis was subtyped from this index case, in the way described above, and for only $N = 6$ of the 21 other patients in the cluster. $M = 3$ other patients at other independent locations in Maine were also examined, forming the reference group. The seven samples from the cluster, including the index case, had the same subtype so that $n = 6$, whereas none of those in the reference group did ($m = 0$). Thus, the profile likelihood function is

$$L(\delta, \pi_p, \pi_c = 1) \propto [\delta + (1-\delta)\pi_p](1-\pi_p)^3$$

This is plotted in Figure 4.11. Even with such a small set of observations, we see that the evidence is rather strong in favour of the cluster, including the index case, being a distinct subgroup for which transmission occurred from the index case ($\delta = 1$).

Further reading Many good introductions to methods in epidemiology are available: for example, Armstrong *et al.* (1992), Checkoway *et al.* (1989), Kelsey *et al.* (1986), Khoury *et al.* (1993), and Lilienfeld and Stolley (1994). For introductions to the standard statistical analyses in epidemiology, see Clayton and Hills (1993), Kahn and Sempos (1989), and Selvin (1991).

For the spread of epidemics, see Anderson and May (1991), Bartlett (1960), Murray (1993), and Shigesada and Kawasaki (1997).

4.7 Exercises

(1) For the weight gains of pregnant women of Section 4.2.2:
   (a) Does allowing the slope to vary among women improve the model?
   (b) Can you find a distribution other than the log normal that fits these data well?
(3) Try to develop a better model for the neoplasm mortality data of Section 4.3.2.

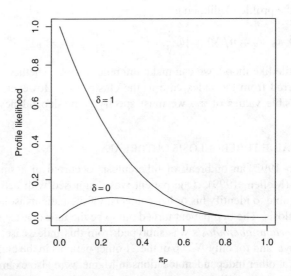

Fig. 4.11. Profile likelihood function for the tuberculosis outbreak in Maine, USA.

(4) In the final model for the hæmolytic uræmic syndrome, as shown in Figure 4.6, there is considerable variability about the mean lines. Check if overdispersion is present.

(5) The most famous study of cigarette smoking and lung cancer was that of Doll and Hill for British physicians. The numbers of cases are given in Table C.3 along with the corresponding person-years at risk, by years of smoking (age minus 20 years) and number of cigarettes smoked per day.

   (a) The standard model fitted to these data is Poisson log linear with log person-years at risk as offset. Fit the additive model (without interaction between years of smoking and number of cigarettes smoked).

   (b) Frome (1983) suggests a nonlinear model based on the amount of carcinogen applied per unit time at a constant rate (d, here, the number of cigarettes smoked) and the time since exposure began (t, here, the years of smoking):

$$\mu = N(\gamma + \alpha d^\theta) t^\beta$$

   where N is the number of person-years at risk for those values of d and t. (For the development of a somewhat similar model in a different context, see Section 9.4.2.) Fit this model as well.

   (c) Which model fits best? Interpret the results.

   (d) Is there any indication of overdispersion? If so, fit an improved model and interpret the results.

(5) An historical cohort study of mortality of workers in an asbestos textile manufacturing plant was sponsored by the USA National Institute for Occupational Safety and Health. The plant was located in Charleston, South Carolina, USA, and had been producing asbestos products, primarily fireproof fabrics and automotive parts, since 1896. The cohort consisted of any white male employed for at least one month between 1 January, 1940 and 31 December 1965. Mortality follow-up continued until 1975.

Exposure measurements were made at the workplace. Air concentrations of asbestos were measured as the numbers of fibres longer than 5 μm per cm^3 of air. For each worker, the cumulative exposure was estimated as the summed product of air concentrations and time in days at the job.

Within this cohort study, 35 individuals died of lung cancer. A case–control study was set up by matching them with other members of the cohort with four controls for each case. The controls were selected by incidence density matching on age at risk. The results, classified by age and exposure, are given in Table C.4.

(a) Develop an appropriate model to describe the dependence of risk of lung cancer mortality on exposure to asbestos.

(b) Age is not a measure of time working in the plant. How can you appropriately enter age into your model?

(3) For the data on cases of measles and chicken pox in Section 4.5.2:

(a) Is it possible to develop a reasonable model based on autoregression?

(b) Which model fits the data better?

(c) Which model provides a better explanation of the processes?

5
Clinical trials

One of the main driving forces behind the development of new statistical methods in recent years has been the importance of *clinical trials* both in public health initiatives and in industry. Public control of the release of new medications by national agencies has led to their more rigorous testing, with the accompanying need for reliable statistical procedures. A long-term goal must be the understanding of *why* a drug works and not just an empirical demonstration that it produces a better result than a placebo or the standard treatment. This will require mechanistic models at all stages of the development process. In this and the following chapters, I shall explore some of the tools that are available.

5.1 Evaluating a new medication

In medical research, clinical trials are the main method used to evaluate the effectiveness of some treatment(s), such as drugs, surgery, physiotherapy, diet, health education, and so on, in curing some illness or improving health. Here, I shall consider the more advanced, and more publicized, stages of this process, before going on, in the following chapters, to look at some of the more fundamental phases of drug discovery and development.

5.1.1 GOALS

Thus, for the moment, the goal will be to evaluate a new treatment, under the most realistic conditions possible, to determine if it will provide significantly better results than the current methods. However, first, we need an overview of the drug development process.

Clinical trials, at least in the more advanced phases, involve patients with a given medical condition and are designed to provide information about the most appropriate treatment for future patients having the same condition. The majority of clinical trials are designed for the evaluation of some specific drug, most often conducted, or at least financed, by a pharmaceutical company.

Early phases of study of a new treatment involve a wide variety of statistical techniques, often nonlinear; these will be covered here and in various other chapters of this text. Later phases with their single 'endpoint' have, as an immediate goal, the decision as to whether or not to introduce the new treatment so that decision-making procedures, such as statistical tests, dominate and the scientific component can often be rather minor.

5.1.2 DESIGNS

Once a potential new therapy has been discovered, a complete study of it requires evaluation of *safety*, *efficacy*, and *quality of life* (Chapter 6). Especially for a drug that is to be commercialized, pre-clinical research begins with animal experiments testing for safety. Assay methodology (Chapter 9) must also be developed at this time in order to be able to detect the drug and measure its concentration. Extensive toxicology testing is carried out to ensure safety before first administration to human beings. For drugs, a preliminary formulation (Chapter 9) is determined.

Then, human experimentation can begin. It can generally be classified into four phases:

(1) *Phase I*: initial study of pharmacology and toxicity, usually with healthy volunteers (a major exception being cancer trials, where treatments can be very aggressive), to determine safety at various doses, including side effects (see Chapters 7 and 8);
(2) *Phase II*: small-scale, often noncomparative, clinical investigation on patients, to screen out ineffective drugs and to determine dose and other characteristics of the therapy;
(3) *Phase III*: full-scale evaluation of an apparently effective treatment in its final form, as compared to a control or to standard treatment;
(4) *Phase IV*: surveillance after approval for commercialization, monitoring long-term adverse effects and quality of life.

The first two phases involve tightly controlled scientific investigation of medical aspects, whereas the third is closer to realistic administration of the therapy once commercialized. The first two are exploratory, providing hypotheses that can be tested with the results of the third. The fourth may often take the form of a sample survey, rather than a trial. Ascertainment of effects on quality of life (Chapter 6) has become an important component of the later phases.

Phase II trials were traditionally often uncontrolled and not blinded; this could bias the results, for example by the enthusiasm of the investigators. Many early studies of this type have suggested that the new treatment is highly effective, only for this apparent benefit to disappear when more carefully tested in Phase III. Thus, the use of randomization is increasing in Phase II studies.

Most trials are parallel with subjects receiving the treatment to which they are randomized over the complete period of the study. However, in some cases, where treatment is short term, without lasting effects, such as for migraine, a cross-over trial may be used. These are also often used in the early phases for pharmacokinetics (Chapter 7) and pharmacodynamics (Chapter 8).

5.1.3 VALIDITY

Internal validity refers to the extent to which conclusions apply to the people actually studied, whereas *external validity* refers to the possibility of generalizing such conclusions to a wider population, whether persons, settings, or times. Clinical trials, when properly conducted, should have good internal validity. Thus, causal relationships can be studied in such closely controlled circumstances, but this will limit generalization of conclusions. Such trials must use volunteers so that there is no guarantee that they are representative of the population to which the results of the trial will be applied. Conclusions drawn from clinical trials to a general population about causal efficacy of a medication constitute a leap of faith with little or no statistical support.

Several major problems can arise in almost any clinical trial. Subjects may not follow the treatment regimen to which they have been assigned, called noncompliance. They may miss some meetings when observations are to be made (missing data) or leave the trial before it is finished (dropouts). All are extremely difficult to handle statistically and can invalidate any conclusions. The reasons for each case of noncompliance, missing data, or dropping out should be documented as completely as possible.

5.1.4 MODELS

A great variety of different models may be used in the analysis of clinical trial data, depending on the primary outcome of interest. For example, if the endpoint is survival, then models for durations (Chapter 6 and Section B.6) will be required. Here, I shall concentrate on one important class of nonlinear models, growth curves (Section 3.1). These can be used to model how some response variable either increases or decreases over the treatment period, hopefully eventually to settle down to some steady state, the asymptote, that is an acceptable condition for the patient.

5.2 Response decline to a stable state

Often in clinical trials, interest centres on how some treatment may improve the condition of patients by reducing some response to a safe, low, stable state. This, then, will be a case of 'negative growth'.

5.2.1 THE AZATHIOPRINE STUDY

Multiple sclerosis patients usually have high levels of immunoglobulins in their cerebrospinal fluid; lymphocytes can occur in the multiple sclerosis plaques in their central nervous system. These are characteristics of an autoimmune disease. Azathioprine (AZ) is a chemotherapy that has been applied successfully in treating other autoimmune diseases, such as lupus and renal transplant rejection. The steroid, methylprednisolone (MP), can also help to induce immunosuppression when used in conjunction with azathioprine.

Heitjan (1991b) analysed a randomized double-blinded clinical trial with three arms in which patients received (1) two placebos (P), or (2) real azathioprine and a placebo, or (3) real doses of azathioprine and methylprednisolone. The primary outcomes were frequency of relapse and rate of deterioration of neurological exam scores; measures of the size and functional capabilities of lymphocyte populations were important secondary outcomes. One of these is considered here.

One way in which the immune system damages target tissues is known as ADCC. In this process, the immune system recognizes a cell target and produces an antibody against it. When the cell becomes coated with this, killer lymphocytes attach themselves to the coating and destroy the cell. Such binding involves F_C receptors (FCR). Absolute FCR (AFCR) is the number of lymphocytes having the F_C receptor in a 1 mm^3 sample of peripheral blood. One goal is to reduce the level of AFCR.

Thus, blood samples were drawn from the 48 patients one or more times prior to therapy, at initiation, and in weeks 4, 8, and 12 plus every 12 weeks thereafter, and this measure of autoimmunity (AFCR) made. Samples taken during relapse were excluded. Treatment with AZ in the trial lasted for up to four years. On the other hand, the MP treatment was an initial series of intravenous infusions of MP followed by decreasing oral doses on alternate days for 36 weeks. Any treatment was reduced or discontinued if toxicities developed that were suspected to be related to it.

The data are reproduced in Lindsey (1999a, pp. 400–413). The responses are plotted in Figure 5.1; they were measured at highly irregular periods in time. Except for the profiles of two or three patients under placebo, all three of the plots seem rather similar, although the placebo group does not approach as closely to the zero level of AFCR as do the two other groups. The responses are generally decreasing in time, except, perhaps, at the very end, and the average profiles appear to be nonlinear.

An additional complication is that the dose of the medication for each patient was varied in time as a function of the patient's condition. AZ was administered orally, starting with a dose of 2.2 mg/kg daily (here scaled to be one unit), all being previously zero up until time zero. The dose was increased monthly in steps of 25 mg until white blood cells were held within a given range, until toxicity developed, or until double the initial dose was reached (although, with good tolerance, even higher doses could be given, at the discretion of the doctor). Thus, doses were often drastically reduced and increased, following the condition of the patient, the changes occurring at irregular periods that did not correspond to the times when the response, AFCR, was measured.

For blinding to be effective, each patient in the complete placebo group was matched with a patient in the other groups and their dose followed that of the paired patient, so that neither the patient nor the physician would know who was on placebo. The data on dose changes are plotted in Figure 5.2.

5.2.2 ASYMPTOTIC AND POLYNOMIAL CURVES

Heitjan (1991b) used a square-root transformation on the AFCR responses with a normal distribution for these data and I followed him in this for the analyses in Lindsey (1999a, pp. 134–142, 170–171). However, these are count data so that a more realistic mechanistic model can be used, although models based on the Poisson distribution fit very badly. I shall use the generalized logistic regression function of Equation (3.22) to describe the change in mean AFCR.

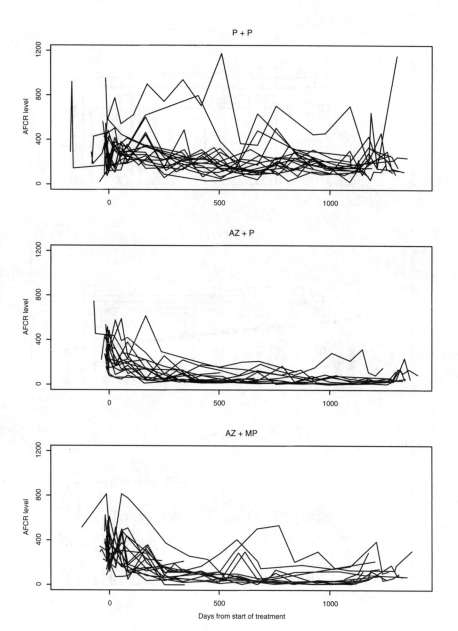

Fig. 5.1. Plots of AFCR level against time in days for the three treatments, for the multiple sclerosis data.

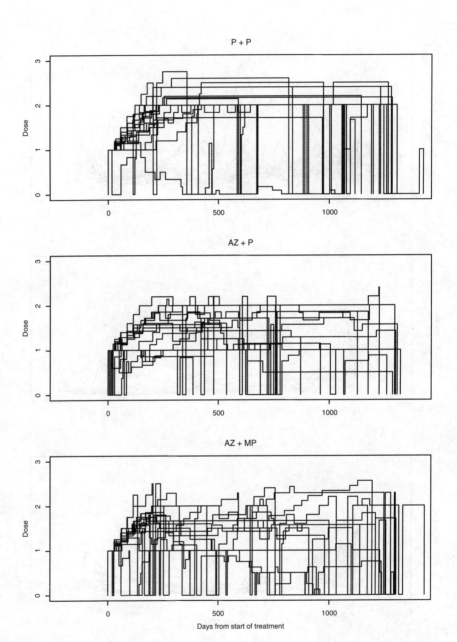

Fig. 5.2. Plots of dose level against time in days for the three treatments of multiple sclerosis.

5.2. RESPONSE DECLINE TO A STABLE STATE

Generalized logistic growth curve Let us first look at some models that do not take into account dependence among observations on the same subject. With this growth curve for the location parameter, the Poisson distribution has an AIC of 43 318.8 compared to 4786.0 for the corresponding negative binomial model. This clearly indicates that overdispersion is present.

With an autoregressive serial dependence, as in Equation (B.12), the negative binomial AIC drops to 4636.9 (γ can be set to unity in the logistic regression model). When α is allowed to depend on treatment, the AIC becomes 4634.2 with the same parameter value for both nonplacebo treatments whereas it is 4633.9 when ι is instead allowed to depend on treatment.

In this study, dose appears to be following a stochastic process that may be interdependent with that for AFCR because the doctor is varying dose in light of previous measurements of AFCR; it is an endogenous time-varying covariate. However, here I follow Heitjan (1991b) in conditioning on the dose at a given time in modelling AFCR. When the ι parameter is also made to depend on dose, for the two nonplacebo groups only, the AIC is 4620.6. One final improvement can be made by letting the negative binomial dispersion parameter depend on time, dose, and treatment, with an AIC of 4612.9.

The estimated regression function, with $\hat{\alpha} = 13.0$ and $\hat{\kappa} = -2.5$, is

$$\mu_t = 13.0 \left\{ 1 + \left[(13.0 e^{-5.56 + (0.44 + 0.318 d)a})^{2.5} - 1 \right] e^{13.0^{-2.5}(t-501)} \right\}^{0.4}$$

where t is time (with mean 501), d is dose, and a is a treatment indicator, being zero for the double placebo and one otherwise. The underlying marginal and individual recursive profiles for three subjects are plotted in Figure 5.3. The estimated value of κ indicates that the shape lies between the Mitscherlich ($\kappa = -1$) and Gompertz curves.

Polynomial curves Inspection of the profile graphs in Figure 5.1 shows that the response tends to rise at the end of the observation period instead of staying at an asymptotic value as predicted by the logistic curve. It is, thus, worthwhile to compare these results to those using a quadratic polynomial (with log link). The latter, with the negative binomial dispersion parameter depending on time (quadratically), dose, and treatment, has an AIC of 4585.9, quite a lot better than the generalized logistic curve. The estimated regression function is

$$\mu_t = e^{5.8 - 0.0017t + 0.0000012 t^2 - 0.00095 at - 0.29 bd}$$

Here, only the AZ plus placebo treatment, indicated by b, involves dose. The underlying marginal and individual recursive profiles, for the same three subjects as in Figure 5.3, are plotted in Figure 5.4.

Normality assumption As mentioned above, both Heitjan (1991b) and Lindsey (1999a) transformed the AFCR responses to normality using a square-root

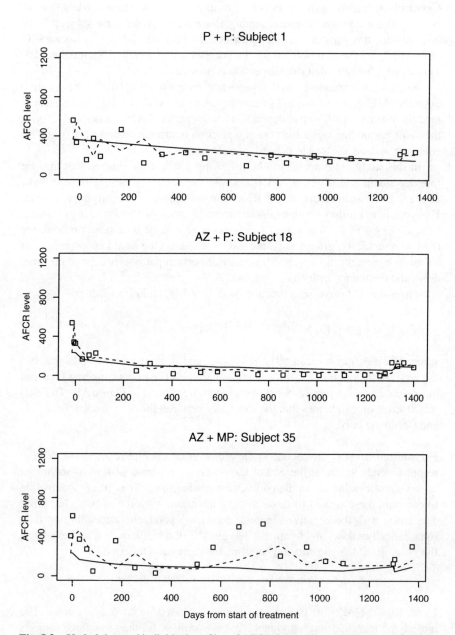

Fig. 5.3. Underlying and individual profiles of AFCR for the three treatments of multiple sclerosis, using the generalized logistic regression with a negative binomial distribution and serial dependence.

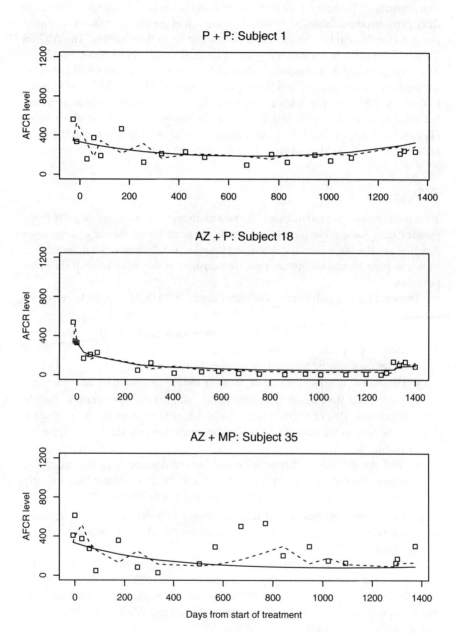

Fig. 5.4. Marginal and individual profiles of AFCR for the three treatments of multiple sclerosis, using the quadratic polynomial regression with a negative binomial distribution and serial dependence.

transformation. However, such a transformation is not strictly correct as there are three zero-response values for which the Jacobian of the transformation is infinite. For a comparison to be possible, let us eliminate these three values. The AIC for the best (quadratic polynomial) negative binomial model above becomes 4567.4. The corresponding best quadratic regression function with a normal distribution, square-root transformation, and autoregression has an AIC of 4548.4. (The AICs in Lindsey, 1999a, p. 136, include the three zero-response observations and have 0.5 missing in the Jacobian and hence are not comparable to those given here.) However, although fitting better, this model is less appealing because of the artificiality of a transformation when a more mechanistic model for counts is available.

5.2.3 CONCLUSIONS

With both regression models fitted, the two treatments showed significantly lower profiles than the double placebo. The conclusions about choice of regression function are the same with the negative binomial distribution as with the square-root-transformed normal distribution, demonstrating the robustness of these approaches.

The result that a polynomial fits better than a growth curve may have several explanations.

- The generalized logistic model with dose may not be flexible enough, because it only allows the asymptote, α, to vary among groups. The rate of decay may also be affected by the type of treatment.
- The dose may affect the rate of decay as well as or instead of the asymptote.
- Some other function of the dose, rather than the present strength, may be important. This might, for example, be a lagged value of the dose, given at some time in the past, or the total dose given up to the time the response is measured.
- Only the difference in treatment, and not the dose, may be important. As long as the patient is closely monitored, and the dose adjusted accordingly, the strength of the dose at a given time may not be important.

Any of these possibilities would require special knowledge from the research workers involved, because the variability in the data would not permit us to choose among them.

The examination of this example shows that a number of different complex models can often be applied to the same data and give relatively comparable fits. Only theoretical considerations, from the branch of research involved, can allow one to distinguish among them. However, each may provide its own illumination on the subject under study.

Further reading Standard introductions to clinical trials are given be Meinert (1986) and Pocock (1983). Matthews (2000) provides a good statistical introduction. Senn (1997) discusses many of the important issues in drug development.

5.3 Exercises

(1) (a) In the azathioprine study, does some other overdispersed count model fit better than the negative binomial distribution?

(b) Where possible, determine if any of the possible models mentioned in the conclusions improve the fit.

(c) Dose is a time-varying covariate that depends on the previous condition of the patient. Develop a suitable model for dose to describe this dependence.

(d) Can you link your model for dose to your model for the response variable?

(e) Subjects dropped out if toxicities developed that were suspected to be related to treatment. Unfortunately, information as to those involved is not available. Is there any indication that dropping out of those subjects with shorter observation periods depended on previous responses, on treatment, or on dose?

(6) A randomized double-blind clinical trial studied the roles of vitamins C and E and a high-fibre diet in reducing rectal polyps in a population at high risk from familial polyposis. This is a rare inherited disease that develops into cancer without preventive treatment. Patients were randomized to take either placebo (22), vitamins C and E (16), or vitamins C and E and high fibre (20). Two baseline counts were made, the second being a 'run-in'. The subjects were then examined every three months over four years and rectal polyps were counted, as shown in Table C.5.

A fair number of observations are missing and certain participants dropped out. Generally polyps were not removed. Nevertheless, polyp counts could decrease, owing either to spontaneous regression or to being hidden from view.

One goal of the study would be to see if polyps are reduced to a lower stable level. Because the treatments are not cures, one cannot expect complete elimination. The same polyps are being counted repeatedly, so that one may expect considerable dependence among the observations on each patient.

(a) Construct a suitable model.

(b) Determine if either of the treatments shows indication of being effective.

(c) Do any particular modelling problems arise because counts of polyps can decrease because they are hidden from view?

(d) Is dropping out occurring randomly?

6
Quality of life

As we have seen, a major goal of clinical trials is to evaluate the effectiveness of some treatment for illness or health problems. Although good health is important, if only defined in a narrow sense of curing a disease or longer life, it may not necessarily lead to increased well-being of a population in all its aspects.

6.1 Effects of medical treatment

Many modern medical treatments have important side effects that can make life difficult while, at the same time, perhaps alleviating or curing the condition being treated. Weighing the relative importance of the many dimensions of improved health is an extremely difficult problem, especially because each can have a different meaning and importance for different people.

6.1.1 GOALS

Medical research has slowly been moving from restricting attention to 'hard' goals such as curing a disease or increasing life span once an incurable disease has occurred to 'softer' goals related to the quality of life during this process. For example, one may ask if a patient should be submitted to an invasive treatment that causes pain or incapacity simply in order to delay the time of death. Thus, such measurements have become an important component of clinical trials (Chapter 5).

Unfortunately, quality is a difficult concept to measure. It may mean different things to different people. Thus, quality of life studies can involve many kinds of measures, often of an ordinal nature. Many of these necessarily imply personal, subjective, value judgements.

Here, I shall concentrate on the analysis of events defined as changes of state and of the times between such events. These are important because the state in which each individual finds him- or herself usually determines the quality of life. Of course, defining the states themselves may be a difficult conceptual problem.

6.1.2 CONSTRUCTING EVENT HISTORY MODELS

Event histories involve the times between events. These may be recurrent events such as migraine, epileptic fits, or infections, or they may involve moves between distinct states, such as catching a disease, being hospitalized, recovering, or dying.

We have seen an example of the second of these, in the epidemiological context, in Section 4.5.1. A subject is said to change *state* and the event is called a *transition* between the states. Several special cases are particularly important.

- Mortality: two states of which the second is absorbing (classical survival analysis).
- Competing risks: transition from one state to any one of several others.
- Recurrent events (the first example mentioned above).
- Alternance between two states.
- Disability: transition through a series of irreversible states (the second example mentioned, if death must be the final result).

Several of these may need to be combined to describe the complete history of subjects.

Model construction depends greatly on how the series of states for individuals is defined; generally, there is no unique structure. Where they are possible, certain assumptions will facilitate model building. A model is *progressive* if all states, except the first, have only one transition into them. Then, the current state defines what states were previously occupied and in what order, but not when the changes occurred. A transition probability is *Markovian* if it only depends on the present state and not on the previous history of the individual. However, it may depend on time; an extension is to allow it to depend on the time since the last event, a special case being the semi-Markov model (Section B.6.3).

Generally, it useful to clarify ideas by constructing a diagram for the states and possible transitions between them. Examples for several common models are shown in Figure 6.1.

A multistate model should not have several transition routes from one state to another; instead several different states may be defined. For example, if subjects in the state of having a given disease may recover either by natural body defences or by medical treatment, either these can be defined as two different recovery states, as in the alternative outcomes model of Figure 6.1, or they are not distinguished at all.

For recurrent events, it is especially important to establish a zero time point. If this is birth, then the time to the first event will generally be quite distinct from subsequent repetitions of the event. Often, it is convenient to start the process from the time of the first event. If this is unknown, the possible models that can be fitted may be limited; for example, a birth process is usually unreasonable because the actual number of previous events is unknown.

6.1.3 MODELS FOR ORDINAL VARIABLES

Ordinal regression models are closely related to binary logistic regression. A major difference is that more than two categories must be compared. However, as the name suggests, these response categories are ordered. Thus, the models cannot be simply based on a standard multinomial distribution which only carries the assumption that they are nominal.

6.1. EFFECTS OF MEDICAL TREATMENT

Recurrent events

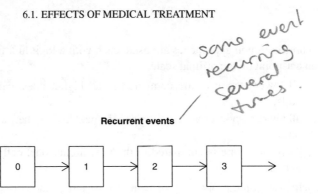

same event recurring several times.

Alternating events

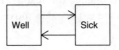

Progressive events

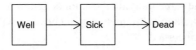

Alternative outcomes

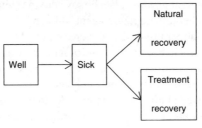

Fig. 6.1. Examples of diagrams for simple event histories.

Three common approaches are used, each with a logit link function. At each given cut-point on the ordinal scale,

(1) all lower responses are compared to all higher ones, called proportional odds;
(2) all lower responses are compared to the next higher one, called continuation ratio;
(3) each lower one is compared to the next higher one, called adjacent categories.

In each case, some probability of being to the left of the cut-point is compared to a probability of being to the right using a logit link. A major assumption of all of these models is that this logit follows the same regression function for all cut-points on the ordinal scale, with only the intercept changing. Notice that, in contrast to the other two, the continuation ratio model is not symmetric so that reversing the scale will change the results; the choice should depend on the direction in which patients are expected to move on the scale.

6.2 Recurrent events

Many illnesses involve some event that recurs at irregular intervals (Figure 6.1): epileptic fits, asthma, infections, and so on. These involve durations between events, but, in contrast to classical survival analysis of times to death, they are repeatable. Because more than one event can occur to each subject, dependence among events on the same individual cannot be ignored. In a quality of life study, the idea is that reducing the frequency of recurrence will improve the quality of life of the person concerned.

6.2.1 THE BLADDER CANCER STUDY

In a clinical trial conducted by the USA Veterans Administration Cooperative Urological Research Group, 116 patients with bladder cancer were randomized to one of three treatment groups: placebo, pyridoxine (vitamin B_6) pills, or periodic instillation of a chemotherapeutic agent, thiotepa, into the bladder. All patients had superficial bladder tumours that were removed transurethrally when they entered the trial. At each discovery of one or more new tumours at a visit, these were removed. The times, in months, between recurrences of tumours were recorded for each patient. Thus, times are between visits when one or several tumours were detected, not between individual tumours (Andrews and Herzberg, 1985, pp. 254–259). One might expect that the risk of further tumours might change depending on the specific history of each patient.

The Kaplan–Meier curves are shown in Figure 6.2, separately for the first and for subsequent recurrence times.

6.2.2 BIRTH PROCESSES

Here, I shall use the dynamic models of Section B.4. These use a gamma mixing distribution. The AICs for a number of such models are presented in Table

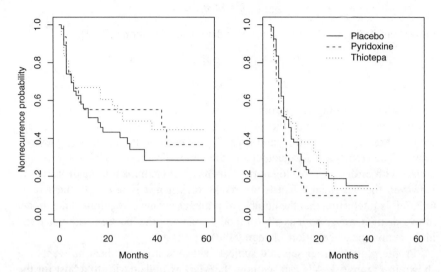

Fig. 6.2. Kaplan–Meier curves for the first (left) and subsequent (right) recurrences of bladder cancer tumours.

Table 6.1. AICs for various models fitted to the bladder tumour data of Andrews and Herzberg (1985, pp. 254–259).

	Independence		Markov update	Count update	Frailty
	Weibull		Weibull mixture		
Null	747.0	698.5	697.5	685.8	707.4
Treatment	746.6	698.9	699.2	685.9	708.6
Treatment+Birth	725.3	699.5	700.1	685.1	708.4
	Log normal		Log normal mixture		
Null	719.5	697.9	685.7	684.5	689.5
Treatment	720.4	698.0	686.5	684.6	691.2
Treatment+Birth	710.5	698.7	685.5	682.5	690.4

6.1. We see that the mixture distributions fit much better than the corresponding Weibull and log normal distributions, and the log normal intensity better than the Weibull (the latter are forms of multivariate Burr distributions). Most of the improvement arises from using a mixture distribution, with its thicker tails.

In no case is there evidence of a treatment effect. On the other hand, there is clearly a longitudinal serial dependence rather than frailty. For these data, this is best modelled by the nonstationary count update

$$\lambda_{1k} = \rho\lambda_{1,k-1} + 1$$
$$\lambda_{2k} = \delta + \Omega(y_k; \kappa) \qquad (6.1)$$

rather than, for example, by a Markov update from Equations (B.44):

$$\lambda_{1k} = \rho^{t_k - t_{k-1}} \lambda_{1,k-1} + (1 - \rho^{t_k - t_{k-1}})\delta + 1$$
$$\lambda_{2k} = \delta + \rho^{t_k - t_{k-1}} \Omega(y_{k-1}; \kappa) + \Omega(y_k; \kappa)$$

Another possibility for introducing time dependence is the birth model; this has μ depending directly on the number of previous events in contrast to the updates where the value of the parameter, λ_1, depends on the number of previous events. The results are also included in the table. The best model has the count update with birth effect in a log normal intensity and gamma mixing distribution. However, the treatment effect is not required: when it is removed, the AIC is 682.6. It is interesting that the number of previous events is required in the model in two distinct ways: both as a birth model changing the location parameter and in the count update equation, changing the dispersion.

Profile plots for four selected subjects with the high numbers of events are shown in Figure 6.3. We can see how the Markov update tries to adjust for the longer periods between events and fails because the following period is often much shorter.

6.3 Change of state

In contrast to recurrent events, where the same event occurs repeatedly, in many circumstances the sequence of events is different, each one signalling the transition to a new state. Here, I shall only consider progressive events (Figure 6.1). Treatment may aim to prolong the period in a more favourable state, where quality of life will hopefully be superior. In certain cases, it is important to predict the eminent possibility of change to the next state so that a new preventive treatment can be implemented as early as possible.

6.3.1 THE ADENOSINE DEAMINASE STUDY

Chronic myelogenous leukæmia accounts for 20–30% of all leukæmia patients in Western countries, with an incidence of about one in 100 000 persons per year. This disease has a chronic or stable phase followed by transition to an accelerated or blast phase that resembles a refractory acute leukæmia. The second phase is usually quickly followed by death.

In a study of this disease, the patients may thus be in one of three ordered states: stable, blast, or dead. The goal is to find a marker for the first transition so that aggressive therapy can be initiated before that transition in order to prolong the chronic phase. One possibility is adenosine deaminase (ADA), an enzyme important in purine catabolism, that has been found in high concentrations in leukæmia cells. This study tried to determine whether patients had high levels of ADA just before entering the accelerated phase (from Klein *et al.*, 1984).

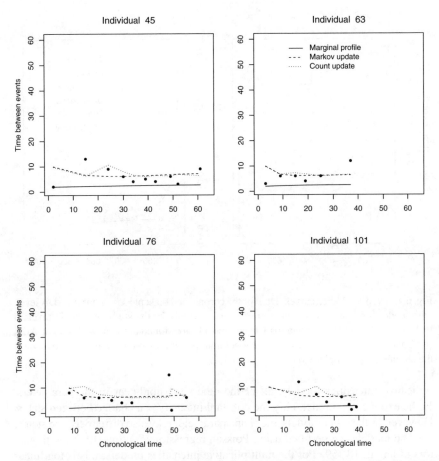

Fig. 6.3. Marginal and individual profiles from the log normal mixture model with count and Markov updates and a birth process for selected individuals.

Here, the state space is ordered, with only two types of transition possible. Note that there are only 38 transition events in this fairly large data set. The Kaplan–Meier curves for the times in the stable and blast states are plotted in Figure 6.4. The level of the enzyme, adenosine deaminase (10^{-8} moles of inosine per hour per million blood cells), in leukæmia cells, is a time-varying covariate that was measured periodically. I shall arbitrarily assume that the value at the beginning of a period holds over the whole period until the next measurement: for a more reasonable model that does not make this assumption, see Kay (1986).

6.3.2 TIME-VARYING COVARIATES

I shall base the analysis on several intensity functions: the exponential, Weibull, gamma, log normal, log logistic, and log Cauchy models. The first two are mul-

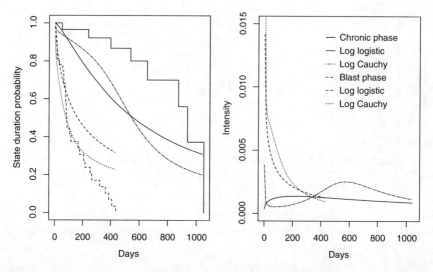

Fig. 6.4. Kaplan–Meier curves (left) for the chronic and blast phases, ignoring ADA level, with model survival curves, and intensity curves (right) for the study of chronic myeloid leukæmia. The log logistic and log Cauchy models are plotted at the mean levels of ADA (8.52 and 21.22×10^{-8} moles of inosine per hour per million blood cells, respectively, for the chronic and blast phases).

tiplicative intensities models; all of the others are nonlinear in the parameters. In the exponential model, only the constant intensity can change between states. However, in the other models, the shape parameter may also differ between states.

The models can be fitted using Poisson regression (Section B.6.2), with vectors of length 18 259. For the multiplicative intensities models, this is log linear with regression function

$$\log(\omega_{ij}) = \beta_{0j} + \beta_{1j} x_{1ij} + \beta_{2j} x_{2ij}$$

where i indexes the individual and j the state. Here, x_{1ij} is log time since the last event for the special case of the Weibull model and x_{2ij} is the level of adenosine deaminase. For the exponential model, $\beta_{1j} = 0$. For the other models, the log intensity involves a nonlinear function that can be calculated from the density and cumulative distribution functions using Equation (B.53).

The AICs for various models, with and without the effect of adenosine deaminase, are given in Table 6.2. The log logistic and log Cauchy distributions fit best. When both parameters are allowed to vary with adenosine deaminase, the difference between states is not necessary (except for the log normal and log logistic intensities). Thus, there is an effect of adenosine deaminase, with no difference in effect between the two states. From the log logistic and log Cauchy models, respectively, the location coefficients (for duration, not intensity) are estimated to

Table 6.2. AICs for various models fitted to the myeloid leukæmia data. ADA stands for adenosine deaminase.

	Exponential	Weibull	Gamma	Log normal	Log logistic	Log Cauchy
Null	273.6	273.3	273.3	272.7	273.4	275.5
Location depends on						
State	272.3	272.6	272.6	272.4	272.8	274.3
ADA	266.3	266.8	266.9	263.4	264.7	268.0
State+ADA	265.4	266.2	266.3	263.5	264.7	260.5
State*ADA	266.4	267.2	267.3	264.4	265.6	261.5
Location and shape depend on						
ADA	—	267.8	253.9	261.6	253.1	253.3
State+ADA	—	268.1	254.1	254.0	252.4	253.9

be -0.097 and -0.152: the risk of changing state increases with higher levels of adenosine deaminase. The corresponding coefficients for the shape parameters are 0.039 and 0.080.

The estimated survival and intensity curves are plotted in Figure 6.4 at mean levels of adenosine deaminase. Recall, however, that these levels are actually changing over time for each subject; the Kaplan–Meier curves ignore the adenosine deaminase level whereas the model curves are for the mean level. Both models give similar results, with the risk of changing from the chronic to the blast phase staying fairly constant over time, *if the adenosine deaminase level were to remain constant*, which it does not. On the other hand, the risk of dying is highest just after the transition to the blast phase and decreases sharply thereafter.

6.4 Transition probabilities

In the study of quality of life, responses are often measured on ordinal scales. Many different approaches to their statistical analysis are slowly becoming available. Here, I shall look at three: ordinal regression (Section 6.1.3) and Markov chains (Section B.5.1) in this section and hidden Markov models for spells (Section B.5.2) in the next.

6.4.1 THE PEPTIC ŒSOPHAGITIS STUDY

To study the efficacy of a new treatment for peptic œsophagitis, a double-blind clinical trial was conducted. The goal was to see if the addition of carbenoxolone to standard medication, an antacid, improved symptoms and endoscopy. A total of 59 patients were randomized, 30 to the control group and 29 to the group given carbenoxolone in addition to the standard medication. Both symptoms and endoscopy were measured on six-point ordinal scales. Here, I only consider the results for reduction of symptoms. This response was measured five times at two-week intervals, as shown in Table 6.3. Lower scores indicate an improved condition. Notice that patients change by at most one point on the ordinal scale

Table 6.3. Symptom scores for 59 patients over eight weeks in a clinical trial for the treatment of peptic œsophagitis (generated by Yudi Pawitan following the description in Hopper and Young, 1988).

Control					Treatment				
\multicolumn{10}{c}{Week}									
0	2	4	6	8	0	2	4	6	8
3	4	4	4	4	4	4	3	3	3
5	5	5	5	5	4	4	3	3	3
2	2	2	1	1	6	5	5	4	3
6	6	5	5	5	3	3	3	3	2
4	3	3	3	3	6	5	5	5	5
5	5	5	5	5	3	3	3	2	2
3	3	3	3	3	5	5	6	6	6
3	3	3	2	2	3	2	2	2	2
4	4	4	3	2	4	3	2	2	2
5	4	4	3	4	5	5	5	5	5
4	4	4	4	4	3	2	2	2	2
4	4	4	4	4	3	2	2	1	1
5	5	5	5	5	6	6	6	6	5
5	4	4	4	4	2	2	1	1	2
5	5	5	4	3	4	4	4	3	2
3	2	2	2	2	3	3	3	3	3
5	5	6	6	6	2	1	1	1	2
6	6	6	6	6	4	4	4	4	4
3	2	2	2	2	4	4	4	4	3
5	5	5	5	5	4	4	3	3	3
4	4	4	3	3	4	4	3	3	3
2	2	2	2	2	4	3	2	2	2
4	3	3	3	3	3	2	2	2	2
3	2	2	1	1	3	3	3	3	3
4	3	3	3	3	3	2	2	1	1
4	3	3	3	3	4	4	3	3	3
5	5	5	5	5	2	1	1	1	1
3	3	3	3	3	3	2	3	2	1
3	3	3	3	2	2	1	1	1	1
6	6	6	6	6					

in a two-week period.

One approach would be to consider an event to be the change between a pair of consecutive points on the scale and to study the duration of time each patient spent at a given level on the scale. The model would be a combination of the models for alternating and for progressive events in Figure 6.1. Here, however, I

6.4. TRANSITION PROBABILITIES

Table 6.4. AICs for the ordinal regression models fitted to the peptic œsophagitis data of Table 6.3.

	Multinomial	Proportional odds	Continuation ratio	Adjacent categories
Treatment	497.3	495.1	494.3	495.2
Time	499.7	499.7	497.9	500.2
Treatment + time	492.0	489.9	487.6	490.5
Treatment * time	494.7	490.2	488.2	490.8

shall approach the problem from another point of view.

6.4.2 ORDINAL REGRESSION

In the peptic œsophagitis study, time and treatment can be used as covariates. The length of time is too short to attempt to fit a nonlinear regression. The results are summarized in Table 6.4. The multinomial model, which does not take into account the ordering of the responses, has also been included. The continuation ratio model consistently fits best. This is not surprising as it has a biological interpretation, measuring the probability of moving one point further along the ordinal scale.

There appears to be both a time trend and a treatment difference. On the other hand, there is no indication of a different time trend under the two treatments. The slope of the time trend is estimated to be 0.119, indicating a progressive move towards the lower end of the scale (improvement). The treatment difference is estimated to be 0.775, showing that the addition of carbenoxolone appears to be superior.

However, these models have the major drawback that they do not take into account the dependence among the five observations on each patient. There are many ways in which this can be done; I shall now look at one.

6.4.3 RANDOM WALKS

In this study, we noted that patients only change by at most one point on the ordinal scale between measurements. We can set up a special case of a Markov chain (Section B.5.1) that uses this information. It is called a random walk with drift. The transition matrix in such models gives the probability of being in a given state, here a point on the ordinal scale, given the state at the previous observation time. For the random walk model, there are only three possibilities:

(1) stay at the same level;
(2) move down one point (improve);
(3) move up one point (deteriorate).

Thus, the transition matrix will be of size 6 × 6, corresponding to the six levels of the ordinal scale, and will be zero except for the main diagonal (stay the same) and the two immediately adjacent minor diagonals (move up or down one point).

There are two parameters, the probability of moving up, say π_u, and of moving down, say π_d, with the probability of no changing being $1 - \pi_u - \pi_d$. Then, the transition matrix is

$$\begin{pmatrix} 1-\pi_u & \pi_u & 0 & 0 & 0 & 0 \\ \pi_d & 1-\pi_u-\pi_d & \pi_u & 0 & 0 & 0 \\ 0 & \pi_d & 1-\pi_u-\pi_d & \pi_u & 0 & 0 \\ 0 & 0 & \pi_d & 1-\pi_u-\pi_d & \pi_u & 0 \\ 0 & 0 & 0 & \pi_d & 1-\pi_u-\pi_d & \pi_u \\ 0 & 0 & 0 & 0 & \pi_d & 1-\pi_d \end{pmatrix}$$

This model has reflecting barriers; the other possibility would be that they are absorbing so that, once an individual reaches an extreme state, he or she stays there, but that is not appropriate in this case. There will also be five further parameters, giving the initial probabilities of being in the various states (summing to one).

I shall fit two models, with the same transition matrix for the two treatments and with different matrices. The AICs are, respectively, 246.9 and 214.7, a big improvement on the previous models. With treatment differences, the estimated probabilities are $\pi_d = 0.1696$, $1 - \pi_u - \pi_d = 0.8023$, and $\pi_u = 0.0281$ for the control and $\pi_d = 0.3155$, $1 - \pi_u - \pi_d = 0.6477$, and $\pi_u = 0.0368$ for the new treatment, addition of carbenoxolone. We see that there is a higher probability of moving down with this treatment. If the initial probabilities are set equal in the two groups, the AIC rises to 245.4, showing that most of the difference between the two groups arises from their initial condition! The probabilities of being in the six categories at week 0 are $(0.00, 0.07, 0.27, 0.27, 0.30, 0.10)$ for the control group and $(0.00, 0.14, 0.34, 0.34, 0.07, 0.10)$ for carbenoxolone so that the control group was considerably worse at initiation.

The stationary marginal distributions (Section B.5.1) are estimated, respectively, to be $(0.83, 0.14, 0.02, 0.004, 0.0006, 0.0001)$ and $(0.88, 0.10, 0.01, 0.001, 0.0002, 0.00002)$. These are quite different from the initial probabilities given above. They predict that, under prolonged application, the carbenoxolone treatment will produce a somewhat higher proportion of patients with the lowest level of symptoms. If the processes were incorrectly assumed to be in a steady state so that these stationary marginal distributions hold from initiation, the AIC rises to 468.0, showing the error in this assumption.

6.5 Analysis of diary cards

In many quality of life studies, patients are asked to fill in a diary card each day giving an evaluation of their state during that day. Generally these evaluations will be placed on some ordinal scale. One special characteristic of such data is that the subjects will often experience spells, being worse during some periods of days than in others. Thus, hidden Markov models (Section B.5.2) may be especially appropriate for the analysis of this type of study.

6.5. ANALYSIS OF DIARY CARDS

6.5.1 THE SEASONAL RHINITIS STUDY

A multicentre, randomized, parallel-group, placebo-controlled, double-blinded, clinical trial was conducted to compare the efficacy and safety of an antihistamine in the treatment of seasonal rhinitis. The doses were in proportions of 0, 1, 2, and 4, and were given once a day during two weeks to adult patients with seasonal rhinitis allergic to grass and/or weed pollen. Thus, patients were randomized to one of the three treatment groups or to placebo.

Five rhinitis symptoms are evaluated daily by each patient on a daily record card: sneezing, runny nose, itchy nose, itchy eyes, and blocked nose. They used a four-point scale, from 0 to 3, corresponding to none, mild, moderate, or severe. These constitute the standard total symptom score (TSS). However, blocked nose is often discarded from analysis of allergy because it is clinically less relevant and treatment is expected to have little effect on it. Nevertheless, it is an important aspect of quality of life.

Subjects visited the investigator's office three times. Randomization occurred at the first visit; the second was a control visit one week after randomization; the third was two weeks after randomization. At each visit, the investigator also scored the five symptoms. These latter data will not be used here.

At the randomization visit (Day 1), each patient evaluated the five rhinitis symptoms and also provided a score for each symptom for his or her status the day before that visit (Day 0). This provides two baseline scores for each symptom. Each patient was supposed to start the medication intake in the evening after the randomization visit and was to take one tablet in the evening each following day for two weeks and was also to fill in the daily record card. Thus, evaluations under treatment started on Day 2. However, five patients did not start immediately with their drug intake but were delayed a few days; for these Day 2 was defined as the day after they started, and the two most recent previous values were used as baseline.

The intention-to-treat population was used for the analysis of these rhinitis symptoms. This includes 470 patients: 119 in the placebo group, 117 in the level 1 group, 116 in the level 2 group, and 118 in the level 4 group. However, several patients were missing baseline data and could not be used in the following analysis, leaving 462 subjects.

6.5.2 SPELLS

In the analysis to be presented here, I shall only consider the blocked nose response. Inclusion of the first baseline value adds little to the models when the second baseline value is in. Hence, I shall only use the latter because this reduces the number of patients with missing baseline data from 25 to eight. The mean response profiles over time for each treatment group are plotted in Figure 6.5. This provides an idea of the change over time, although averaging ordinal responses is not really meaningful.

Ordinal regression models (Section 6.1.3), assuming independence among ob-

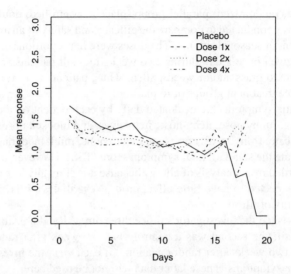

Fig. 6.5. Mean profiles for the blocked nose ordinal response for the four treatment groups. (At days 19 and 20, there is only one individual in the placebo group.)

servations on each subject, indicate that treatment, baseline, and a linear effect of time should be included in the model, with a different slope for time under placebo than for the three doses. The proportional odds model has an AIC of 6484.4 and the continuation ratio 6517.3.

Nonlinear logistic growth curve regression functions for time do not fit as well. This probably indicates that the study was not conducted over a long enough time so that the patients reached a stable state.

Two-state hidden Markov models take dependence due to spells into account and fit much better. Because responses are occasionally missing, continuous-time models must be used, assuming that those values are missing at random. With these models, a different slope under placebo is no longer necessary. The proportional odds model now has an AIC of 5380.4 and the continuation ratio 5366.3. (Reversing the scale for the continuation ratio model gives 5414.1; the proportional odds model is symmetric.) However, this model may be further simplified. In one of the states (number 2), the treatment effect is not required so that only time and baseline are present. This reduces the AIC to 5364.3.

The intensity transition matrix is

$$\begin{pmatrix} -0.067 & 0.067 \\ 0.052 & -0.052 \end{pmatrix}$$

yielding a probability transition matrix for one day of

$$\begin{pmatrix} 0.937 & 0.063 \\ 0.049 & 0.951 \end{pmatrix}$$

The corresponding stationary probabilities in the two states are 0.44 and 0.56.

In the first hidden state, the coefficients for the three doses, as compared to placebo, are estimated respectively to be -0.174, -1.125, and -0.713. The slope for time is 0.119 and the baseline effect is -1.376. Comparisons are 'better' as opposed to 'worse' so that negative values indicate worse on the scale. Thus, in this state, treatment has a negative effect as does baseline, but the patients improve over time, whether under placebo or active treatment, as can be seen in Figure 6.5.

In the second state, the slope for time is 0.030 and the baseline effect is -1.266. Here, treatment has no effect, change over time is smaller, and baseline has a similar effect to that in state 1. Note that treatment has no direct effect on change of state in this model. In state 1, it influences change of score, not change of state directly.

With the covariates set to zero at day 2 (that is, someone on placebo with a baseline score of 0 on the first day of treatment), the probabilities of being in the four categories for the two states are

State	Score			
	0	1	2	3
1	0.899	0.098	0.003	0.001
2	0.055	0.771	0.150	0.023

The first state corresponds to spells when the patients are feeling better, at least with respect to blocked nose, having little or no problem with this symptom. This implies that the probability of moving to a worse score is estimated to be higher under treatment than under placebo. (Remember that a patient with score 0 can only remain stable or get worse, but this is true under both placebo and treatment.) The probability of being in state 1 is plotted over time for the first eight patients in Figure 6.6. In periods when a patient is feeling less well with respect to this symptom (state 2), treatment has no effect on blocked nose, as compared to placebo. We see that the changes between states vary widely among patients.

Naturally, the possibility of this small adverse effect of this medication on quality of life through a blocked nose will have to be checked by further studies.

Further reading Two useful reviews of modelling event histories are Clayton (1988) and Hougaard (1999). More detailed discussion is provided in Hougaard (2000).

For an alternative approach to the analysis of ordinal diary card data, see Lindsey *et al.* (1997).

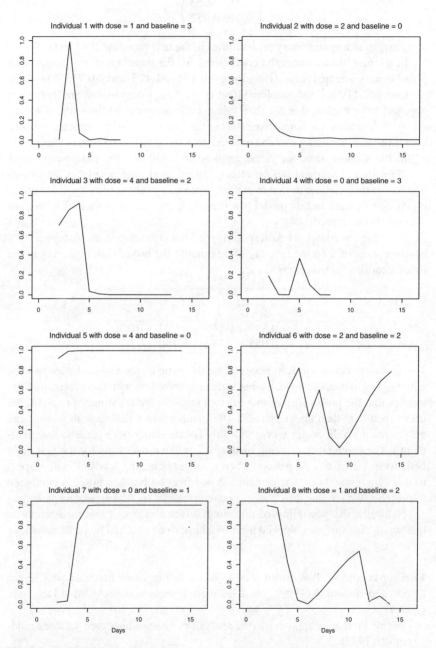

Fig. 6.6. Probability of being in state 1, where treatment has a strong negative effect, for the first eight subjects.

6.6 Exercises

(1) Kidney patients using a portable dialysis machine may have recurrent infections. These occur at the point of insertion of the catheter. When this happens, the catheter must be removed and the infection cured, after which the catheter can be reinserted. There can be right censoring if the catheter must be removed for other reasons. Patients were followed for two recurrence times, one or both of which might be censored. Age, sex, and type of disease (GN, AN, PKD, or other) are available as risk factors, as shown in Table C.6.
   (a) Which factors are most closely related to risk of infection?
   (b) Is the risk of a second infection higher than that of the first one?

(3) A pre-clinical study looked at the time to appearance of mammary cancer tumours in rats when treated with retinyl acetate. A number of animals were injected with a carcinogen for mammary cancer and then given retinyl acetate to prevent the cancer. After 60 days, those still free of tumours were randomly assigned to the two treatments, 23 animals continuing the retinoid prophylaxis and 25 acting as a control. The rats were palpated for tumours twice weekly, with observation ending 182 days after the initial carcinogen injection. The data for 48 female rats under two treatments are reproduced in Table C.7.
   (a) The presence of one or more tumours may induce further tumours. Does this 'snowball' effect appear in these data?
   (b) Is there any evidence of differences among the rats, such as a frailty effect?

(3) One possible cost-effective alternative to long-term bioassays for testing the carcinogenic potential of chemicals is to use skin painting of genetically engineered mice. Certain strains of knockout mice have been genetically designed to under-express genes regulating normal cell death so that these mice are susceptible to developing tumours. Other transgenic strains over-express tumour-inducing oncogenes so that they are also susceptible to tumours. The strain involved here is Tg.AC. These mice have a low background rate of skin papillomas but are sensitive to known nongenotoxic carcinogens.

Skin-painting studies last 20 to 30 weeks (in contrast to two years for traditional bioassays) and provide more information from each animal because tumour progression and multiplicity are observed over time instead of only at death.

The Laboratory of Environmental Carcinogenesis and Mutagenesis of the USA National Institute of Environmental Health Sciences conducted such a study for benzene. Female Tg.AC mice were exposed either to acetone or to a low dose (400 μl) of benzene. The former had previously been found to have no carcinogenic effect. Papilloma counts were made each week for 20 weeks. No positive counts appeared before week 6; one animal died in each group. The results are shown in Table C.8. From these data, we clearly see that papilloma could spontaneously disappear from some mice.

(a) Develop a model to describe the appearance of new papilloma.

(b) Does this indicate a difference between the two groups?

(c) Can you extend your model to allow for disappearances?

(4) Is there any evidence that a completely different intensity function is required for each of the two states in the adenosine deaminase study?

(5) A clinical trial was conducted to study intensification therapy combined with a high-dose combination chemotherapy in the treatment of acute non-lymphoblastic leukæmia in adults. Patients were assigned to one of three groups. All subjects received the same treatment for the first 186 days. Then, because the first group had been treated prior to the development of the intensification programme, they could not be treated with this therapy. The second group were eligible to receive the therapy but did not, whereas the third group received it. Times, in days, from remission to relapse and from relapse to death were recorded, as shown in Table C.9. Notice that treatment is time-varying because it only starts after six months.

(a) What influence does therapy have on remission and survival?

(b) Thirteen additional subjects were lost before the end of the 186 days. Their survival times were 24, 68*, 76, 85, 90, 95, 119*, 124, 151, 158*, 172, 182, and 182*, the four indicated by an asterisk being censored. Can you incorporate this information into your model?

(3) In another study, leukæmia patients who had attained remission were followed to subsequent relapse and possible death. Entry to the study was staggered so that termination of the study resulted in censoring after various lengths of observation. The results for 15 patients are shown in Table C.10.

(a) Does the same distribution adequately describe both times to relapse and to death?

(b) Do any of the parameters of the distribution of times to death depend on the time to relapse?

(3) Breast cancer patients in a hospital in London, England, were being treated for spinal metastases. They were followed over a five-year period, with their ambulatory state being recorded before treatment began, and at 0, 3, and 6 months, and 1, 2, and 5 years. Their ambulatory status, defined by whether or not they could walk unaided, is shown in Table C.11.

(a) What are the probabilities of transition between the two ambulatory states?

(b) Do they evolve over time?

(c) What is the risk of death?

(4) For the peptic œsophagitis study:

(a) Fit a hidden Markov chain (Section B.5.2) with two states.
(b) Which type of ordinal regression fits best in this model?
(c) Do the results have any biological interpretation?

7
Pharmacokinetics

Pharmacokinetics involves the study of the course of absorption, distribution, metabolism, and elimination of some substance in a living body over time, usually relating it to the dose given. Thus, it is not concerned with what a drug does to the body, but only with how the drug moves through the body.

7.1 Studying drug concentrations in the body

In order to model the concentration of some substance in the body over time, information must be collected from the body. Most often the substance of interest cannot be measured directly at the site of action so that its concentration in the blood or plasma is usually recorded.

7.1.1 GOALS

Pharmacokinetics is an especially important aspect of the development of drugs. Plasma drug levels often show a strong relationship to clinical response, efficacious or toxic, and therefore can act as an important surrogate endpoint. Pharmacokinetics is a valuable component in the determination of optimal doses and dosing schedules.

Data-rich studies In a Phase I study (see Section 5.1.2), a small number of healthy volunteers is usually given one or more different doses of a new drug and, each time, blood samples are taken at frequent intervals to determine the profile of the concentration of the drug in the plasma. Often cross-over trials are used. This is an experimental, *data-rich* situation in which dosing levels, at least with respect to toxicity, can be found. On the other hand, actual patients will generally be required in order to determine minimal effective doses. However, the subjects involved in such early studies may not be very representative of the population that may eventually be treated with the medication.

Some of these studies will use single increasing dose protocols to determine the range of tolerable doses, followed by repeated dosing to find out how to maintain concentrations in the body at a useful level. Influences of food, concurrent medication, age, and sex may also be checked. Subsequently, often in Phase II, the effects of renal and hepatic insufficiencies are studied.

Population studies In the later phase trials, many patients are involved in more routine clinical analyses, generally in parallel trials, so that usually only one or a few observations can be made on each. Hopefully, these subjects will be more representative of the target population for the medication than those in earlier phase trials, even though they are not sampled randomly for that population. Analysis of such a data-poor situation is called *population pharmacokinetics*. However, care must be taken in drawing conclusions because the patients are volunteers.

In both types of studies, some nonlinear regression function can be used to describe the change in concentration over time (Section 3.2.1). However, some of the statistical problems are quite different in the two cases. Phase I work is usually tightly controlled so that administered doses and sampling times are accurately known whereas in later phase trials this may not be so. The early trials are primarily to determine the basic shape of the concentration curve over time at different doses, whereas the later ones are often oriented more towards determining possible variations in the curves among subjects. The latter information may be used to develop individualized dosage regimens so that information on relevant covariates is particularly important.

7.1.2 COMPARTMENT MODELS

As we saw in Section 3.2.1, one way to construct a mechanistic model for such processes is to divide the system into *compartments* and to assume that the rate of flow of the substances between these obeys first-order kinetics.

For example, a three-compartment model might correspond to blood, soft tissue, and muscle, plus the outside environment from which the substance comes and to which it is eliminated. In such models, the substance under study is assumed to be well mixed in all compartments and to have identical kinetic behaviour within each one.

When a medication is introduced into the body, it is metabolized in some way, producing a new substance called the metabolite. Thus, in some studies, two substances need to be studied, the parent drug and its metabolite.

Once a model for one dose has been established, that for multiple dosing can theoretically be predicted by superposition. However, this only works if the differential equations are linear, that is when the model parameters are independent of dose. If they vary with dose or time, superposition cannot be used. In such cases, concentrations are not changing proportionally with dose. Such characteristics of a drug can create difficulties for prescription so that they are usually checked closely in the early stages of drug development. Discovery of nonproportionality may lead to abandoning the development of a drug.

Basic models A drug may be administered by intravenous bolus or infusion, orally, or subcutaneously. A bolus is an instantaneous injection directly into the blood stream, whereas an infusion is a constant introduction into the blood stream over a specified period of time. In contrast, a subcutaneous dose is injected under the skin, not directly into the blood. An orally taken drug may be administered in the form of liquid solution, powder, tablets, pills, or capsules (Section 9.5).

Parameter interpretation   Once an appropriate regression function, such as the open first-order, one-compartment model of Equation (3.24) or the zero-order, one-compartment model of Equation (3.27), is derived, the parameters need to be interpreted in the specific context of pharmacokinetics.

The volume of distribution (L), usually denoted by V, converts total drug dose in the compartment into the measured concentration. Thus, it is a proportionality constant relating the amount of drug in the body to the serum concentration. This is a nominal volume that is determined by the physiological volume of blood as well as by whether or not the drug binds to plasma protein (albumin) or tissues. A drug with high volume is usually highly bound to protein whereas one with small volume is bound to tissue outside the vascular area. Larger volume generally corresponds to lower concentration; smaller individuals usually have smaller volume, although there is generally a great deal of individual variation for most drugs.

The absorption, k_a, and elimination, k_e, rate parameters (1/h) for a drug are constants describing the speed with which these two processes operate so that the amount removed from the body is proportional to the amount in the body. However, for a metabolite, k_a will rather be a formation rate because it is not being absorbed.

Derived parameters   Other parameters of medical interest, such as the mean *time to peak*, T_{max}, and the average *maximum concentration*, C_{max}, can easily be calculated. For example, for the open first-order, one-compartment model, the former is

$$T_{\max} = \frac{1}{k_a - k_e} \log\left(\frac{k_a}{k_e}\right) \qquad (7.1)$$

and the latter is the concentration at T_{max}, obtained by substituting this value into Equation (3.24). The mean *area under the curve* (AUC) can be calculated by numerical integration using the estimated parameter values.

A drug in the body is usually eliminated either by the liver or by the kidneys. Generally, this is done by metabolizing the drug into some other form. *Clearance* is the volume of a compartment cleared of the substance in unit time: here, $V k_a$. More generally, for any compartment system, it is defined as the dose divided by the AUC. This is the volume of blood from which the drug has been eliminated in unit time; it describes how efficiently the drug is being eliminated.

Bioavailability is the proportion of an administered drug dose that actually arrives in the blood stream, and hopefully also to the site of action.

Simultaneous models   Under the above assumptions, these compartment model functions can be estimated independently for the parent drug and the metabolite

(Model 1 in Figure 7.1). However, metabolite concentration must obviously depend on previous availability of the parent drug.

Interdependence of parent and metabolite In developing a new model, let us assume ingestion and retain Equation (3.24) for the parent. However, we need to set up a differential equation for the mean metabolite concentration, $\mu_m(t)$, relating it to that for parent, $\mu_p(t)$. (In what follows, I shall use the index, m, to distinguish metabolite parameters and p for parent drug.) Let us call this new predicted metabolite concentration, joint with drug concentration, $\mu_{mj}(t)$. Then, its rate of change will be given by

$$\frac{\mathrm{d}\mu_{mj}(t)}{\mathrm{d}t} = -k_{me}\mu_{mj}(t) + k_{mf}\mu_p(t) \qquad (7.2)$$

where we now have total parent drug elimination, $k_{pe} = k_{pde} + k_{mf}$ with k_{mf} the rate of formation of metabolite and k_{pde} the rate of direct elimination of the parent, not through metabolite formation. Solving these equations, we obtain the following model for the concentration of metabolite in the blood:

$$\mu_{mj}(t) = \frac{k_{pa}k_{mf}d}{V_m(k_{pa} - k_{pe})} \left[\frac{e^{-k_{me}t} - e^{-k_{pe}t}}{k_{pe} - k_{me}} - \frac{e^{-k_{me}t} - e^{-k_{pa}t}}{k_{pa} - k_{me}} \right] \qquad (7.3)$$

In this latter model, V_m and k_{mf} are not separately identifiable so that we set $V_m = V_p = V$ when estimating Equations (3.24) and (7.3) simultaneously. Hence, this model (called Model 2 in Section 7.2.4 below) has five parameters (not counting dispersion parameters): k_{pa}, k_{pe}, k_{mf}, k_{me}, and V. It is also illustrated in Figure 7.1.

First-pass metabolism In the models described so far, we assume that the drug is well mixed in the blood. A third model allows for first-pass metabolism before the drug becomes completely mixed. On absorption, the parent drug may go directly, say, to the liver where a part of it is immediately metabolized. This first-pass metabolism is analogous to simultaneous absorption of a bolus of drug and bolus of metabolite. Thus, for the metabolite, we now have a combination of Equations (3.24) and (7.3) yielding

$$\mu_{mfp}(t) = \pi\mu_m(t) + (1 - \pi)\mu_{mj}(t) \qquad (7.4)$$

where π is the proportion of the drug directly metabolized through a first pass.

Thus, $\mu_m(t)$ is a standard one-compartment model for metabolite, independent of parent, that is that part metabolized immediately; $\mu_{mj}(t)$ is the concentration of metabolite formed more slowly from metabolism of the circulating parent drug. In order to maintain mass balance, Equation (3.24) for the parent drug must also be multiplied by $1 - \pi$. Then, this model (called Model 3 in Figure 7.1 and in Section 7.2.4 below) has seven parameters: k_{pa}, k_{pe}, k_{ma}, k_{mf}, k_{me}, V, and π. It may be biologically appropriate that k_{ma} either is or is not equal to k_{pa}.

7.1. STUDYING DRUG CONCENTRATIONS IN THE BODY

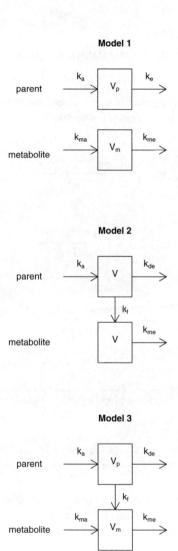

Fig. 7.1. Various compartment models for parent drug and metabolite. Model 1: parent and metabolite independent. Model 2: simultaneous fit. Model 3: simultaneous fit with a first-pass component. Parameters are as defined in Equations (3.24), (7.3), and (7.4).

Notice that any parent drug metabolized in the first pass will not be available for action in the body.

7.1.3 STATISTICAL MODELS

Let us now look more closely at some statistical aspects of the analysis of pharmacokinetic data.

Distributions Some of the possible skewed distributions that might be considered to describe variation in concentration around the compartment model function include the Weibull,

$$f(y;\mu,\phi) = \frac{\phi y^{\phi-1} e^{-(y/\mu)^\phi}}{\mu^\phi} \tag{7.5}$$

gamma,

$$f(y;\mu,\phi) = \frac{\phi^\phi y^{\phi-1} e^{-\phi y/\mu}}{\mu^\phi \Gamma(\phi)} \tag{7.6}$$

log normal,

$$f(y;\mu,\phi) = \frac{e^{-[\log(y)-\log(\mu)]^2/(2\phi)}}{y\sqrt{2\pi\phi}} \tag{7.7}$$

log Cauchy,

$$f(y;\mu,\phi) = \frac{1}{y\pi\sqrt{\phi}\{1+[\log(y)-\log(\mu)]^2/\phi\}} \tag{7.8}$$

and log Laplace.

$$f(y;\mu,\phi) = \frac{e^{-|\log(y)-\log(\mu)|/\phi}}{2y\phi} \tag{7.9}$$

Here, μ is some location parameter that may not be the mean and ϕ is a dispersion or shape parameter that is not the variance of the concentration. The first of these parameters, μ, will vary over time according to one of the compartment models described above.

One useful generalization of some of these distributions is the generalized gamma distribution,

$$f(y;\mu,\phi,\lambda) = \frac{\lambda \phi^\phi y^{\phi\lambda-1} e^{-\phi(y/\mu)^\lambda}}{\mu^{\phi\lambda} \Gamma(\phi)} \tag{7.10}$$

When the family parameter $\lambda = 1$, this yields a gamma distribution, when $\phi = 1$, a Weibull distribution, and when $\lambda \to \infty$, a log normal distribution.

Response transformation Traditionally, nonlinear least squares is used to estimate the parameters in compartment models. Generally, a log transformation is applied resulting in a log normal distribution for the concentration, as in Equation (7.7). This induces an implicit relationship between the variance of concentration and its mean.

Thus, if $\log[\mu(t)]$ is used for the location regression function, it refers to the mean of the log concentration, $\sum \log(y_i)/n = \log(\prod y_i^{1/n})$. Hence, in such a model, $\mu(t)$ is the geometric mean of concentration. The arithmetic mean for the log normal distribution is then given by $\exp\{\log[\mu(t)] + \phi(t)/2\}$, where $\phi(t)$ is the variance function for log concentrations. The geometric, and not the arithmetic, mean is following the compartment model.

In other words, when log concentration is used with any distribution, the rate and volume parameters can only be directly interpreted in terms of the geometric mean (if it exists) concentration, or by some conversion of the location parameter. The arithmetic mean concentration will depend not only on these parameters but also on those in the dispersion function (see Section 1.3.3).

Nonconstant dispersion Often, in nonlinear least squares estimation, the variance is made a direct function of the mean. This has no clear biological interpretation but follows from the empirical fact that the variability must be smaller when the mean is close to zero. Suppose that the nonlinear regression for the mean (or, more generally, some location parameter) can be written

$$\mu(t) = h(t, \boldsymbol{\theta})$$

which, as we saw above, will usually be some compartment model. Then the change in variance parameter might, for example, be assumed to be given by

$$\phi(t) = \sigma^2 h(t, \boldsymbol{\theta})^\kappa \qquad (7.11)$$

where $\boldsymbol{\theta}$ is a parameter vector common to the two equations. In this function, κ might be estimated but has often been set to two (Davidian and Giltinan, 1995, pp. 245, 264; Wakefield, 1996).

A major problem with this approach is that the changing form of the variance regression function will directly influence that of the mean, with the only flexibility coming from κ. Thus, if the assumed relationship between the mean and variance does not hold, the estimates of the parameters in the regression function for the location parameter can be greatly distorted.

Instead, I shall allow the dispersion parameter (in any chosen distribution) to vary independently of the location parameter with a regression function of a similar form to the compartment model for the location parameter, say Equation (3.24), but with different 'volume' and 'rate' parameters, and an extra power parameter, κ, similar to that in Equation (7.11):

$$\phi(t) = \left[\frac{k'_a d}{V'(k'_a - k'_e)} \left(e^{-k'_e t} - e^{-k'_a t} \right) \right]^\kappa \qquad (7.12)$$

We gain added flexibility but at the expense of a number of additional parameters. Recall that this form of equation yields two symmetric solutions (Section 3.2.1) so that, when used in combination with a similar one for the location parameter, it gives a likelihood function with four maxima of equal size.

Recall, finally, that a non-normal distribution with a constant dispersion parameter nevertheless has a nonconstant variance (Section 1.2.3).

Random effects In Phase I studies, as in all clinical trials, the subjects involved are volunteers; they are not a random sample from the target population. Nevertheless, random effects models are systematically used in order to account for individual differences. This can be justified as a mathematical technique for constructing multivariate distributions (Section B.1). However, one of the main statistical arguments for random effects, generalizing to a wider population, does not hold: the participants do not represent a larger patient population and generalization must be based on nonstatistical arguments.

One of the important goals of such studies is to detect possibly harmful effects on certain individuals so that it is crucial not to attenuate the reactions of extreme responses. However, the shrinkage estimates obtained from random effects models carry the assumption that all individuals are similar so that the extremes are pulled towards a common mean; this is true even if the mixing distribution is asymmetric and/or heavy tailed. In exploratory studies of a new drug, this is not a reasonable assumption; instead, we are trying to detect dissimilar individuals. Thus, such estimates can give dangerously misleading conclusions, possibly hiding extreme effects of the drug on certain individuals that should be detected as early as possible in the drug development process. The issue can be of even more concern in Phase III, where sparse data must often be collected because of practical and financial constraints but where the larger sample size may include extreme subjects not available in earlier studies.

Even with a reasonable number of observations per individual, distortions can occur if normally distributed random effects are imposed on the data when, for example, a thicker tailed distribution would be more appropriate. On the other hand, a random effects model has the advantage of simplicity because only one parameter is required instead of one per subject in a fixed-effects model. It also provides one method of introducing dependence amongst the responses on each subject (but see Section 7.2.5). However, these are only advantages if the chosen mixing distribution is appropriate.

Nondetectable values A further problem that occurs in pharmacokinetic studies is that low concentrations of the drug are difficult to detect in the blood. Any assay (Chapter 9) to be used can only detect some known minimal quantity of the substance. Thus, the smallest responses are nondetectable (ND) and hence left censored. If this is not taken into account in the model, it can have considerable impact on the parameter estimates obtained, and on the shape of the resulting concentration profile curves, as we shall see. For these ND values that are left-censored observations, the cumulative distribution function can be used instead of the density (Wakefield and Racine-Poon, 1995). This is the same type of procedure as is used in models for right censoring of survival data (Section B.6.1).

7.2 Parent drug and metabolite

Sophisticated nonlinear modelling techniques are widely used in pharmacokinetics. However, pharmacokinetic modelling usually makes strong assumptions about variability in the data, assuming a normal or log normal distribution. Here, I shall look closely at these assumptions and show that they are not always warranted. I shall also show that a surprising amount of information can be drawn from pharmacokinetic data when parent drug and metabolite are modelled simultaneously.

7.2.1 THE FLOSEQUINAN STUDY

Flosequinan (7-fluoro-methyl-3-methylsulphinyl-4-quinolone) was found to be useful in the management of patients with chronic heart failure in early clinical trials (Wynne *et al.*, 1985; Gallo *et al.*, 1993; Hinson *et al.*, 1994). It was thought to act by dilation of venous capacitance and arterial resistance vessels, so that cardiac preload and afterload were reduced. In other words, it was an orally active peripheral vasodilator meant to lower blood pressure. However, a long-term study demonstrated that there might be increased mortality in patients taking the drug (Kamali and Edwards, 1995), so that it was withdrawn from the market in the United Kingdom in April 1993.

The Phase I study that I shall analyse here looked at pharmacokinetic dose proportionality using 50, 100, and 150 mg doses in 18 healthy volunteers from whom informed written consent to participate was obtained. It was conducted in the summer of 1988 after approval by a local research ethics committee.

Blood samples were taken at 0, 0.5, 1, 1.5, 2, 3, 4, 6, 8, 10, 12, 24, 36, 48, 72, and 96 hours after dosing. Concentrations of flosequinan and of its pharmacologically active metabolite, flosequinoxan, were measured (see Wynne *et al.*, 1985, for the assay methodology). Patient demographics and clinical chemistry and biochemistry at baseline are also available: the baseline covariates are sex, age, height, weight, serum creatinine, bilirubin, alkaline phosphatase, ALT, AST, and gamma gt. Although the study design was a three-period, three-dose crossover, with a two-week washout between periods, I shall not use these aspects of the data here.

As can be seen in the left graph of Figure 7.2, time to peak concentration for the drug is less than one hour. Two of the volunteers have higher profiles, especially at the low dose level. These are the lightest and youngest members of the group. The peak metabolite concentration occurs somewhat later than that of the drug, as shown in the right graph of Figure 7.2, although considerable

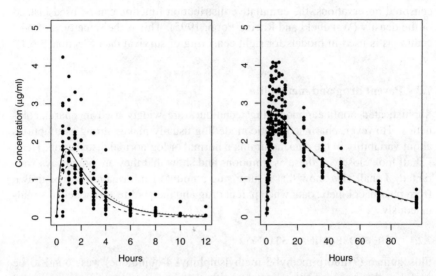

Fig. 7.2. Fitted regression lines from the log normal model for the geometric (dashed) and arithmetic (dotted) means, along with that for the arithmetic mean from the gamma distribution for the flosequinan concentration and from the normal model for the metabolite concentration (solid). Notice the different time scales in the two graphs.

concentration was already present at one-half hour. However, the elimination phase is also much longer, with a half-life of about 38 hours. The metabolite could still be detected in most volunteers after four days whereas the drug itself was undetectable after 24 hours. (As can be seen in Figure 7.2, considerable concentrations of the drug were still found in two subjects after 12 hours.)

7.2.2 MODELLING THE PARENT DRUG

In modelling the drug, flosequinan, I shall only use concentrations up to 24 hours because all subjects had an ND value starting at this time.

Independence assumption Let us begin with a simple, and unrealistic, model to show how distributional assumptions are affected by changes in the regression functions fitted.

Constant dispersion I shall take Equation (3.24) to describe the location parameter in the distributions listed above (plus the normal distribution), but momentarily leave the dispersion parameter fixed and ignore subject differences. Recall that the variance of the concentration will not be constant even though the dispersion parameter is held constant in all of these distributions, except the normal distribution.

7.2. PARENT DRUG AND METABOLITE

Table 7.1. Parameter estimates and AICs for various models for flosequinan concentrations. (The prime indicates parameters in the variance function.)

Parameter	Normal	Log normal	Log Cauchy	Log Laplace	Weibull	Gamma
			Constant dispersion			
$\widehat{k_{pa}}$	1.83	1.77	1.82	1.79	2.03	2.11
$\widehat{k_{pe}}$	0.61	0.45	0.56	0.51	0.33	0.32
$\widehat{V_p}$	46.47	79.32	60.92	65.71	75.64	75.42
$\hat{\phi}$	0.25	0.94	0.20	0.71	0.92	0.97
AIC	2198.7	2113.3	2093.6	2077.6	2159.8	2162.3
			Dispersion regression			
$\widehat{k_{pa}}$	1.16	1.29	1.66	1.43	1.66	2.90
$\widehat{k_{pe}}$	0.80	0.63	0.56	0.63	0.55	0.41
$\widehat{V_p}$	36.86	54.96	57.12	54.50	43.73	59.75
$\widehat{k'_a}$	5.60	3.52	∞	533.3	2.20	1.05
$\widehat{k'_e}$	0.21	2.70	10.08	4.22	0.68	0.45
$\widehat{V'}$	195.39	1969.6	0	0	4.80	17.29
$\hat{\kappa}$	1.279	−0.080	−0.018	−0.025	0.249	1.117
AIC	2110.0	2053.9	2085.1	2045.5	2042.0	2003.7
		Dispersion regression and fixed effects				
$\widehat{k_{pa}}$	2.22	2.40	3.35	2.65	7.15	4.19
$\widehat{k_{pe}}$	0.43	0.49	0.50	0.52	0.47	0.48
$\widehat{V_p}$	63.41	64.46	57.18	58.10	52.18	57.69
$\widehat{k'_a}$	1449.7	0.54	1.10	0.98	0.79	0.43
$\widehat{k'_e}$	0.26	0.18	0.17	0.19	0.25	0.43
$\widehat{V'}$	657.21	17.2	6.51	10.58	13.07	10.70
$\hat{\kappa}$	0.896	−1.478	−1.578	−0.698	0.865	1.875
AIC	1996.2	1915.8	1858.6	1853.6	1833.5	1817.7

The parameter estimates and AICs are shown in the first panel of Table 7.1. Note that, because all models in a given panel have the same number of parameters, the comparison of AICs on a line is directly in terms of (minus log) likelihoods, the penalty being the same for all distributions. Recall, also, that the parameters for the location regression function in a 'logged' distribution have a different interpretation than the others.

The three 'logged' distributions have similar parameter estimates for the regression and fit better than the gamma and Weibull distributions, which also have similar estimates. Both the log Cauchy and log Laplace distributions, which fit best, are thick tailed; the tails appear to be absorbing the variability not allowed for because the dispersion is constrained to be constant.

Time-varying dispersion Now, I shall model the changing dispersion using the regression function in Equation (7.12). The results are displayed in the middle panel of Table 7.1. Note that we cannot expect the regression functions for the dispersion parameter to be similar for different distributions because the dispersion, ϕ, has a quite different interpretation in each case. I have not constrained the parameters in the two regression functions (for a given probability distribution) to be identical in the traditional way; we can see that they are estimated to be quite different, showing that the constraint imposed by Equation (7.11) is inappropriate.

The ranking of the fits of the distributions has also drastically changed; the gamma distribution is now clearly superior to the others. For example, the latter predicts the observations much better, making them $\exp(2042.0 - 2003.7) = 4.3 \times 10^{16}$ times more probable than the next most likely model, that based on the Weibull distribution. Of course, this does not imply that it is a *good* model, only that it is better than the others. The parameter estimates for the location regression still differ considerably among distributions and are quite different from those obtained when the dispersion was held constant showing the influence of inappropriately modelling the dispersion.

Recall that the location models for the normal and gamma distributions are directly comparable, being based on (arithmetic) mean concentration and that the one for the log Laplace also has a direct interpretation in terms of the median. In contrast, the classical log normal model is one of the more difficult to interpret in terms of arithmetic mean concentration, although it is direct for the geometric mean.

It is interesting to compare the regression function for the mean of the gamma distribution with that obtained in the traditional way (but without individual effects for the moment) from the log normal distribution. Both its arithmetic and geometric means are plotted for the highest dose level in the left graph of Figure 7.2, along with that for the arithmetic mean from the gamma distribution. The gamma regression line rises more sharply and shows the peak concentration to occur somewhat earlier and higher. As would be expected from skewed distributions, the geometric mean from the log normal distribution is considerably smaller than the arithmetic mean. This should be taken into consideration when interpreting the curves.

Fixed effects From the study of a variety of models that cannot be presented here, the scientists involved suspected that much of the individual variability might be due to differences in volume (V_p). Let us then add a fixed effect (α_i) for this parameter

$$\log(V_i) = \nu + \alpha_i$$

α_i being the difference from the average log volume of the volunteers (indexed by i) in the trial. (In other words, I am using the 'conventional' constraint so that $\sum_i \alpha_i = 0$.) The results are presented in the lower panel of Table 7.1. Again, the

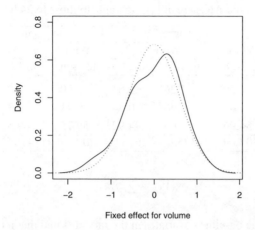

Fig. 7.3. Kernel density estimation of the variability of volume among individuals (solid line) and the corresponding normal distribution (dotted line).

gamma distribution fits best. Here, the parameter estimates for this model have not changed greatly from those without the fixed effects. That for volume is the transformed average of individuals, instead of being marginal to individuals, as before.

The fixed-effects parameter estimates can be viewed as estimating a nonparametric mixing distribution. I can apply a kernel density estimation to them to see its form, as shown in Figure 7.3. Note, however, that the form of this distribution depends completely on the volumes of those people who happened to have volunteered and, from a strictly statistical point of view, tells us little about the distribution of volumes in any larger population. From the graph, we see that a normal mixing distribution might not be an adequate representation of the distribution of (log) volumes in the sample.

Inspection of the individual fixed-effects estimates (on the log scale) is of interest to see if any extreme values of estimated volume, $\widehat{V_p}$, have been recorded. Here, all values except two are within about $\exp(\pm 0.75)$ of the estimate in Table 7.1; those have values $\exp(-1.31) = 0.27$ and $\exp(1.02) = 2.77$ times the transformed average log volume in the group of volunteers. The first, with small estimated volume, is the youngest female who is relatively slender. The second, with the largest volume, is the shortest, lightest male who is also very slender.

Covariates I shall now replace the fixed effects for volume in the gamma model by a regression in the individual covariates recorded:

Table 7.2. Parameter estimates with and without allowing for left censoring. Without censoring, the ND values are set to 0.02. The models to 12 h have fewer observations so that the AICs are not comparable to those to 24 h.

	Log normal			Gamma		
Censoring	With	Without		With	Without	
Period	to 24 h	to 12 h	to 24 h	to 24 h	to 12 h	to 24 h
$\widehat{k_{pa}}$	1.29	2.26	2.61	2.90	2.20	3.04
$\widehat{k_{pe}}$	0.63	0.40	0.34	0.41	0.34	0.18
$\widehat{V_p}$	54.96	82.66	94.92	59.75	69.52	101.59
AIC	2053.9	(2395.8)	2603.0	2003.7	(2416.2)	2609.5

$$\log(V_i) = \sum_j \beta_j x_{ij}$$

where j indexes the baseline covariates in the model. I find that inclusion of sex, age, bilirubin, gamma gt, and creatinine clearance improves the model, whereas body mass index, AST, ALT, and alkaline phosphatase do not. Weight is also a good predictor and the model including it instead of creatinine clearance was almost as good as my chosen model. The parameter estimates in this model are 0.481 for males versus females, 0.0303 for age, 0.0490 for bilirubin, -0.0390 for gamma gt, and -0.0055 for creatinine clearance. The AIC of 1817.7 for the fixed effects rises to about 1896.6, when they are replaced by these five variables; this can be compared to 2003.7 for the model fitted above that ignored individual differences completely. Thus, these five variables account for considerably more than one-half of the individual differences in volume.

The fit could be further improved by allowing for variation of the rate parameters among the subjects, but I shall leave this until I have a more satisfactory model below.

ND values Consider now the effect on the models of having allowed for left censoring of the ND concentrations. Of the 594 concentrations recorded up to 12 hours, 217 were left censored, as were all 54 of those for 24 hours. In the above models, the cumulative distribution function (≤ 0.04) has been used for these observations. Let us look at the effect of ignoring this and setting the left-censored values to 0.02, one-half of the nondetection limit.

The estimates for the concentration curve, with and without ignoring the values for 24 hours, are shown in Table 7.2. We see that they change considerably when left censoring is ignored. (In contrast, the model allowing for censoring does not change at all if the values at 24 h are ignored.) In addition, the AICs indicate that the models without left censoring fit very much more poorly. When the ND values for 24 hours are included, the models not accounting for left censoring fit extremely poorly. As an example of the change in shape of the concentration

7.2. PARENT DRUG AND METABOLITE

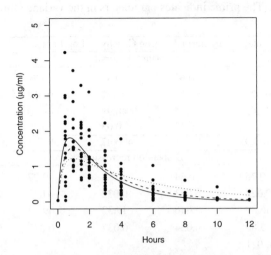

Fig. 7.4. Fitted regression lines from the gamma model with left censoring (solid), as plotted in Figure 7.2, and without allowing for left censoring (ND values set to 0.02) for observations to 24 h (dashed) and only to 12 h (dotted), for the flosequinan concentration.

profiles, the three curves for the gamma distribution at the highest dose level are plotted in Figure 7.4.

We see, as might be expected, that the curves that do not allow correctly for left censoring drop more slowly for small concentrations. In particular, when the observations at 24 hr are used, forcing the ND values to equal 0.02 makes the data no longer follow a one-compartment model, underestimating the elimination rate and forcing a reduction in the peak concentration.

7.2.3 MODELLING THE METABOLITE

For this drug, the pharmacokinetics of the metabolite is extremely important because it has an active pharmacological effect (Kamali and Edwards, 1995). As can be seen from the right graph of Figure 7.2, the metabolite is eliminated relatively slowly so that we can expect the parameters in the model to have considerably different values than for the parent drug. It might even require a quite different model.

I shall follow through the same steps in model development as for the parent drug. The parameter estimates and log likelihoods for the models with constant dispersion are shown in the first panel of Table 7.3. We immediately see that the elimination rate, k_{me}, is estimated to be much smaller than for the drug, reflecting the fact that it is eliminated more slowly. The volume estimate, $\widehat{V_m}$, is fairly similar to that for the parent, $\widehat{V_p}$.

Here, the Weibull distribution fits best. However, when the dispersion parameter is allowed to vary with dose and time (middle panel), the normal distribution

Table 7.3. Parameter estimates and AICs for various models for the metabolite concentrations. (The prime indicates parameters in the variance function.)

Parameter	Normal	Log normal	Log Cauchy	Log Laplace	Weibull	Gamma
			Constant dispersion			
$\widehat{k_{ma}}$	0.70	0.67	0.87	0.79	1.23	0.85
$\widehat{k_{me}}$	0.023	0.023	0.022	0.022	0.021	0.022
$\widehat{V_m}$	46.49	47.64	48.98	49.10	45.96	47.46
$\hat{\phi}$	0.16	0.13	0.03	0.25	3.51	8.96
AIC	4104.0	3994.5	4006.7	3942.2	3933.8	3957.5
			Dispersion regression			
$\widehat{k_{ma}}$	0.76	0.64	0.85	0.77	0.87	0.76
$\widehat{k_{me}}$	0.022	0.023	0.022	0.022	0.022	0.022
$\widehat{V_m}$	46.89	47.46	49.32	49.14	43.70	46.81
$\widehat{k'_a}$	5.80	0.034	0.037	0.037	0.051	0.051
$\widehat{k'_e}$	0.021				0.038	0.029
$\widehat{V'}$	215.6	0.266	0.014	0.081	0.145	0.412
$\hat{\kappa}$	1.899	−0.637	−0.516	−0.290	0.290	0.678
AIC	3830.1	3871.7	3989.2	3895.1	3863.1	3846.9
		Dispersion regression and fixed effects				
$\widehat{k_{ma}}$	0.67	0.63	0.87	0.78	0.87	0.72
$\widehat{k_{me}}$	0.023	0.023	0.022	0.022	0.022	0.023
$\widehat{V_m}$	46.98	47.44	47.30	47.29	45.81	47.34
$\widehat{k'}$	0.0002	0.040	0.061	0.048	0.045	0.042
$\widehat{V'}$	0.0012	0.707	0.062	0.364	0.422	0.771
$\hat{\kappa}$	−0.598	−1.088	−0.928	−0.540	0.533	1.146
AIC	3684.4	3630.2	3582.0	3563.0	3541.7	3577.8

is superior and the gamma second. For the metabolite, the two 'rate' parameters in the dispersion regression were almost identical for the 'logged' distributions, so that I have used the simplified expression of Equation (3.25) for them.

The results for the normal and log normal distributions are compared for the high dose level in the left graph of Figure 7.2. Here, the curves are much more similar than for the drug because the distribution is less skewed. However, this lack of skewness would probably no longer be true if the metabolite had been measured until it reached a nondetectable level, some time after 96 hours.

When the fixed effects for individuals are introduced into the model, the Weibull distribution again gives the best fit. If I apply kernel density estimation (not shown), the shape is again not too close to normality. Here, all of the fixed-effects estimates for variation in log volume are much smaller than for the drug, lying in between about ±0.35, even though the estimated volumes are of similar size for both parent drug and metabolite. As well, the two individuals with the extreme values in the parent drug model are not the same ones having the extreme values here.

If I replace the fixed effects by the individual covariates, we find that, of the variables mentioned above, sex, age, bilirubin, alkaline phosphatase, gamma gt, and creatinine clearance are retained in the model, with estimates -0.111 for sex, 0.0165 for bilirubin, -0.00091 for alkaline phosphatase, 0.00846 for gamma gt, and 0.00464 for creatinine clearance. The AICs of 3541.7 (Weibull) and 3577.8 (gamma) for the fixed-effects models rise to 3675.4 (gamma) when they are replaced by these five variables; this can be compared to 3830.1 for the normal model fitted above that ignores individual differences completely. Thus, these variables again account for more than half of the individual differences in volume.

7.2.4 SIMULTANEOUS MODELLING

Independence assumption Consider now how the curves change when I model the parent drug and the metabolite simultaneously.

Interdependence model I shall first use Equation (7.3), corresponding to Model 2 in Figure 7.1. The gamma distribution proves to give the best fit among the distributions considered, now simultaneously for the two substances. (For example, gamma AIC, 5911.1, log normal AIC, 5981.0.) The curves for flosequinan are shown in the left panel of Figure 7.5. We see that now the absorption is estimated to be much more rapid and that the peak concentration is estimated to occur earlier and to be much higher, the result of an implausible assumption in the model. Note that the peak lies in the first half-hour time period, before the first post-dose measurement was taken. This change of peak occurs because the absorption rate is estimated to be much higher than when the drug is modelled alone, as can be seen in the top panel of Table 7.4.

Consider next the curves for the metabolite, also shown in Figure 7.5. Here, there is much less difference, with the peak concentration occurring slightly later. The rate and volume parameters have not changed much, as can be seen in the bottom panel of Table 7.4.

The modification to the parent drug concentration curve arises from taking into account the fact that, as mentioned above, a fairly high concentration of metabolite is already present at the first post-dose measurement time of one-half hour. Under this model, this implies that the parent drug must have been absorbed very quickly. Note also that the estimated drug elimination rate, $\widehat{k_{pe}}$, is virtually identical to the estimated metabolite forming rate, $\widehat{k_{mf}}$, indicating that there is (almost) no direct elimination of the drug ($\widehat{k_{pde}} \doteq 0$).

For these two models, the estimated values of $T_{\max}$ and $C_{\max}$ for the parent drug at the highest dose level are given in Table 7.4, along with the estimated AUCs. We see that $T_{\max}$ is estimated to be much earlier and $C_{\max}$ to be higher, as could be seen in Figure 7.5. As well, the mean AUC is estimated to be somewhat

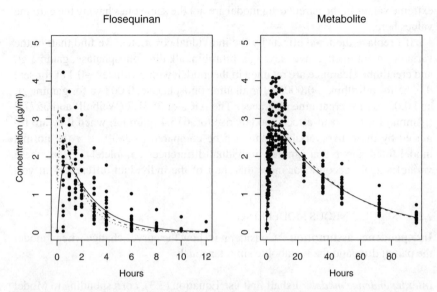

Fig. 7.5. Fitted regression lines from the model for the flosequinan and metabolite concentrations at a dose of 150 mg when modelled jointly but without the first pass, using a gamma (dashed) and log normal (dotted) distribution, along with that when each is modelled alone with a gamma distribution (solid), as plotted in Figure 7.2.

Table 7.4. Parameter estimates for flosequinan and metabolite concentrations from the gamma models, when estimated alone and jointly. For the first-pass model, Equation (3.24) is multiplied by $1 - \hat{\pi} = 0.47$ to obtain $\widehat{C}_{\max}$ and $\widehat{\mathrm{AUC}}$, which is equivalent to dividing V_p by this value.

Parameter	Alone	Joint	First pass
		Flosequinan	
$\widehat{k_{pa}}$ (1/h)	2.90	52.90	2.43
$\widehat{k_{pe}}$ (1/h)	0.41	0.51	0.42
$\widehat{V_p}$ (L)	59.75	44.56	31.80
$\widehat{T}_{\max}$ (h)	0.80	0.089	0.88
$\widehat{C}_{\max}$ (μg/ml)	1.80	3.22	1.74
$\widehat{\mathrm{AUC}}$ (μg h/ml)	6.06	6.65	6.02
		Metabolite	
$\widehat{k_{ma}}$ (1/h)	0.76	—	1.12
$\widehat{k_{mf}}$ (1/h)	—	0.51	0.42
$\widehat{k_{me}}$ (1/h)	0.022	0.024	0.023
$\widehat{V_m}$ (L)	46.81	44.56	31.80
AIC	5850.6	5911.1	5840.8

7.2. PARENT DRUG AND METABOLITE

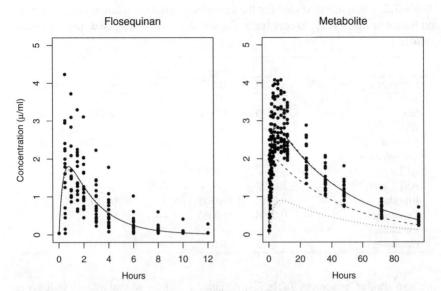

Fig. 7.6. Fitted regression lines from the model for the flosequinan and metabolite concentrations at a dose of 150 mg when modelled jointly, including a first pass, with a gamma distribution. The parent drug curve coincides with that when it is modelled alone, as plotted in Figure 7.2. The metabolite shows the first pass (dashed) and after mixing (dotted), their sum yielding the dot–dashed line. The (solid) curves are when each is modelled alone as in Figure 7.2.

larger under the joint model.

When either volume (V_p) or drug elimination (k_{pe}) is given a different value for each subject to allow for variability in these parameters among them, the estimate for drug absorption (k_{pa}) explodes. This is due to the lack of information about drug concentration in the first half-hour, when the peak is theoretically occurring.

First-pass model The first-pass metabolism forces the parent model to act as if the parent is absorbed very rapidly and at a high concentration. This is model mis-specification: the mixing assumption does not hold in a first-pass situation.

Hence, I shall next look at how the curves change when I introduce the first pass into the simultaneous model for the parent drug and the metabolite (Model 3 in Figure 7.1). I shall fix the volume to be the same for both compounds and the elimination rate to be the same for both routes of elimination of the metabolite.

The gamma distribution (AIC 5840.8) proves to give the best fit among the distributions considered (log normal AIC, 5927.1). The curves for flosequinan are plotted in the left graph of Figure 7.6. The parameter estimates are shown in the last column of Table 7.4 and are quite similar to those in the original independence model, except for V which is smaller. $T_{\max}$, $C_{\max}$, and the estimated mean AUC

Table 7.5. Parameter values for the covariates fitted simultaneously, measured on the logarithmic scale except for π, for which the logit was used. (Sex: male 0, female 1)

	$\widehat{V}$	$\widehat{k_{pa}}$	$\widehat{k_{mf}}$	$\widehat{k_{ma}}$	$\widehat{k_{me}}$	$\widehat{\pi}$
Intercept	3.48	−1.59	−0.617	−0.0049	−3.96	−0.124
Age	—	—	0.0283	—	—	—
Sex	—	−1.75	−0.545	—	0.0992	−0.451
BMI	—	—	—	—	—	—
Alkaline phosphatase	—	—	—	—	0.00068	—
ALT	−0.0116	—	−0.0097	—	—	—
AST	—	0.122	—	—	—	—
Bilirubin	—	0.0482	0.0506	—	0.0108	—
Creatinine clearance	—	0.0204	−0.0065	—	—	—
Gamma gt	—	—	−0.030	—	−0.0048	—

are also similar, as seen in Table 7.4. Again, $\widehat{k_{pe}} \doteq \widehat{k_{mf}}$ so that $\widehat{k_{pde}} \doteq 0$, leaving six parameters in the compartment model.

The corresponding curves for the metabolite with the first pass are also shown in Figure 7.6. As can be seen from the last column of Table 7.4, the first-pass formation rate of the metabolite, k_{ma}, is much higher than that after mixing, k_{mf}. The proportion of the drug immediately metabolized by the liver (first pass) is estimated to be $\hat{\pi} = 0.47$. This value is only weakly supported by an absolute bioavailability study in healthy volunteers which estimated the mean absolute bioavailability of flosequinan to be 72%. I shall discuss this further below, once I have a final model.

Covariates I can now make a more complete investigation of the usefulness of covariates in explaining the variability in the parameters. It might be expected that gender and body mass index (BMI) could be related to drug volume, that age and the liver enzymes, ALT, AST, alkaline phosphatase, and gamma gt, might be related to metabolite forming rate, and that creatinine clearance might be related to metabolite elimination rate.

After trying the covariates in various combinations, I have found a number to improve the fit of the model, reducing the AIC from 5840.8 to 5444.8. Those retained are summarized in Table 7.5. No parameter depends on BMI and k_{ma} does not depend on any covariate. Although $\log(k_{ma})$ has a large standard error, eliminating this parameter from the model, which implies also removing π, that is returning to Model 2, raises the AIC to 5694.3, indicating that it cannot be removed. Setting $k_{pa} = k_{ma}$ raises the AIC to 5470.0 but changes little the values in Table 7.5. The poorer fit occurs because k_{pa} depends on a number of covariates whereas k_{ma} does not; this shows that the data do not support their being set equal.

7.2. PARENT DRUG AND METABOLITE

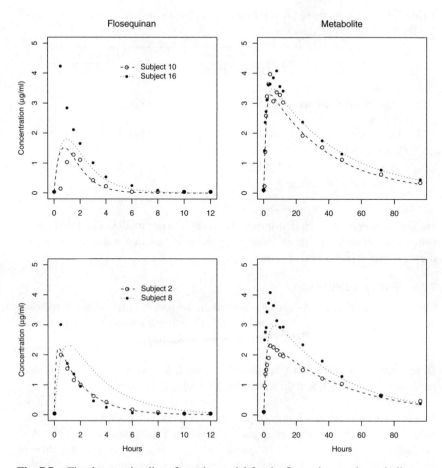

Fig. 7.7. Fitted regression lines from the model for the flosequinan and metabolite concentrations at a dose of 150 mg when modelled jointly, including a first pass, with a gamma distribution and the covariates. Top panel: the two extreme subjects for parent drug; bottom panel: the two extreme subjects for metabolite.

Introduction of covariates to allow for variability among subjects does not alter the choice of distribution (for example, log normal AIC, 5584.9). On the other hand, allowing the volume to be different for parent and metabolite slightly improves the model (AIC 5440.5) and shows that only metabolite volume depends on ALT. Thus, none of the covariates for volume found necessary when the parent drug was modelled alone (Section 7.2.2) are retained here.

The predicted individual profile curves for the four most extreme subjects are plotted in Figure 7.7. For these subjects, the model with these covariates appears to follow better the metabolite curve than that for the parent drug. However, the departures from the fitted curves show that the concentrations for these individuals

Table 7.6. AICs for three models fitted separately to the parent drug and metabolite for the flosequinan data.

	Parent drug		Metabolite	
	AIC	Parameters	AIC	Parameters
Log normal random coefficients	2025.7*	8	3826.7	8
Gamma fixed effects	1817.7	24	3578.7	24
Generalized gamma autoregression	1682.5	7	3305.5	7

*158 eliminated observations

are not following an open first-order, one-compartment model. The fitted curves follow the observations more closely for the more average subjects. I address these problems in the next section.

7.2.5 SERIAL DEPENDENCE

Let us first see what results are obtained when the parent drug and the metabolite are modelled separately, but allowing for dependence among the responses of each subject, before continuing with the joint modelling.

Drug and metabolite fitted separately I shall first look at some traditional random effects models and then at autoregression.

Random effects models For flosequinan, with a random coefficient for volume only and the variance depending on the mean as in Equation (7.11), the AIC is 2148.7 whereas I obtain 2126.7 with my more flexible variance function in Equation (7.12). With all three parameters random, the value is 2038.9 with a constant variance and 2025.7 with variance depending on the mean.

For the metabolite, with a random coefficient for volume and the variance depending on the mean, the AIC is 4036.8 whereas I have 3900.0 with my more flexible variance function. With all three parameters random, the value is 4263.7 with a constant variance and 3826.7 with variance depending on the mean.

In all of these models, which are those traditionally used (fitted here using nlme), one is assuming a log normal distribution. The AICs of the best models are reproduced in the first line of Table 7.6 and the parameter estimates for the $\mu(t)$ function in the first column of Table 7.7. Here, the ND values have been set to 0.02 for the parent drug and 0.05 for the metabolite. For flosequinan, all values after the first ND have been eliminated, a total of 158 of the 648 observations because nlme cannot handle left censoring and because including them with small fixed values greatly distorts the form of the curve.

When a gamma distribution is fitted with a different volume for each subject (the fixed effects), the models are much improved, as can be seen in the second

7.2. PARENT DRUG AND METABOLITE

Table 7.7. Parameter estimates from the three models of Table 7.6. Those for the log normal distribution are for the geometric mean concentration whereas the others are for the arithmetic mean.

	Log normal random coefficients	Gamma fixed effects	Generalized gamma autoregression
	Parent drug		
$\widehat{k_{pa}}$	1.71	4.19	2.21
$\widehat{k_{pe}}$	0.55	0.48	0.41
$\widehat{V_p}$	18.57	57.68	39.10
	Metabolite		
$\widehat{k_{ma}}$	0.72	0.72	0.69
$\widehat{k_{me}}$	0.023	0.023	0.022
$\widehat{V_m}$	1.50	47.32	42.01

line of Table 7.6. The corresponding parameter estimates are given in the second column of Table 7.7. However, this is a much more complex model because of the large number of parameters (although the AIC has been penalized for this).

In this and the following models, ND values have been treated as left censored, with an unknown value less than 0.04 for the parent drug and less than 0.1 for the metabolite. Thus, no observations are eliminated and the AICs for flosequinan are not strictly comparable to those for the standard model given above. (Those for the log normal distribution with random coefficients are too small because of the 158 eliminated observations.)

Autoregression In all of the models fitted so far, I have assumed that each individual has a specific first-order, one-compartment curve, but with some or all parameters varying among individuals. Instead of this, I shall now use a serial autoregressive model, as in Equation (B.12), with the generalized gamma distribution of Equation (7.10). In this way, we can see more directly how well the gamma assumption above holds, as compared to the classical log normal assumption.

In using such an autoregressive model, we assume that the substance (parent drug or metabolite) has an underlying curve but that subjects can deviate from it. The prediction of the path of a given individual at each time point can be improved by using the deviation from the underlying curve at the previous time point. This new model fits much better than any of the previous ones, primarily because of the autoregression, not the generalization of the gamma distribution. Thus, subject concentrations appear to be wandering rather erratically about the underlying first-order, one-compartment curve.

The final AICs are given in the last line of Table 7.6 and the parameter estimates in the third column of Table 7.7. For flosequinan, $\hat{\lambda} = 1.4$ and, for the

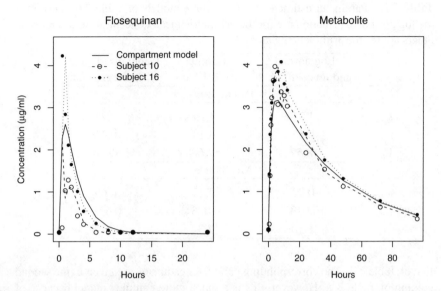

Fig. 7.8. The fitted generalized gamma model for flosequinan and its metabolite and the observed and fitted curves for two individuals at dose 150 mg.

metabolite, $\hat{\lambda} = 1.8$ in Equation (7.10), so that the two distributions show considerable departures from the gamma distribution ($\lambda = 1$), but the log normal ($\lambda \to \infty$) is clearly rejected. The dispersion, ϕ, varies over time so that we cannot easily make a comparison with the Weibull distribution.

The predicted individual profile curves can be plotted for each subject. Those for the highest dose for two subjects are plotted in Figure 7.8, along with the underlying compartment model curves. For both parent and metabolite, the model tracks the individual subject curve rather well, although it is, of course, always one step behind the observations in detecting deviations from the underlying compartment model.

In both the random and fixed-effects models, each subject is assumed to have a smooth concentration curve of the same basic shape, with only one or more parameters varying among subjects. Once on that curve, a subject is assumed not to be able to deviate from it for the period of the study. In contrast, the serial autoregressive model attempts to track individual deviations from the compartment model. Empirically, in this study, the link between an observation and the previous deviation is stronger for the metabolite than for the parent drug, as can be seen by the estimate of ρ: it is smaller for the drug at 0.69 as compared to 0.97 for the metabolite.

The above models can be improved somewhat by including some of the available covariates but I shall instead first go on to the more complex joint models.

7.2. PARENT DRUG AND METABOLITE

Table 7.8. Parameter values for the covariates fitted simultaneously, measured on the logarithmic scale except for π, for which the logit was used. Asterisks indicate additional covariates that were retained in the model without autoregression but that are not necessary here; see Table 7.5. (Sex: male 0, female 1)

	$\widehat{V}$	$\widehat{k_{pa}}$	$\widehat{k_{mf}}$	$\widehat{k_{ma}}$	$\widehat{k_{me}}$	$\widehat{\pi}$
Intercept	3.30	1.04	−0.932	0.351	−3.99	−0.225
Age	—	—	0.0122	—	—	—
Sex	—	−0.86	−0.096	—	0.0829	−0.845
BMI	—	—	—	—	—	—
Alkaline phosphatase	—	—	—	—	*	—
ALT	*	—	*	—	—	—
AST	—	0.047	—	—	—	—
Bilirubin	—	*	*	—	0.0157	—
Creatinine clearance	—	*	*	—	—	—
Gamma gt	—	—	−0.0221	—	*	—

Simultaneous modelling For the simultaneous model of the parent drug and the metabolite, I shall proceed directly to that with covariates. Introducing the serial autoregression into the gamma model with covariates fitted above reduces the AIC from 5444.8 to 4937.6. However, a number of covariates are no longer necessary; this is not surprising as the previous model did not adequately take into account the dependencies among the observations on a subject. Removing them reduces the AIC to 4931.3. Introducing the generalized gamma distribution further improves the fit without changing the covariates required; the AIC is 4880.5.

Again, $\hat{\lambda} = 1.5$, some distance from a gamma distribution, but clearly rejecting a log normal distribution. (This is confirmed by fitting the classical log normal model with autoregression; it has an AIC of 5316.9, a very much worse fit.) The autoregression parameters are $\hat{\rho} = 0.66$ for the parent and 0.97 for the metabolite.

The parameters retained in this final model are summarized in Table 7.8, with those newly eliminated being indicated. The standard errors are generally larger, and the effects smaller, than those in the model without autoregression. This is the general result of more adequately allowing for dependency among repeated measurements on each subject. The first-pass effect, π, is now estimated to be 0.44 (males) and 0.26 (females).

The predicted individual profile curves for the same four most extreme subjects as plotted in Figure 7.7 are given here in Figure 7.9 for the serial autoregression model. The underlying compartment models that the subjects are supposed to be following, given their covariate values, do not change as much with these covariates as when autoregression was not used. On the other hand, the individ-

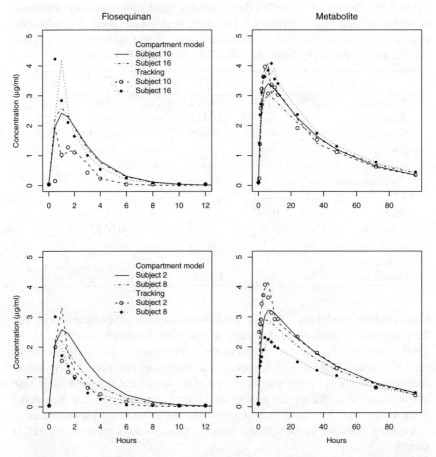

Fig. 7.9. Fitted regression lines from the model for the flosequinan and metabolite concentrations at a dose of 150 mg when modelled jointly with a generalized gamma distribution and the covariates. Top panel: the two extreme subjects for parent drug; bottom panel: the two extreme subjects for metabolite.

ual predicted (tracking) curves, taking into account the subject's previous history, follow the observations much better.

7.2.6 CONCLUSIONS

The amount of parent drug reaching systemic circulation is related both to the fraction of drug absorbed via the gut and to the fraction metabolized at the first pass. This is normally estimated in absolute bioavailability studies where both oral and intravenous (IV) formulations are administered. Comparison of AUCs enables the fraction of oral dose reaching systemic circulation to be established. As mentioned earlier, an absolute bioavailability study of flosequinan in healthy volunteers estimated the mean absolute bioavailability to be 72%. If all loss of parent drug resulted from first-pass metabolism this would correspond to a π value of 0.28, close to the values 0.44 (males) and 0.26 (females) estimated by my model with covariates and serial autoregression. It is likely, however, that a proportion of parent drug is not observed in the blood stream because not all of the oral formulation is absorbed making 0.28 an underestimate of π (the first-pass effect). In practice, the absorption and first-pass effects are rarely disentangled, but the model proposed here enables the magnitude of the first-pass effect to be estimated.

This analysis also illustrates how conventional parent–metabolite models ignore the first pass and carry the assumption that concentrations are perfectly mixed; this is not the case initially when absorbed drug is presented immediately to the liver. As we saw above, this model mis-specification can have major effects on predictions, particularly perturbing predicted parent concentration–time profiles. Some approaches first fit the parent model independently, then at a second stage use the (fixed) parent predictions to model metabolite levels. Such a method may also be misleading and may underestimate the initial peak metabolite levels which may be important in relation to pharmacodynamic effects.

In the joint models, I considered two possibilities: that the metabolite appearance rate (k_{ma}) equals that of the absorption rate of parent (k_{pa}) or that the two parameters are different. The former is intuitive because, during first pass, a proportion (π) of absorbed parent is converted into metabolite which appears in systemic circulation. However, k_{pa}, in reality, represents the rate of presentation of parent to the liver and k_{ma} incorporates the metabolic process. The model fits support the latter scenario, and as expected, the estimate of k_{ma} is less than that of k_{pa}.

7.3 Repeated dosing

Most drugs are not administered just once to a patient. For example, a medication may need to be taken several times a day. The idea is to keep the concentration in the body high enough to have the desired therapeutic effect but low enough to avoid toxicity. Hence, the shape of the curves for a given dose, as studied above, is very important. But the reactions of patients under repeated dosing can also be important. In most repeated dosing studies, concentrations are only measured once or twice at each dose administration, around peak time, so that detailed information about the shape of the curve is not available. The following study did not have these repeated dosing goals but its design makes the results closely related to such studies.

7.3.1 THE PROPOXYPHENE STUDY

In a study to investigate the relationship between the shape of plasma concentration curves of propoxyphene and the route of administration, four normal subjects were assigned to various sequences according to a four-period cross-over design.

The four methods of administration were: A, 150 mg propoxyphene hydrochloride orally; B, 225 mg propoxyphene napsylate orally; C, 25 mg propoxyphene hydrochloride intravenously; and D, 50 mg propoxyphene hydrochloride intramuscularly. These doses had been selected to induce approximately equal peak plasma concentrations of propoxyphene. After the oral administration, subjects sat, stood, or lay on their right sides for at least one hour. Notice that only treatment C enters directly into the blood.

Each subject fasted for at least eight hours prior to administration and for nine hours after. The drug was given to a subject, in its different forms, four times at successive 24 hour intervals so that there was no washout period. Two such sequences of the four treatments, in different orders, were given to each subject, with an interval of 10 days between them. The orders were ABCD and DCBA for subject 1, BDAC and CADB for subject 2, CADB and BDAC for subject 3, and DCBA and ABCD for subject 4. As shown in Table 7.9, plasma concentration was measured at 0, 1/12, 1/4, 1, 2, 3, 6, 9, and 24 hours, with the 24 hour measurement corresponding to the 0 hour measurement of the next day. The concentration is zero at time zero beginning each four-day sequence. The individual profiles over the four days are plotted in Figure 7.10.

7.3.2 TRACKING PATIENTS

I shall use the first-order, one-compartment model of Equation (3.24) for all treatments except C, for which I shall take the zero-order model of Equation (3.27). Because there is no washout period, the subjects often begin treatment on the second, third, and fourth days with propoxyphene still in the blood, as can be seen in Table 7.9. For this reason, I shall add the two models together during the first six hours of any new treatment, except on day 1. (A carry-over effect might also be introduced as an additional variable.)

We may expect that the absorption rate would differ most among the four means of administration, and indeed this is the case. The results for various distributional assumptions, and a serial autoregression model as in Equation (B.12), are shown in the first column of Table 7.10, assuming that the dispersion parameter stays constant. We see that the log Cauchy distribution is better than the gamma or Weibull distributions. When the volume and/or the elimination rate are also allowed to vary among treatments, the fit is not improved.

However, as we have already seen, it is usually unreasonable to assume that the dispersion remains constant over time, as I did in these models. Thus, I shall now let this parameter vary, following the same function as for the location parameter, but with an estimated constant included in it; I shall also allow the parameters in this dispersion function to have different values than those in the location function. The resulting AICs are given in the second column of Table 7.10. We see that the best-fitting distribution changes dramatically, now being the gamma distribution. For this model, the absorption rate can be set equal for treatments A and B, with an AIC of 1686.8.

Table 7.9. Concentrations of propoxyphene (μg/l) in the plasma of four normal male volunteers, each in two four-day periods. Time zero of the second, third, and fourth days is time 24 hours of the previous day. Treatment order is ABCD and DCBA for subject 1, BDAC and CADB for subject 2, CADB and BDAC for subject 3, and DCBA and ABCD for subject 4. Two apparent errors in the original table have been corrected. (Rodda et al., 1971)

1/12	1/4	1	2	3	6	9	24=0
			Subject 1				
0.0	0.0	11.8	50.6	47.6	25.6	15.0	0.0
4.0	6.1	25.8	94.5	74.2	50.9	21.7	9.6
114.9	125.2	72.5	65.3	37.8	37.0	15.1	7.0
36.8	63.9	97.5	118.3	109.0	77.6	36.2	10.7
37.0	63.4	111.8	115.6	121.4	84.4	50.0	20.7
227.8	136.1	122.4	87.2	88.7	44.7	47.8	7.9
6.9	7.5	46.4	94.4	84.7	50.3	30.6	8.9
8.9	9.6	55.6	121.4	97.6	66.7	32.7	8.9
			Subject 2				
3.9	5.2	20.4	47.8	48.6	23.1	15.5	0.0
47.8	79.5	177.2	117.5	126.1	62.2	59.0	9.0
16.4	13.3	47.2	89.2	85.9	62.9	41.3	7.4
130.9	76.0	111.2	88.2	38.9	35.6	36.9	11.5
114.4	183.5	70.8	94.8	33.6	27.2	11.3	4.5
4.5	4.4	4.9	103.9	46.7	36.6	17.6	5.5
88.9	123.2	140.4	118.3	100.8	73.5	41.3	10.5
12.0	11.7	39.8	102.0	105.2	63.2	41.0	10.6
			Subject 3				
100.0	97.7	93.2	43.4	32.8	33.7	15.5	4.8
5.3	5.3	18.5	83.2	54.6	60.5	24.2	7.2
42.3	57.9	100.5	96.4	88.1	50.6	32.7	7.0
10.0	9.8	36.9	71.1	109.0	49.5	27.6	7.5
0.0	0.0	8.8	19.5	58.1	63.4	33.0	8.0
73.2	86.2	149.4	148.4	120.8	83.9	38.2	8.4
5.8	6.6	16.5	83.6	53.3	35.2	28.1	0.0
104.0	90.9	66.8	44.1	47.0	54.2	25.5	4.3
			Subject 4				
18.1	37.9	67.8	60.0	48.5	41.0	38.8	12.1
71.2	195.8	118.8	69.0	62.4	48.1	25.3	14.3
10.4	11.0	54.7	157.2	203.9	132.1	67.0	23.9
23.0	23.7	150.0	257.0	183.6	131.5	100.0	30.4
0.0	0.0	123.9	161.2	145.4	84.6	51.1	9.4
9.5	11.7	33.8	147.0	213.3	82.0	79.1	18.4
98.7	103.3	93.1	70.4	49.2	40.6	26.1	15.6
134.9	128.7	99.6	93.7	112.0	85.9	22.5	19.5

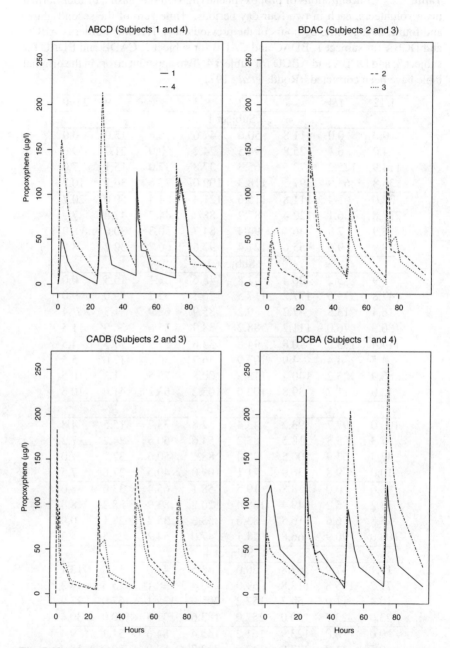

Fig. 7.10. Individual observed response profiles of propoxyphene over four days from Table 7.9.

Table 7.10. AICs for various serial dependence models for first-order, one-compartment models, with different absorption rates, for the propoxyphene data of Table 7.9.

	Constant dispersion	Dispersion function
Normal	1765.8	1701.1
Gamma	1755.3	1687.2
Weibull	1749.1	1706.4
Log normal	1817.8	1753.4
Log logistic	1797.6	1737.2
Log Cauchy	1746.3	1734.3

The underlying mean profiles and the individual profiles for the first sequence of four days for each subject are shown in Figure 7.11. The underlying profile curve follows the responses much better for the first day, no matter what treatment was used, than for the other three days when the carry-over effect is present. Although different compartment models are used for treatments C and D, their underlying profiles have fairly similar shapes. On the other hand, we see how the individual predicted profiles attempt to track the measurements, with a one-observation delay, and how they succeed in following the fourth subject who has much higher plasma concentrations than the other three.

From this combined zero- and first-order model with a gamma distribution and dispersion function, the volume is estimated to be 0.0078 for A, B, and D, and 0.00079 for C, the absorption rates to be 0.577 for A and B and 4.707 for D, and the elimination rate to be 0.105 for all four treatments. The normed profile likelihood for V for A, B, and D and k_{pe} (the same of all treatments) is plotted in Figure 7.12. Finally, the serial dependence parameter is estimated to be $\hat{\rho} = 0.90$.

This cross-over design without washout periods decidedly was not the best way to investigate the shape of plasma concentration curves.

Further reading Standard texts on pharmacokinetics include Gibaldi and Perrier (1982) and Notari (1987); see also Bauer (1983). Gutfreund (1995) gives a useful introduction to the basic principles of kinetics. Matis and Kiffe (2000) provide applications of compartment models to stochastic processes of birth, death, and migration; they also present stochastic models that do not carry the assumption of uniform mixing (exponential passage times) in each compartment.

7.4 Exercises

(1) The steroid, prednisolone, was suspected of showing high-risk potential for therapeutic nonequivalence due to differences in bioavailability in its commercially available 5 mg tablet form. A study was conducted to verify this *in vitro* and *in vivo*. The results for the latter study, comparing two tablets, are reproduced in Table C.12.

Is there any evidence of difference between the two types of tablets?

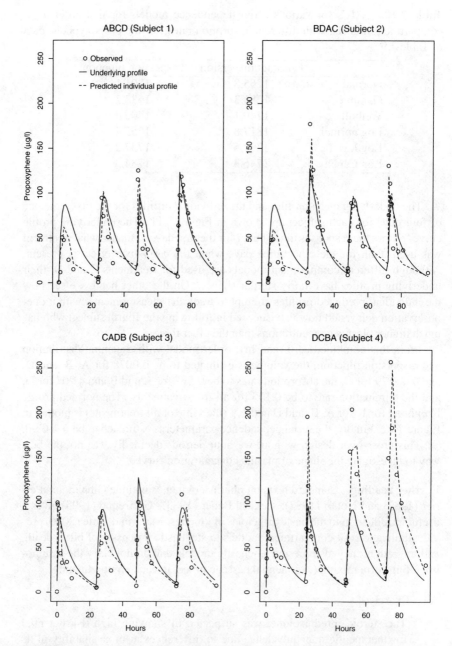

Fig. 7.11. Estimated underlying response profiles of propoxyphene over four days from the gamma distribution with the combined zero- and first-order, one-compartment models and a dispersion function. The observed responses and the predicted individual profile for the first sequence from each subject are also shown.

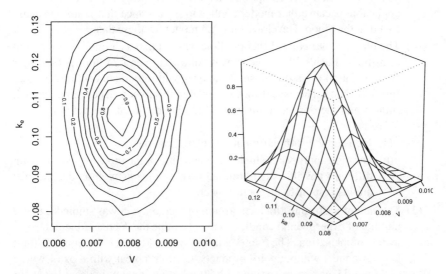

Fig. 7.12. Normed profile likelihood for k_{pe} and V (for treatments A, B, and D), propoxyphene study.

(2) A bolus intravenous injection of the same dose of indomethicin was given to each of six human volunteers to study the kinetics of its absorption, elimination, and enterohepatic circulation. Plasma concentration of indomethicin was subsequently measured at 11 time points, as in Table C.13.
  (a) Fit a suitable compartment model to these data.
  (b) Develop appropriate stochastic elements for the model by considering different possible distributional assumptions as well as dependence among responses on each subject.

(3) In a Phase I clinical trial, an oral dose of Sho-seiryu-to was administered to each of eight healthy male volunteers. Blood concentrations of ephedrine were measured over the following 24 hours with the results as shown in Table C.14.
  (a) Fit a suitable compartment model to these data.
  (b) Develop appropriate stochastic elements for the model by considering different possible distributional assumptions as well as dependence among responses on each subject.

(3) In a study of blood glucose levels, six student volunteers at Surrey University, UK, were fed test meals on different days at different times. These levels (mg/10 l) were recorded at times -15, 0, 30, 60, 90, 120, 180, 240, 300, 360, and 420 minutes relative to the time of the meal. The meals were given at six different times of the day and night: 2:00, 6:00, 10:00, 14:00, 18:00, and 22:00. The data are reproduced in Table C.15.

The first-order, one-compartment model of Equation (3.24) is not directly applicable because that model applies to a substance that is not normally found in the blood. Develop a suitable model for these data.

(4) The pharmacokinetics of theophylline was studied as a possible treatment of asthma. Each of 12 subjects was followed over a 24 hour period after administration of an oral dose of the drug with blood concentrations measured 11 times. The exact times varied among subjects. The weight of each subject and the dose administered were also recorded, as shown in Table C.16.

  (a) Fit a suitable compartment model to these data.
  (b) Develop appropriate stochastic elements for the model by considering different possible distributional assumptions as well as dependence among responses on each subject.

(3) The rate of gastrointestinal absorption of Declomycin was studied under a number of experimental conditions to determine the decrease due to heavy-metal complexation. The four conditions were: A, after eight hours fasting; B, after a meal without dairy products; C, after a meal with 8 oz of whole milk; and D, coadministration with 20 ml of aluminium hydroxide gel. In each group, 300 mg of Declomycin were administered orally, with the results shown in Table C.17.

  (a) Fit appropriate models to determine which parameters vary under the various treatment conditions.
  (b) What is the proportional reduction in total absorption when milk is taken with a meal as compared to fasting?
  (c) What is the reduction with aluminium hydroxide gel?
  (d) Compare these to the situation of a meal without dairy products.
  (e) As stated in Table C.17, these are averages. There were six volunteers in the fasting group and four in each of the other groups. What would be the advantages of having the individual data for all participants instead of just mean values?

(6) Let us consider possible improvements to the models for propoxyphene in Section 7.3.

  (a) Try the generalized gamma distribution to see how well the distributional assumptions are suited to these data.
  (b) Can the fit be improved by using a dynamic model (Section B.4) instead of the serial autoregression?

(3) A second study of propoxyphene used the same design (but without the measurement at two hours). Here, the doses were selected to induce approximately equimolar levels instead of equal peak plasma concentrations. The four doses were: A, 65 mg propoxyphene hydrochloride orally; B, 100 mg propoxyphene napsylate orally; C, 65 mg propoxyphene hydrochloride

intravenously; and D, 65 mg propoxyphene hydrochloride intramuscularly. The results are shown in Table C.18.
- (a) Develop an acceptable model for these data.
- (b) Can the same type of model as used above in Section 7.3 be applied here?
- (c) Compare your results to those in the text and to those from the previous question.

8
Pharmacodynamics

Whereas pharmacokinetics involves the study of the concentration of some substance in the body, pharmacodynamics looks at the reaction of the body to that substance. Thus, pharmacodynamic models attempt to relate changing concentrations of some substance in the body to some pharmacological effect.

8.1 Studying the effects of drugs on the body

Pharmacodynamics can be considerably more difficult than pharmacokinetics for several reasons:
- Responses are often not continuous measurements such as concentrations, often being counts or ordinal values.
- Few mechanistic models have been developed for such responses.
- Pharmacodynamic responses depend on concentrations of the substance of interest in the body so that, ideally, the pharmacokinetic and pharmacodynamic models should be developed simultaneously, with appropriate interrelationships.

Not all aspects of this complexity can be treated here.

8.1.1 GOALS

Pharmacodynamics looks at dose–effect relationships. Demographic (age, sex), biological, genetic, environmental, and disease factors, as well as concurrent medication, may influence pharmacodynamics. Thus, the goal is to establish the dose–effect relationship as it varies with these factors so that the medication can be prescribed optimally to different individuals.

Ideally, the physiological response to a drug is related to its concentration at the site of action. This poses a major practical problem in that the drug effect usually takes place in organs or tissues so that drug concentration cannot be sampled at that effect site. As in pharmacokinetics, drug levels can generally only be measured in plasma or serum. If plasma concentration is used, a further practical problem is that there may be a time lag between its changes and those at the site of action. One solution to this is to attempt to maintain the drug at a steady state in the body.

Often, no suitable mechanistic models are available, as in pharmacokinetics, so that more empirical modelling may have to be done. In simple cases, changes in pharmacodynamic reaction can be modelled over time with only dosing information but without serum concentrations being available. A second possibility is to model the concentrations and reactions separately. The most complex approach is to model them jointly. Here, models are required both for the dose–concentration and the concentration–effect relationships. This becomes even more difficult if the metabolite is also active.

8.1.2 RESPONSE VARIABLES

Often, the relevant reaction of the body will not be a continuous measurement. For example, it may be a count (such as the number of coughs in a given unit of time) or an ordinal variable (Section 6.1.3) recorded on some appropriate scale. In making a choice, factors such as clinical relevance, ease of measurement, and variability and sensitivity of the response should be taken into account.

Count data are often recorded in clinical trials. If the observations are longitudinal, few statistical methods have been available to account adequately for the dependencies, especially with complex designs, such as cross-over studies having several counts made in each period. Classical approaches often attempt to allow for the overdispersion and correlation among responses by *ad hoc* corrections such as modifying the standard errors by means of the coefficient of dispersion and/or using generalized estimating equations.

For ordinal data, models allowing for dependence among responses are only slowly becoming available. (For analyses using ordinal models, see Sections 6.4 and 6.5.)

8.2 Continuous response

Normality is a common assumption for continuous response data. Here, I shall examine closely this assumption for a clinical trial involving the treatment of gastric acidity.

8.2.1 THE GASTRIC pH STUDY

To evaluate the dose of an H_2 receptor antagonist required in the treatment of gastric pH, six patients were given five different doses plus placebo in varying orders, following a cross-over design. The dose levels of 10, 20, 40 80, and 160 mg were selected following results from studies of animal reactions and also from Phase I rising-dose trials. No serious, irreversible adverse effects had been recorded at any of these dose levels in previous studies. Each new dose administration was only begun after a washout period of one week to ensure that the previous dose had been completely eliminated.

Gastric pH level was measured immediately before administering the drug, and at 2, 4, 6, 8, 10, and 12 hours after. In the original study, the statisticians concluded that the responses were reasonably normally distributed with constant variance (Ekholm *et al.*, 1989). A clinically important response would be one raising the gastric pH level over 3 for two consecutive recordings. No adverse effects were recorded at the lower doses, but at 160 mg all patients except number 3 experienced intolerable diarrhoea or abdominal cramps.

The data are given in Table 8.1 and the individual profiles are plotted in Figure 8.1. We see that there is a great deal of variability in the responses and that only the two highest doses bring the pH above 3.

8.2.2 REGRESSION FUNCTIONS

In contrast to pharmacokinetic data, here we have little prior information available to help us in constructing a regression function to describe the response profiles. Compartment models are of little aid because we are not interested in how the acid determining the pH is flowing in and out of the stomach. Nevertheless, the general shape of a sums of exponentials function may be useful to start an empirical search for a suitable function. However, all pH levels are at least 1 so that I shall modify slightly the function in Equation (3.24):

$$\mu(t) = 1 + \frac{dk_a}{V(k_a - k_e)} \left(e^{-k_e t} - e^{-k_a t}\right) \quad (8.1)$$

Note that the parameters, V, k_a, and k_e, will no longer have the mechanistic interpretations of a compartment model. When this function is fitted to these data, we discover that the two 'rates' are virtually identical. This leads to the simplified function

$$\mu(t) = 1 + \frac{kdte^{-kt}}{V} \quad (8.2)$$

derived from Equation (3.25), that fits as well but has one less parameter.

However, this still does not provide an exceptionally good fit. An improvement is obtained by using, instead,

$$\mu(t) = \exp\left(\frac{kdte^{-kt}}{V}\right) \quad (8.3)$$

where the addition of one is no longer necessary. This still does not follow the changing doses adequately. A final modification gives

$$\mu(t) = \exp\left(\frac{kte^{-kt}}{V_d}\right) \quad (8.4)$$

where V_d is a distinct parameter value for each dose level. Thus, the pharmacodynamic response is not varying 'linearly' with dose. This can be seen in the individual profiles of Figure 8.1 where the two highest dose levels give considerably higher responses.

8.2.3 GAUSSIAN COPULAS

Cross-over designs such as this involve two levels of nesting (Section B.1). Because of the observed irregularities in the response profiles, an autoregression

Table 8.1. Gastric pH measured in a cross-over design involving six patients each given six doses (mg) of an H_2 receptor antagonist and measured seven times over 12 hours. (Ekholm *et al.*, 1989)

		\multicolumn{7}{c}{Time (h)}						
Dose	Period	0	2	4	6	8	10	12
0	1	1.4	1.8	1.8	1.4	1.4	1.2	1.1
10	2	2.6	1.6	1.4	2.6	1.0	1.3	1.5
20	3	2.5	1.9	1.4	1.9	1.0	1.4	1.9
40	4	1.4	1.0	2.9	2.7	3.1	2.3	1.5
80	5	1.0	2.4	4.8	5.3	5.4	3.2	1.5
160	6	1.0	2.3	5.0	5.4	4.2	3.7	3.4
0	6	1.0	2.0	1.4	2.2	1.0	1.0	1.0
10	5	1.6	1.0	1.0	1.7	1.0	1.3	1.6
20	4	1.4	1.5	1.0	1.9	2.7	1.8	1.0
40	3	1.0	2.2	3.4	2.3	3.3	1.7	1.0
80	2	1.9	1.9	5.5	4.9	4.0	2.5	1.4
160	1	1.0	1.0	5.9	6.1	3.2	2.5	2.4
0	4	1.6	2.4	1.0	1.3	1.3	1.6	2.5
10	1	1.0	3.3	1.0	1.0	2.0	1.8	1.6
20	5	1.4	1.5	3.1	2.6	3.5	2.2	1.0
40	2	1.0	1.2	3.8	4.0	2.5	1.7	1.0
80	6	1.6	2.5	5.0	5.3	4.7	3.4	2.5
160	3	1.3	2.4	5.0	3.4	3.8	2.2	1.0
0	5	2.0	1.0	1.0	1.0	1.0	1.0	1.0
10	3	2.2	1.2	1.5	1.6	1.0	1.3	1.6
20	1	1.3	1.0	1.0	1.0	2.2	2.5	2.9
40	6	1.0	1.9	4.3	3.4	2.2	2.6	3.2
80	4	1.0	4.0	6.4	6.4	3.7	2.8	2.4
160	2	1.7	1.3	5.1	4.5	3.6	2.6	1.8
0	2	2.6	1.0	1.0	2.3	1.0	1.0	1.0
10	4	1.7	2.1	1.0	1.0	1.9	1.4	1.0
20	6	1.8	1.4	2.3	2.3	2.0	1.6	1.3
40	1	2.6	1.9	2.2	4.0	2.1	1.5	1.0
80	3	1.0	2.6	5.6	5.1	3.8	3.0	2.7
160	5	1.2	2.7	5.0	4.9	5.8	3.1	1.0
0	3	1.0	1.7	1.3	1.0	1.3	1.2	1.0
10	6	1.8	1.0	1.4	3.2	1.7	1.3	1.0
20	2	1.0	1.1	1.8	1.8	2.1	2.2	2.2
40	5	1.0	2.0	3.6	2.7	4.4	3.0	1.7
80	1	1.0	2.1	5.1	4.5	3.9	2.7	1.4
160	4	1.0	3.7	4.5	5.1	4.6	2.8	1.8

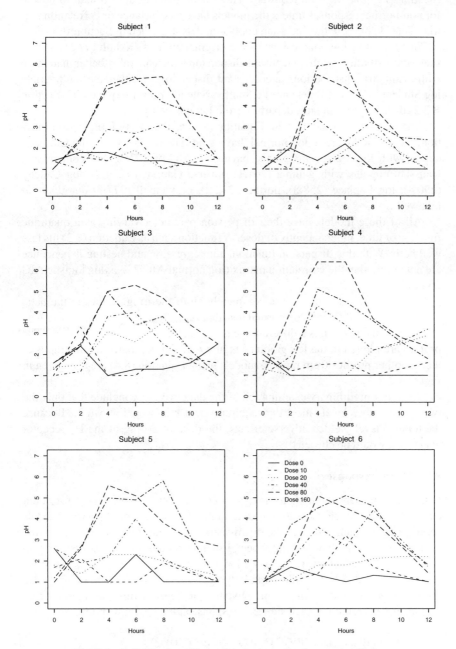

Fig. 8.1. Individual profiles at the six doses for the gastric pH data.

(Section B.2) may also be required. These combinations are difficult to handle for non-normal responses unless the models have a covariance or correlation matrix. Thus, I shall use the Gaussian copula models described in Section B.3.

In contrast to the conclusions of the original authors (Ekholm *et al.*, 1989), skewed distributions with nonconstant dispersion fit considerably better than those with symmetric distributions and constant dispersion. Neither the multivariate log Student t (Section B.3.1) nor the multivariate log power-exponential (Section B.3.2) distribution indicates departure from log normality.

The best–fitting models, with Equation (8.4) as the location regression function, are the multivariate log normal, having an AIC of 257.3, and the Gaussian copula with log logistic marginals, having an AIC of 257.2. For comparison, Gaussian copulas with gamma (261.1), inverse Gaussian (274.7), log Cauchy (290.4), log Laplace (258.3), normal (272.2), or Weibull (277.3) marginals fit less well.

All of these models have their dispersion parameter varying as a quadratic function of time, independently of dose. A function such as Equation (8.3) fits less well here. With this dispersion function, autoregression and nesting dependence are not required in the correlation matrix (log normal AIC 257.5; log logistic AIC 258.3).

These models do not capture completely all of the irregularities in the data. The saturated multivariate log normal distribution with autoregression has an AIC of 249.8. This model has a different mean for each dose–time combination. The profiles are plotted in the left graph of Figure 8.2. For comparison, the graphs of the smoother profiles from my two models using Equation (8.4) are also given in Figure 8.2.

As in our preliminary examination of the data, we can conclude that only the two highest dose levels meet the requirement of raising pH above 3. Because the highest level yielded adverse effects, the dose of 80 mg of the H_2 receptor antagonist would be chosen.

8.3 Count response

I shall now present methods to analyse a complex cross-over design for count data with many levels of nesting through the development of stochastic models appropriate for such data. For the overdispersion, I shall use a negative binomial distribution. For the longitudinal aspect, I shall introduce an autoregressive effect into the models (Section B.2). As we have already seen several times (Sections 4.2, 5.2, 7.2, and 7.3), this allows underlying 'population' curves to be produced for individuals with the same covariate values, at the same time giving individual profile curves predicting each subject's response at the next time point.

8.3.1 THE CAPSAICIN COUGH CHALLENGE STUDY

Nonproductive cough is common and significantly reduces the quality of life. It is, however, difficult to treat because of the lack of appropriate pharmacological

8.3. COUNT RESPONSE

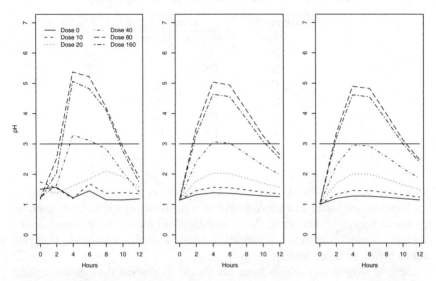

Fig. 8.2. Arithmetic mean profiles from the saturated model (left), arithmetic mean profiles from the log normal model (centre), and geometric mean profiles from the log logistic model (right) for the gastric pH data.

agents, and this lack of compounds may be linked to the difficulty in assessing the activity of anti-tussive agents for human beings.

Cough is a reflex action triggered by either mechanical or chemical stimulation of irritant receptors and specialized sensory afferent nerve fibres located in bronchial mucosa. Chronic cough can be attributed to a number of underlying pathological, physiological, and pharmacological conditions including, but not limited to, chronic obstructive pulmonary disease (COPD), asthma, post-viral infection, and angiotensin-converting enzyme (ACE) administration. In order to understand both contributing factors and to investigate the effects of novel products and existing pharmaceutical medicines, numerous experimental cough models have been devised in man and animal species, using a variety of chemical mediators to induce a cough reflex.

Anti-tussive agents can only be evaluated in individuals who cough. The cough can result from a natural disease (viral infection) or it can be induced with a tussive agent. In the Phase I evaluation of an anti-tussive, it is usual to induce cough using an appropriate agent. This allows a more rigorous control over the study since post-viral cough is unpredictable and will inevitably resolve with time.

Capsaicin is an extract of chilli peppers that directly stimulates nonmyelinated sensory C-fibre nerve endings. It has been used as an inhaled aerosol in many investigations directly to stimulate a cough reflex in human beings (see Millqvist, 2000). The effect is dose dependent, short acting, and reproducible in subjects sensitive to the stimulus. It is also well tolerated and has been used to stimulate

Table 8.2. Treatment structure for the cough study.

Treatment label	Time −30 min	Time 0 min
A	Y	X_1
B	PY	X_1
C	Y	X_2
D	PY	X_2
E	PY	Z
F	PY	PX
G	Y	PX

cough in pædiatric subjects. Repeated stimulation with high doses of capsaicin has been shown to induce tachyphylaxis over a period of 40 minutes, but response returns to normal within hours. Most investigations record cough counts as the reaction to increasing doses of capsaicin solution inhaled with a single breath from a breath-actuated inhaler.

Several simplistic methods have been used to analyse data obtained from cough studies using a tussive agent. These include

- measuring the threshold dose of the tussive agent which induces cough;
- counting the number of coughs to increasing doses of the tussive agent; and
- measuring the dose of tussive agent that produces more than three coughs, but less than five coughs.

However, more complex and realistic nonlinear models should often also be appropriate.

The aim of this Phase I double-blinded, placebo-controlled, cough study trial was to compare the responses to two doses of a drug, X (X_1 and X_2), in attenuating capsaicin-induced cough in the presence or absence of drug Y. For comparison, drug Z at a single dose was also included in the trial. Drug Y, or its placebo PY, was taken orally 30 minutes before the (X or Z) treatment was applied. In addition to these five treatments, a placebo for X taken after PY and after Y was also included. The structure of all seven treatments is given in Table 8.2.

The 24 subjects in the trial were healthy males and females who received the treatments according to the seven-period cross-over design given in Table 8.3. As will be seen there, subjects 16 and 23 were actually observed for eight periods, their last treatment being repeated. (In the presentation of the models, I shall ignore this, although I use these data in the analysis.) Between each pair of treatment periods, there was a washout period of three days.

On each study day, a subject took the oral dose of Y or PY 30 minutes before taking the test drug. Then, one and five hours later, the series of capsaicin challenges was given. For these, each subject took four tidal-breath inhalations, one minute apart, of the capsaicin vehicle at each of four increasing concentrations (1, 3, 10, and 30 μM). The series at different concentrations were begun at 20 minute

8.3. COUNT RESPONSE

Table 8.3. Cross-over design for the cough study.

Subject	\multicolumn{8}{c}{Period}

Subject	1	2	3	4	5	6	7	8
1	C	G	A	F	B	E	D	
2	F	A	B	C	E	D	G	
3	D	B	E	A	F	G	C	
4	A	C	F	G	D	B	E	
5	G	E	D	B	A	C	F	
6	B	D	G	E	C	F	A	
7	E	F	C	D	G	A	B	
8	C	E	B	F	D	G	A	
9	B	C	F	G	E	A	D	
10	E	F	C	D	A	B	G	
11	G	B	A	E	F	D	C	
12	A	G	D	C	B	F	E	
13	F	D	E	A	G	C	B	
14	D	A	G	B	C	E	F	
15	F	A	D	C	B	E	G	
16	D	B	A	E	F	G	C	C
17	B	G	C	A	D	F	E	
18	E	D	F	B	G	C	A	
19	C	F	E	G	A	B	D	
20	G	E	B	D	C	A	F	
21	A	C	G	F	E	D	B	
22	G	A	F	C	D	B	E	
23	B	C	A	F	G	E	D	D
24	E	G	B	A	C	D	F	

intervals. The recorded response is the number of coughs in the one minute period after each inhalation. Therefore, each subject produced 32 counts in each period: four for each of the four concentrations of capsaicin at each of one and five hours. Note that no pharmacokinetic information is available.

These data have a complex clustering structure with several levels of nesting:

(1) individual subjects;
(2) periods within individuals, with a three-day washout between them;
(3) set of challenges at one and at five hours within periods;
(4) four levels within a challenge;
(5) four one-minute counts within a level;
(6) the individual cough events within the one minute, aggregated as a count.

I shall handle level (6) using overdispersion models and levels (4) and (5) using autoregression over the 16 minutes of cough recording (in fact, embedded in an 80 minute period). I shall analyse separately the challenges at one and five hours within a period and allow for a trend in coughing over the periods, assuming that washout is adequate so that there is no other dependence.

Besides the baseline cough count measurement, available covariates included sex, age, height, weight, pulse rate, systolic and diastolic blood pressure, and an atopic allergen test. All of these were only measured at baseline.

8.3.2 OVERDISPERSED AUTOREGRESSION

The usual model for such count data is the Poisson distribution. However, with a risk of overdispersion, other more complex models, such as the negative binomial distribution, may be more appropriate. I shall consider both of these possibilities.

The average number of coughs in a minute may depend on various factors. Let $\mu_d(t)$ be some nonlinear function describing how this mean number of coughs changes over time, t, and with challenge level, d. For the change in the frequency of coughing with the escalating challenge level, one may expect a curve with an asymptote, perhaps of an S-shaped form, because there will be an upper physical limit to the number of coughs possible in one minute. On the other hand, we only have four observed points on the curve, the four challenge levels, so that little information is available about its exact shape.

I have found empirically that a growth curve of the logistic form fitted best of those tried:

$$\mu_d = \frac{\alpha + \delta d}{1 + \gamma d}$$

$$= \frac{\alpha + \delta e^{\log(d)}}{1 + \gamma e^{\log(d)}}$$

(8.5)

where d is the series of four increasing concentrations of capsaicin. The effects of the seven treatment combinations can be introduced in various ways. I tried treatment

(1) acting additively on the mean (that is, on α);
(2) affecting the slope through γ; and
(3) acting multiplicatively on the whole expression.

The third of these proved empirically to give the best fit.

This resulted in the final form of the nonlinear regression function, whereby Equation (8.5) was multiplied by an exponential function to allow for changes in the mean over the 16 minutes of challenge and over the seven periods of the complete trial, as well as the effects of treatment and covariates:

$$\mu_d(t) = \left(\frac{\alpha + \delta d}{1 + \gamma d}\right) e^{\eta t + \Sigma_j \beta_j x_j}$$

(8.6)

where the x_j represent period, treatment, and the covariates. This can be interpreted as a standard log linear model for count data (the second factor) nonlinearly adjusted for changing challenge level by multiplying it by the logistic growth curve of Equation (8.5).

8.3. COUNT RESPONSE

Table 8.4. Poisson and negative binomial autoregression models for hour one. First line: fit of the full model, as in Equation (8.6), with treatment, height, diastolic blood pressure, baseline, period, and time, plus the interactions of time with period, baseline, and concentration. Second to seventh lines: fit after removal of various individual effects or interactions from the full model.

	Poisson	Negative binomial
Full model	3269.9	3264.8
Removing		
Treatment	3277.0	3271.2
Height	3278.4	3271.4
Diastolic pressure	3271.5	3266.2
Concentration*Time	3279.7	3274.6
Baseline*Time	3270.4	3265.6
Period*Time	3272.1	3267.1

8.3.3 ANALYSING THE CHALLENGE–RESPONSE CURVE

The investigators were interested in the effects of covariates in order to determine what kinds of healthy subjects should be used in such Phase I trials. Let us, however, first look at a model with fixed effects for subject. The Poisson model has an AIC of 3205.4 at one hour and 3335.1 at five hours. A negative binomial distribution does not improve the fit, indicating that overdispersion is not present. These results can be compared with a 'null' model containing no covariates distinguishing among individuals; this has, respectively, AICs of 3314.2 and 3401.1. Thus, the differences among subjects are more apparent at one hour than at five hours.

Let us now replace the fixed subject effects by the available covariates. The results of fitting various models are summarized in Tables 8.4 and 8.5 for hours one and five respectively. In the full model at one hour, there is some overdispersion so that the negative binomial model is required whereas there is no evidence of overdispersion at five hours. On the other hand, more covariates are required at five hours. The available covariates explain about 50% of the variability at five hours but only about 40% at one hour.

The model at one hour can be simplified by combining some of the treatment groups but these combinations do not have any medical meaning. The treatments A, B, and C are most different from placebo, whereas those for D, E, and G are intermediate between the former and placebo. At five hours, treatment appears not to be required in Table 8.5. However, if treatments A, B, and G are together contrasted with all of the others, including placebo (F), the AIC is reduced.

With full placebo (F) as point of comparison, the treatment contrasts at one hour are A -0.412, B -0.341, C -0.302, D -0.2016, E -0.151, and G -0.246. Thus, A, B, and C induce the least coughing. At five hours, they are A -0.194, B -0.190, C -0.096, D -0.003, E -0.039, and G -0.165. The difference in cough rate among treatment groups is considerably less at this later time point.

Table 8.5. Poisson and negative binomial autoregression models for hour five. First line: fit of the full model, as in Equation (8.6), with treatment, height, weight, systolic blood pressure, baseline, period, and time, plus the interactions of time with period, baseline, and concentration. Second to eighth lines: fit after removal of various individual effects or interactions from the full model.

	Poisson	Negative binomial
Full model	3367.6	3368.6
Removing		
Treatment	3367.4	3368.2
Height	3379.8	3380.2
Weight	3379.8	3380.7
Systolic pressure	3370.0	3370.9
Concentration*Time	3376.3	3377.2
Baseline*Time	3368.3	3369.2
Period*Time	3369.6	3370.6

Sex was significant when included in the models alone but was no longer required when height was included. The only other significant covariate at hour one is diastolic blood pressure. At hour five, systolic fits slightly better than diastolic blood pressure; weight is required here as well as height. There is a linear change over time with period as well as with time of the challenge: one to 16 minutes, ignoring the gaps between changes in challenge level. The interactions of baseline and of challenge concentration with time are also significant.

The autoregression parameter is estimated to be 0.44 at one hour and 0.43 at five hours. These values are surprisingly close and show that only moderate dependence is present.

The challenge curve parameters are respectively $\hat{\alpha} = -3.19$, $\hat{\delta} = 5.55$, and $\hat{\gamma} = -0.016$ at one hour and $\hat{\alpha} = -2.52$, $\hat{\delta} = 4.58$, and $\hat{\gamma} = -0.013$ at five hours. The main effects of time are respectively $\hat{\eta} = -0.037$ and $\hat{\eta} = -0.056$ and of period -0.219 and -0.161, with interactions between the two, 0.0090 and 0.0077. The baseline effect is estimated to be 0.061 and 0.035 at one and five hours respectively. As might be expected, subjects with higher baseline values cough more. However, these effects decrease with time: respectively, -0.0028 and -0.0023.

The most significant effects arise from the size of the person: height (m) with estimates respectively -1.115 and -1.391 at one and five hours. At the latter time point, weight (kg) is also significant: 0.015. Shorter and heavier people cough more, the former being closely connected with sex. The normed profile likelihood graph for the relationship between these two parameters at hour five is plotted in Figure 8.3, showing that they are virtually unrelated. As well as size, blood pressure affects coughing so that people with higher pressure cough less: at hour one, diastolic blood pressure (mmHg) gives -0.0062, whereas at hour five, systolic blood pressure (mmHg) gives -0.0061. The inclusion of the results of the atopic allergen test failed to improve the fit of the model and the results are

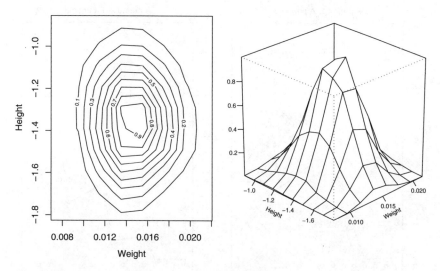

Fig. 8.3. Normed profile likelihood for the coefficients of height and weight at hour five, for the cough challenge escalation study.

not presented here.

As an illustration of how the model describes the data, mean and individual profiles for treatments A and F in both orders in consecutive periods for a given individual at one hour are shown in Figure 8.4, again ignoring the gaps between changes in challenge level. Note, however, that these curves depend on the height, diastolic blood pressure, and baseline counts of the individuals involved.

8.3.4 CONCLUSIONS

The model developed here handles a complex cross-over design with six levels of clustering involving longitudinal count data. It uses the negative binomial distribution to account for overdispersion, when present, and an autoregressive process to allow for individual variations about the mean curves.

Such models have several major advantages. Average differences in responses can be compared, as in the usual models, to check for treatment differences and the influence of covariates. At the same time, the autoregressive structure allows the model to update dynamically the mean so as to track individual subjects, providing predictions of the response at the next observation point. This also provides a benefit in the interpretation of the average differences as measures of precision of the parameter estimates allow for the dependencies in the data.

The presence of overdispersion in the model with covariates instead of fixed effects indicated missing explanatory covariates. The need for them in the model at one hour but not at five hours seemed to indicate a short-term effect. This led

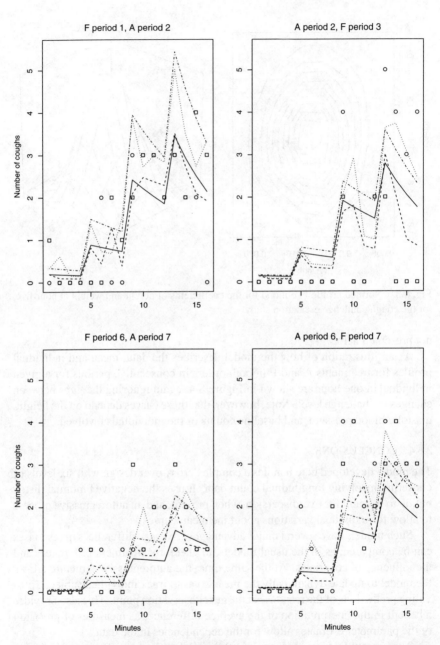

Fig. 8.4. Mean profiles at one hour (A: solid; F: dot–dashed) with corresponding individual profiles (A: dashed; F: dotted). Top row: subjects 15 and 22; bottom row: subjects 6 and 20.

us to investigate differences due to allergy but, as mentioned above, the inclusion of the atopic allergen test as an additional covariate did not improve the model.

As well, this model allows us to understand better the mechanisms by which people are induced to cough and how these change over time and with varying levels of challenge. They allow us to determine what aspects of the phenomenon are influenced by the various treatments, as well as by the covariates. In Equation (8.6), these affect the overall shape of the curve, and not simply the level or the slope separately.

Further reading   See the references given at the end of Chapter 7.

8.4   Exercises

(1) In the challenge escalation study of coughing in Section 8.3:
   (a) Do any of the parameters of the dose–response curve depend on the covariates?
   (b) How does the fit of a dynamic model (Section B.4) compare to that of the autoregression?

(2) In a two-period study, five rabbits were exposed to increasing doses of phenylbiguanide under placebo and an MD_5-antagonist, MDL 72222. The change in blood pressure was recorded at each dose level. The data are shown in Table C.19. (Pinheiro and Bates, 2000, pp. 438–439, call this a cross-over design but the treatments were apparently always given in the same order, placebo before antagonist.)
   (a) Develop a suitable model for these data.
   (b) Discuss what advantages would have been obtained if a cross-over design had been used.

9
Assays and formulations

Medical statistics does not only involve directly medical (human) problems. More chemical aspects are also important and raise interesting nonlinear modelling issues. In this chapter, I shall look at two of these that occur at opposite ends of the development process: the analysis of assays, needed at the beginning, and the development of formulations for the administration of a medication, required once its value has been established.

9.1 Assays

In drug development, one must be able to measure the concentration of a new molecule in samples taken from the human body. Thus, one important step is the derivation of suitable *assays* for measuring the level of the drug in serum, plasma, or other supports. Thus, all of the measurements used in pharmacokinetics (Chapter 7) depend on the availability of such procedures.

9.1.1 GOALS

Bioassay is a procedure for estimation of the concentration of a substance by comparing its effect on some biological material, such as animal tissue, to that of a standard product. In a direct assay, the concentration is varied and some response is measured. In an indirect assay, only some variable related to the event of interest can be measured. For example, in a quantal assay, only the numbers of responses at each dose level are counted.

Here, I shall primarily be interested in methods for measuring the concentration of proteins. Two important special types of proteins are antibodies (immunoglobulins), produced in uncountable numbers of different forms by the immune system as a defence against infection, and enzymes, highly specific protein catalysts.

Assay methods are based on measurement of the activity of the protein of interest; this involves recording its responses at several standard concentrations. A dose–response curve is estimated and this is used to determine protein concentrations in unknown samples. Thus, because the concentration of the protein contained in the support cannot be measured directly, a two-step procedure must be used to estimate it. First, a calibration curve is estimated for a series of known concentrations, as we shall do in this chapter; then, this equation is inverted for use in finding the unknown concentrations.

9.1.2 METHODS

To separate out a protein of interest and measure its level, several standard methods are available. The most common are

- liquid chromatography at high pressure (HPLC) if the drug is of low molecular weight;
- radioimmunoassay (RIA);
- enzyme-linked immunosorbent assay (ELISA).

However, assays may also have to be developed that measure directly the biological activity of a protein. The degree of antigen binding of a polypeptide, such as an antibody, is not always a good measure of biological activity.

Calibration of a protein in a sample involves measuring a signal. The known monotone relationship between signal and concentration can then be used to obtain an estimate of concentration.

High-pressure liquid chromatography In HPLC, the compound of interest, in liquid solvent, is pumped under high pressure through a stainless steel column very uniformly packed with small (3 to 10 μm in diameter) particles of a resin such as silica gel. Separation occurs according to the length of time spent in the column. The column effluent is monitored, often using ultraviolet light, showing peaks at different times corresponding to the different components. Although much faster than conventional column chromatography, this method often does not have sufficient specificity and sensitivity to detect proteins in complex biological matrices.

Radioimmunoassay In RIA, the signal is a radioactive count: both the protein and its marked isotope are assumed to behave similarly with respect to the antibody to be used in the assay. Fixed amounts of radio-labelled protein and of antibody are added to several test tubes. The latter, in large excess over the protein concentration, binds to the protein. Several known concentrations of unlabelled protein are added to the tubes to generate standard curves. This unlabelled protein competes with the radio-labelled protein for binding to the antibody until equilibrium, the level of bound radioactive material thus depending on the level of unlabelled protein. At equilibrium, the bound complex is precipitated and counts per minute recorded using a gamma counter. Because the relationship between the quantity of linked antibody and radioactive protein and the dose of unlabelled protein varies with the experimental conditions, a new calibration curve is generally calculated for each assay.

Enzyme-linked immunosorbent assay Antibodies can be labelled with fluorescent dyes and used to detect and quantify specific molecules. However, their sensitivity as a probe for assaying a given protein can be enhanced by signal amplification. An unlabelled primary antibody attaches to the protein of interest. Then, a group of labelled secondary antibodies bind to the primary antibody. This is most sensitive if the secondary antibodies have an enzyme attached to them: each molecule of enzyme acts catalytically to produce thousands of molecules of some detectable product.

This is the principle of an ELISA; the signal is an enzyme that is subsequently measured by having it react with the appropriate substrate. The protein is incubated on a microtitration plate. Then, the primary antibody solution is added and it is incubated again. Finally, immunoconjugate is added, followed by further incubation. At equilibrium, substrate is added causing a colorimetric reaction proportional to the quantity of protein present: the absorbance, fluorescence, or optical density is measured at the appropriate wavelength for the substrate.

Other, more specialized, assays, such as the Ames microsome assay described in Section 9.4, are also used.

9.2 Colorimetric enzyme assay

In colorimetric enzyme assays, as in all assays, interest often centres particularly on reproducibility, both among replicates on a given day and among days.

9.2.1 ASSAY METHODOLOGY

The colorimetric enzyme assay of an acid phosphatase was performed using the substrate disodium p-nitrophenyl phosphate, for which it has a high affinity. The reactions were performed in a 0.1 molar sodium acetate–acetic acid buffer at pH 4.8 and temperature 25°C using a controlled-temperature water bath. Each vial contained 1 cm^3 of buffer with 25 μg of enzyme and 1 cm^3 of buffer with the substrate at one of the following concentrations: 0.026 38, 0.052 76, 0.1055, 0.1407, 0.2111, and 0.4221 $\times 10^{-3}$ M. After ten minutes of incubation, 3 cm^3 of 1 M NaOH was added to stop the reaction. This produces sodium p-nitrophenate, which has a yellow colour. The absorbance of this product was measured in a spectrophotometer against a reagent blank at 410 nm.

A number of replicates at each of the above sets of concentrations were performed on each of five different days (Passaribu et al., 1999).

9.2.2 MICHAËLIS–MENTEN FUNCTION

The Michaëlis–Menten model of Equation (1.7) gives the initial velocity of an enzyme-catalyzed reaction as a function of substrate concentration. Let us rewrite this function as

$$\mu_s = \frac{V_{\max} s}{K_m + s} \quad (9.1)$$

where μ_s is the mean initial velocity at substrate concentration s, $V_{\max}$ is the maximum velocity (in practice, divided by a calibration constant), K_m is the Michaëlis

Table 9.1. AICs for Michaëlis–Menten model fitted to the acid phosphatase assay with various distributional assumptions and parameters varying over days.

	Normal	Student t
Constant V_{max} and K_m		
Independent	1140.5	1134.7
Random intercept	1134.7	1129.3
Different V_{max}		
Independent	1111.1	1105.9
Random intercept	1112.1	1106.9
Different K_m		
Independent	1114.7	1108.9
Random intercept	1115.7	1109.9
Both different		
Independent	1096.1	1087.3
Random intercept	1096.9	1088.3

constant. The asymptote, V_{max}, is reached when the enzyme–substrate system is saturated. The Michaëlis constant is the substrate concentration when the velocity is equal to one-half the maximum, also called the EC_{50}. Generally, the substrate concentrations, s, can be fixed by the experimenter to a high degree of precision.

9.2.3 ANALYSIS OF THE ACID PHOSPHATASE ASSAY

If I fit the Michaëlis–Menten model to the data, I obtain the results summarized in Table 9.1. I have allowed the variance to change with concentration, also following Equation (9.1) but with different parameter values than for the mean, as discussed in Section 7.1.3.

From Table 9.1, there are clear differences in parameter values among the five days. As well, a heavier-tailed distribution than the normal is required. On the other hand, once the differences among days are accounted for, a random intercept is no longer necessary. There is no indication that a skewed distribution, log normal or log Student t, is required; these models fit considerably more poorly.

This model can be further improved by allowing the parameters of the variance function also to be different among days. Then, the Student t distribution is no longer necessary. The AIC for the normal distribution is 1078.1. The estimates of V_{max} for the five days are, respectively, 0.217, 0.263, 0.237, 0.246, and 0.230, whereas those for K_m are 0.0591, 0.0836, 0.0572, 0.0701, and 0.0710. The values of V_{max} are not significantly different for days 3 and 4, and those of K_m for days 1 and 3 and for days 4 and 5. This simplification (with a simpler variance function) reduces the AIC to 1073.9.

The resulting mean curves for this final model are plotted in Figure 9.1, separately for each day. The normed profile likelihood for V_{max} and K_m, both at day 1, is plotted in Figure 9.2, showing that contours are close to elliptical shape.

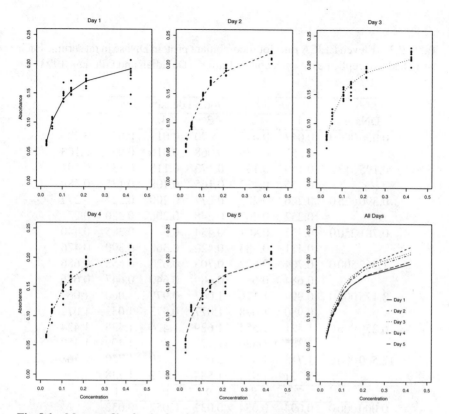

Fig. 9.1. Mean profiles for the five days of the acid phosphate study with the observations.

There is a great deal of variability in parameter values across days. As well, the variance is not the same each day. It would be wise to check closely this assay procedure.

9.3 DNase assay

In the development of an ELISA for recombinant protein DNase, 11 experiments were performed using rat serum. Duplicate absorbance measurements were recorded at each of several standard concentrations as shown in Table 9.2.

9.3.1 GENERALIZED MICHAËLIS–MENTEN FUNCTION

A standard regression function that is used for such assays takes the logistic form (Section 3.1.3), but with an added intercept:

$$\mu_s = \mu_\infty + \frac{\mu_0 - \mu_\infty}{1 + e^{\beta_1[\log(s) - \beta_2]}} \tag{9.2}$$

where s is the concentration and μ_s the corresponding mean optical density. Here, μ_0 is the mean at zero concentration, μ_∞ is that at 'infinite' concentration, β_1

Table 9.2. Eleven ELISA runs for recombinant protein DNase in rat serum. Each assay had two replicates at each concentration. (Davidian and Giltinan, 1993)

DNase	Optical density					
	1	2	3	4	5	6
0.000 000 0	0.047	0.045	0.070	0.011	0.035	0.086
	0.057	0.050	0.068	0.016	0.035	0.103
0.195 312 5	0.159	0.137	0.173	0.118	0.132	0.191
	0.155	0.123	0.165	0.108	0.135	0.189
0.390 625 0	0.246	0.225	0.277	0.200	0.224	0.272
	0.252	0.207	0.248	0.206	0.220	0.277
0.781 250 0	0.427	0.401	0.434	0.364	0.385	0.440
	0.411	0.383	0.426	0.360	0.390	0.426
1.562 500 0	0.704	0.672	0.703	0.620	0.658	0.686
	0.684	0.681	0.689	0.640	0.647	0.676
3.125 000 0	0.994	1.116	1.067	0.979	1.060	1.062
	0.980	1.078	1.077	0.973	1.031	1.072
6.250 000 0	1.421	1.554	1.629	1.424	1.425	1.424
	1.385	1.526	1.479	1.399	1.409	1.459
12.500 000 0	1.715	1.932	2.003	1.740	1.750	1.768
	1.721	1.914	1.884	1.732	1.738	1.806
	7	8	9	10	11	
0.000 000 0	0.094	0.054	0.032	0.052	0.032	
	0.092	0.054	0.043	0.094	0.043	
0.195 312 5	0.182	0.152	0.142	0.166	0.142	
	0.182	0.148	0.155	0.164	0.155	
0.390 625 0	0.282	0.226	0.239	0.259	0.239	
	0.273	0.222	0.242	0.256	0.242	
0.781 250 0	0.444	0.392	0.420	0.439	0.420	
	0.439	0.383	0.395	0.439	0.395	
1.562 500 0	0.686	0.658	0.624	0.690	0.624	
	0.668	0.644	0.705	0.701	0.705	
3.125 000 0	1.052	1.043	1.046	1.042	1.046	
	1.035	1.002	1.026	1.075	1.026	
6.250 000 0	1.409	1.466	1.398	1.340	1.398	
	1.392	1.381	1.405	1.406	1.405	
12.500 000 0	1.759	1.743	1.693	1.699	1.693	
	1.739	1.724	1.729	1.708	1.729	

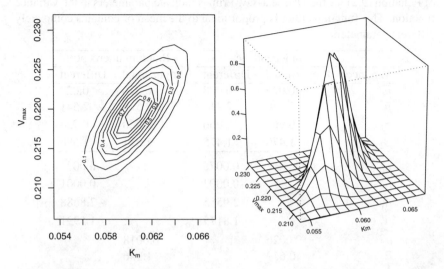

Fig. 9.2. Normed profile likelihood for V_{max} and K_m, both at day 1, for the acid phosphate study.

is the slope, controlling the steepness of the dose–response curve, and β_2 is the logarithm of the concentration yielding a response half-way between those at zero and at infinite concentrations, the log EC_{50}.

This function is a generalization of the Michaëlis–Menten model in Equation (9.1). It can be reparametrized as

$$\mu_s = \frac{V_{max} s^{\beta_1} + K_m V_0}{K_m + s^{\beta_1}} \tag{9.3}$$

with $K_m = e^{\beta_2}$, $V_{max} = \mu_\infty$, $V_0 = \mu_0$, and the concentration is power transformed. In Equation (9.1), $V_0 = 0$ and $\beta_1 = 1$.

9.3.2 ANALYSIS OF THE RAT SERUM

When the generalized Michaëlis–Menten curve is fitted, a multivariate normal distribution fits better than the log normal. There is little evidence of the need for a heavier-tailed distribution. For independent observations, the AIC is 926.9 with a constant variance and 891.5 when the variance varies as in Equation (9.2) but with different parameters than the mean. These values are reduced respectively to 901.9 and 822.1 when a random intercept for the 11 experiments is introduced. In standard analyses (for example, Davidian and Giltinan, 1995, pp. 22–23, 134), the variance is made to depend directly on the mean, as in Equation (7.11). The AICs are raised respectively to 902.1 for independence and 843.4 with a random intercept, with two fewer parameters.

Table 9.3. Parameter estimates from several models using the logistic function of Equation (9.2) for the DNase assay. Primes indicate parameters in the variance function. This function either is proportional to the mean or contains completely different parameters.

	Independence		Random intercept	
Variance	Proportional	Different	Proportional	Different
$\widehat{\mu_0}$	0.026	0.028	0.026	0.022
$\widehat{\mu_\infty}$	2.410	2.413	2.526	2.541
$\widehat{\beta_1}$	0.961	0.966	0.920	0.924
$\widehat{\beta_2}$	1.470	1.475	1.571	1.596
$\widehat{\mu'_0}$		0.0078		0.0073
$\widehat{\mu'_\infty}$		0.0007		0.0001
$\widehat{\beta'_1}$		−2.9555		−2.8688
$\widehat{\beta'_2}$		1.8175		1.5991
σ^2	0.0026		0.0018	
$\widehat{\kappa}$	0.629		1.346	
$\widehat{\delta}$			0.00065	0.00059
AIC	902.1	891.5	843.4	822.1

The parameter estimates are given in Table 9.3. We see that, although the more flexible variance function and the random intercept yield models fitting better, the parameter estimates in the logistic regression function for the mean differ very little among the four models. Notice that $\widehat{\beta_1}$ is fairly close to one and $\widehat{\mu_0}$ fairly close to zero so that the model might possibly be simplified to the Michaëlis–Menten function. The normed profile likelihood surface for the two other parameters, μ_∞ and β_2, is plotted in Figure 9.3.

The (marginal) mean profile is plotted in Figure 9.4, along with the observed responses from the first three experiments. The increase in variability with concentration can clearly be seen. Because the main interest in such studies is the precision of the estimates, it is important to have an adequate model, including that for the variability.

9.4 Ames *Salmonella* microsome assay

The following description follows closely that given by Krewski et al. (1993), who provide an excellent case study of the application of mechanistic models.

9.4.1 ASSAY METHODOLOGY

In genetic toxicology, the Ames *Salmonella* microsome assay is the most widely used and best validated method of testing for mutagenicity. Cells are cultured in a soft agar containing trace amounts of histidine to allow residual growth of auxotrophic bacteria. This is designed to detect reverse mutations from auxotrophic

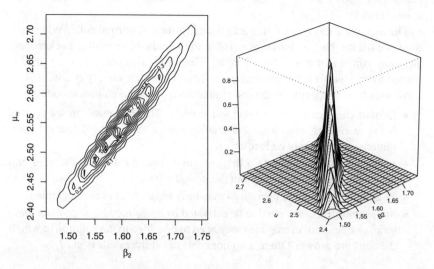

Fig. 9.3. Normed profile likelihood for the log EC_{50} and asymptote parameters for the ELISA study of recombinant protein DNase. (Contours from 0.1 to 0.9 by steps of 0.1. Lower peaks are an artifact of the plotting algorithm.)

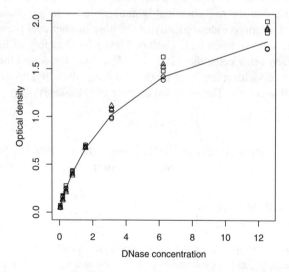

Fig. 9.4. Mean profile for the ELISA study of recombinant protein DNase with observations from the first three experiments.

Salmonella cells requiring histidine for growth (His$^-$) to histidine-independent prototrophic cells (His$^+$). Certain strains of *Salmonella* can also have spontaneous mutations.

The agar plate has an opaque background formed of normal cells. When mutation occurs, the His$^+$ colonies are visible to the naked eye on this background. They may contain from 10^6 to 10^8 cells. The number of colonies on a plate is counted by eye with a light microscope or by an electronic colony counter.

Various factors specific to the test chemicals must be taken into account:

- Certain chemicals can be toxic to the cells. This can result in fewer cells being at risk of mutation. The background may be less dense or fewer mutant colonies may be formed.
- Stable chemicals will retain their original concentration on the agar and have the same effect throughout the period of study.
- Volatile or degradable chemicals may only have effect at the beginning.
- Some chemicals may need to be activated by some metabolic process: bacterial or mammalian enzymes may need to be added to the solution in which the cells are grown. Often, a homogenate of rat liver cells is used.

9.4.2 MECHANISTIC MODELS

If a mechanistic model can be developed to describe the dose–response relationship, the slope of the initial, approximately linear, component will indicate the mutagenic potency.

Let us, first, assume that sufficient histidine is present for k generations of cells to survive and that there is a constant time between generations (cell divisions). Suppose that the test chemical is mutagenic for m generations and cytotoxic for n generations independently of the dose of chemical present and that these two effects are independent. Each cell has a local supply of histidine that cannot be used by other cells; there is no histidine diffusion across the plate.

Setting $m = k$ yields a family of models for the probability, $\Pr_V(m,n)$, that a plate has a visible colony. The expected number of colonies is

$$\mu = N \Pr_V(m,n) \tag{9.4}$$

where N is the number of cells originally plated. The function $\Pr_V(m,n)$ obeys a difference equation with a rather complex solution. A special case of interest is

$$\Pr_V(m,n) = \begin{cases} \pi_M(1-\pi_D) & m=n=1 \\ \frac{\pi_M(1-2\pi_D)_+}{(1-p_D)_+} & m=1, n=\infty \end{cases} \tag{9.5}$$

where the $+$ subscript indicates that the quantity in parentheses is set to zero if it is negative. Here, π_M is the probability of mutation and π_D the probability of cell death. The probability that all descendants of a given cell become extinct within s generations because of toxicity, $\Pr_E(s)$, follows the recursive relationship

9.4. AMES *SALMONELLA* MICROSOME ASSAY

$$\text{Pr}_E(s) = \pi_D + (1-\pi_D)[\text{Pr}_E(s-1)]^2 \qquad 0 \le s \le n \qquad (9.6)$$

with initial condition, $\text{Pr}_E(s=0) = 1$.

Now let us change slightly the assumptions so that histidine can diffuse across the plate. Cell division will continue until histidine is exhausted or all cells die. Toxic and mutagenic effects last throughout the experiment. Let N_T be the total number of cell divisions that can be supported by a given amount of histidine (including the number of cells initially present). The resulting equation is

$$\begin{aligned} \mu &= N_T \pi_M (1-\pi_D)\{1-[Q(\infty)]^2\} \\ &= \frac{N_T \pi_M (1-\pi_D)(1-2\pi_D)_+}{(1-\pi_D)} \end{aligned} \qquad (9.7)$$

This ignores the possibility that all normal cells become extinct before all histidine has been consumed; this probability will be very small unless $\pi_M + \pi_D \ge 0.5$.

If the test chemical has toxic effect only for a short time, for example, the first generation of cell divisions, and if there is only enough histidine for one generation, then $N_T = N$ and

$$\mu = N\pi_M(1-\pi_D) \qquad (9.8)$$

irrespective of the time during which mutations induced by the test chemical might occur. On the other hand, if a mutation arises that gives protection against an enzymatically mediated toxic effect, then

$$\mu = N_T \pi_M (1-\pi_D) \qquad (9.9)$$

We can now construct models for π_M and π_D. If we assume single-hit kinetics, then they are related to dose, d, by

$$\pi_M = 1 - e^{-\beta'_0 - \beta'_1 d} \qquad (9.10)$$
$$\pi_D = 1 - e^{-\beta_2 d} \qquad (9.11)$$

with $\beta'_0, \beta'_1, \beta_2 > 0$. Substituting these into Equation (9.8), we obtain

$$\begin{aligned} \mu &= N(1-e^{-\beta'_0 - \beta'_1 d})e^{-\beta_2 d} \\ &\doteq (\beta_0 + \beta_1 d)e^{-\beta_2 d} \end{aligned} \qquad (9.12)$$

the approximation in the second line applying because π_M is small. Here, $\beta_i = N\beta'_i$ has been used because N is not estimable. An identical function arises from Equation (9.9). For long-term toxicity, we obtain

$$\mu \doteq (\beta_0 + \beta_1 d)(2 - e^{-\beta_2 d})_+ \qquad (9.13)$$

Toxic effects may be nonlinear at low doses. This can be accommodated by raising the dose to a power in the last term of the functions.

Table 9.4. Four Ames *Salmonella* microsome assays from the study by the International Programme on Chemical Safety. (Krewski *et al.*, 1993)

Air particles TA100 +S9		Diesel particles TA98 −S9		1-Nitropyrene TA100 +S9		TA100 −S9	
Dose	Counts	Dose	Counts	Dose	Counts	Dose	Counts
0.00	188 180	0.00	43 42	0.00	145 157	0.00	169 159
0.25	202 181	0.06	355 344	0.75	324 304	0.75	359 426
0.50	199 242	0.13	537 496	1.50	531 522	1.50	679 571
1.00	262 280	0.25	884 755	3.00	764 717	3.00	572 716
1.50	332 313	0.40	776 599	4.50	782 638	4.50	649 423
2.00	373 443	0.50	484 552	6.00	453 619	6.00	299 129

Krewski *et al.* (1993) also describe a number of nonmechanistic models in common use by statisticians.

The regression functions developed here describe mean counts. At least in certain situations, the variance among plates may be greater than the mean of each plate so that the Poisson assumption will not hold and overdispersed models will be necessary. This may occur because the mean number of revertants varies among plates.

9.4.3 THE INTERNATIONAL PROGRAMME ON CHEMICAL SAFETY STUDY

The International Programme on Chemical Safety sponsored a study to estimate the mutagenic potency of three complex mutagenic mixtures and two positive controls. The mixtures were a coal-tar solution, a sample of particulate matter from ambient air in Washington, DC, USA, and particles from heavy-duty diesel engine exhaust. The positive controls were benzo(a)pyrene and 1-nitropyrene. The USA National Institute of Standards and Technology prepared aliquots from each sample and sent them to 20 laboratories throughout the world. Two replicate extracts were to be prepared from each sample and each bioassayed twice at five positive dose levels plus an unexposed control with two replicate plates at each dose. *Salmonella* strains TA98 and TA100 were to be used, with and without metabolic activation using S9. This yielded over 1000 experimental results. Four selected data sets are shown in Table 9.4.

Krewski *et al.* (1993) used a quasi-likelihood method of estimation and fixed the power of the dose at two in the second term of the regression functions. Here, I have used the Poisson, negative binomial, and Consul distributions and estimated the power of dose. In many cases, I obtain quite different parameter estimates than they did. In contrast to the results of Krewski *et al.* (1993), here in all cases, Equation (9.13) gave a negative estimate of β_2, indicating an unacceptable model, although the curve did appear reasonable.

For the air particles, a standard log linear Poisson model, with no indication of overdispersion, fitted best; the linear model used by Krewski *et al.* (1993) fitted considerably less well. For the other three sets of assays, overdispersion was present, with the negative binomial better than the Consul distribution. For these, the power of dose was estimated to be between 1.7 and 2.4 in Equation (9.12). The estimated curves, along with the observed data points, are plotted in Figure 9.5.

The parameter estimates for Equation (9.12) were reasonably similar to those given by Krewski *et al.* (1993). However, the standard errors, with the power of dose fixed at two, were considerably different. These differences may arise because they were not using probability models upon which likelihoods could be based.

9.5 Determining formulations

Once a drug has been shown to be active for the pharmaceutical effect sought and nontoxic at the dose levels required, it must be packaged so that patients can use it. Drug delivery refers to how a medication is pharmaceutically designed to improve therapeutic efficacy by controlling how the drug gets to the target site. Generally, we can distinguish injection, inhalation, oral ingestion, infusion, and transdermal delivery.

9.5.1 DEVELOPING DELIVERY SYSTEMS

In developing a drug delivery system, problems that have to be attended to include
  (1) instability of the compound;
  (2) solubility in water;
  (3) short half-life, requiring frequent administration;
  (4) lack of oral bioavailability, due to degradation by gastrointestinal enzymes;
  (5) the relationship to meals;
  (6) prolonged exposure required to attain efficacy;
  (7) nonlocal action, as the compound reaches organs or tissues that are not the locus of the disorder; and
  (8) dangerous side effects, usually associated with peak drug concentration.

Careful selection of the formulation can have a major effect on the *in vivo* activity of the compound.

The development process for the drug delivery system of a new medication involves
  (1) a small feasibility study of compatibility between the drug and the formulation;
  (2) optimization of the formulation;
  (3) production of clinical samples;
  (4) scaling up for sufficient production to carry out clinical trials;
  (5) submission for registration; and
  (6) market production.

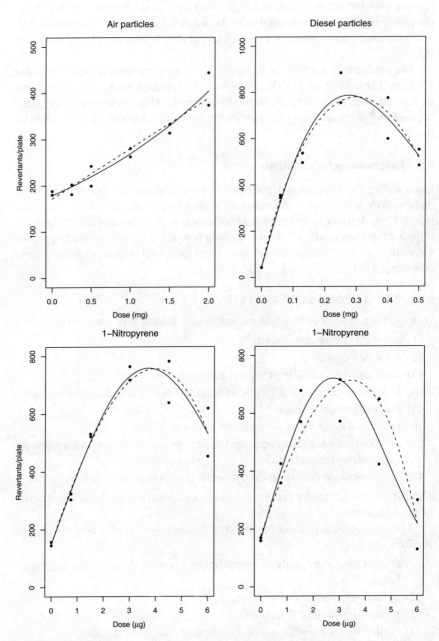

Fig. 9.5. Mean profiles for the four assays from the International Programme on Chemical Safety study. For the air particles, linear (dashed) and log linear (solid) curves. For the other assays, Equation (9.12) (solid) and Equation (9.13) (dashed).

9.5. DETERMINING FORMULATIONS

Formulations that ease the patient's task will have a major advantage. For example, a superior formulation may reduce the dose schedule from four times daily to once a day or allow inhalation instead of injection.

For tablets, pills, and capsules that are ingested, the time necessary for them to dissolve in a liquid is of interest. Much effort has been expended in the determination of the dissolution characteristics of solid doses of medications. Dissolution rates may differ between formulations and shapes, but also among brands, factories, and even batches. They also depend on the solvent, *in vitro* in a beaker or *in vivo* in the stomach and intestine, on the temperature, and on the amount of agitation.

9.5.2 TRANSPORT MODELS

Let us assume that the basic shape of the pill is retained over time, as it dissolves, and that the mass remains proportional to volume. Then, the surface area, say A_t, at time t will be related to the mean mass, m_t, as $A_t \propto m_t^{2/3}$. Oblong slabs, short cylinders, and ellipsoids can be expected to satisfy these conditions (Crowder, 1996). Special forms of diffusion models are required (Section 3.2.2).

One possible assumption is that the instantaneous rate of loss of mass is proportional to the surface area and to the difference between the current concentration of the solution, c_t, and the saturated concentration, c_s:

$$\frac{dm_t}{dt} = -k_1 A_t (c_s - c_t) \tag{9.14}$$

If $c_t/c_s \ll 1$, this yields

$$\frac{dm_t}{dt} = -k_2 m_t^{2/3} \tag{9.15}$$

with solution

$$k_2 t = m_0^{1/3} - m_t^{1/3} \tag{9.16}$$

the cube-root law, where m_0 is the initial mass of the pill.

If the liquid is agitated, this model does not work well. If we assume that the thickness of the stagnant film of solvent on the solid surface is proportional to the square root of the mean volume diameter, then $k_1 \propto m_t^{-1/6}$ so that

$$k_3 t = m_0^{1/2} - m_t^{1/2} \tag{9.17}$$

If, instead, we assume Fick's law of diffusion (Murray, 1993, pp. 234–235, 246) with $c_s - c_t$ constant over time,

$$\frac{dm_t}{dt} = -k_4 \sqrt{A_t}(c_s - c_t) \tag{9.18}$$

so that

$$k_5 t = m_0^{2/3} - m_t^{2/3} \qquad (9.19)$$

These models can be generalized by adding an unknown parameter:

$$t = \frac{1}{k}\left[1 - \left(\frac{m_t}{m_0}\right)^\kappa\right] \qquad (9.20)$$

Crowder (1996) further generalizes this by adding an intercept:

$$\mu_j = \beta + \frac{1}{k}\left[1 - \left(\frac{m_j}{m_0}\right)^\kappa\right] \qquad (9.21)$$

where μ_j is the mean time by which the proportion, m_j/m_0, of the mass is remaining. If $\kappa \to 0$, then

$$\mu_j = \beta - \frac{1}{k}\log\left(\frac{m_j}{m_0}\right) \qquad (9.22)$$

These functions yield dissolution curves derived from the differential equations describing transport phenomena at the solid–liquid interface. They attempt to model physical and chemical laws controlling the properties and behaviour of the substances involved. Unfortunately, in practice, the apparatus used can influence the results. For example, stirring and agitation may vary among machines or over time.

9.5.3 PILL DISSOLUTION RATES

To study the effects of type of storage on the dissolution of pills, the times taken for various fractions of a pill to disappear were recorded. The results for four different methods of storage, with respectively six, four, four, and three pills, are shown in Table 9.5.

When I fit Equation (9.21) to these data, I find that β has the same estimate for groups 2, 3, and 4, different from that of the first group but that k varies more, with only groups 2 and 4 having the same estimate. Assuming independence, the AIC is 245.2 for a multivariate normal distribution and 232.8 for a multivariate log normal distribution. In the latter, an exponential link function is used. Allowing for a serial autoregression (Section B.2) reduces these respectively to 143.3 and 117.4. Including a random intercept raises the AIC in both cases. There is also no indication of heavier tails, either the multivariate power-exponential or Student t distributions.

The parameter estimates are $\hat{\beta} = 12.71$ for group 1 and 9.89 for the other three groups, $\hat{k} = 0.046$ for group 1, 0.037 for groups 2 and 4, and 0.031 for group 3, and $\hat{\kappa} = 0.71$ for all groups. The estimate of κ is closest to that for Fick's law of Equation (9.19), but with an additional intercept term. The normed profile likelihood surface for κ and k for the first group is plotted in Figure 9.6.

The mean profiles are plotted in Figure 9.7. The individual profiles for the first

9.5. DETERMINING FORMULATIONS

Table 9.5. Times for given fractions of pills to dissolve. The four groups with, respectively, six, four, four, and three pills, were stored in different ways. (Crowder, 1996)

	Fraction				
0.9	0.7	0.5	0.3	0.25	0.1
13	16	19	23	24	28
14	18	22	26	28	32
19	24	28	33	33	39
13	17	21	25	26	29
14	16	19	23	25	27
13	16	19	23	24	26
13.0	17.0	21.5	26.0	27.8	33.5
11.5	15.5	20.5	24.5	26.7	31.3
10.4	14.4	18.4	23.5	25.1	29.6
11.1	15.1	19.0	23.6	24.7	28.7
11.7	16.9	22.0	27.6	29.2	34.5
13.5	18.7	24.9	30.0	31.8	37.5
12.0	17.1	22.7	28.4	30.2	35.8
12.1	16.7	21.1	26.8	29.0	33.8
11.0	14.5	19.0	24.5	26.0	32.0
14.0	19.0	24.0	30.0	31.5	39.0
11.0	14.0	17.5	22.0	23.5	29.5

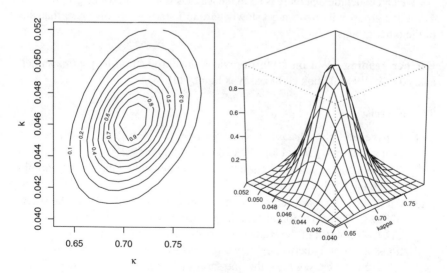

Fig. 9.6. Normed profile likelihood for κ and k for the first group for the pill dissolution data. (Contours from 0.1 to 0.9 by steps of 0.1.)

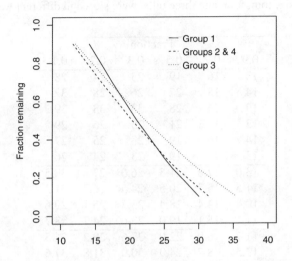

Fig. 9.7. Plots of profiles showing the mean fraction of pills remaining over time in the four groups.

two pills of each group are shown in Figure 9.8, illustrating how the autoregression follows the individual deviations from the mean profiles. The autoregression coefficient is estimated to be 0.97, with variance of 0.0109 for the log times.

We can conclude that there is no evidence of difference between groups 2 and 4, but that group 3 dissolves most slowly. Group 1 starts to dissolve later than any of the other groups.

Further reading   Watson (1999) provides an introduction to pharmaceutical analysis. A classical book on bioassay is Finney (1978).

9.6 Exercises

(1) For the acid phosphatase assay of Section 9.2, is the model improved by fitting the more general logistic curve of Equation (9.2)?

(2) For the DNase assay of Section 9.3, can the model be satisfactorily simplified to the Michaëlis–Menten model?

(3) An ELISA test was used to detect anticoronavirus antibodies in the serum of cows. The results for one cow in two different months are shown in Table C.20. The object of the study was to estimate the change in the concentrations of antibody between the two months. This is done by estimating the relative potency, say κ, of the one serum with respect to the other. This is defined such that one unit of serum in May produces the same response as κ units in June. In doing this, we assume that the two serums contain the

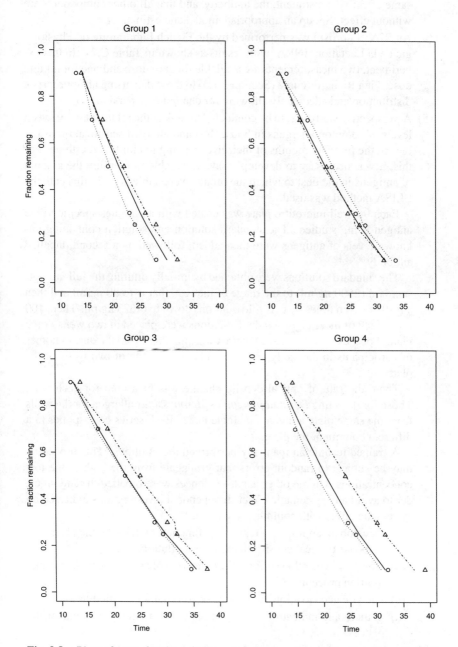

Fig. 9.8. Plots of mean fraction of pills remaining over time in the four groups with the individual profiles for the first two pills in each group.

same effective constituent, the antibody, and that all other components are without effect. Set up an appropriate model and estimate κ.

(4) An RIA of cortisol was performed by the French Laboratoire de Physiologie de la Lactation, INRA, with results as shown in Table C.21. In this experiment, two measurements are available for zero dose and one for infinite dose. Fit a Richards curve (Section 3.1.3) to these data using an appropriate distribution and adequately allowing for changing dispersion.

(5) A prospective study was to be conducted to look at the relationship between levels of common allergens in house dust and allergen sensitization of babies in the first few months of their lives leading to childhood asthma. For this, it was necessary to develop assays to be able to measure the amount of antigens in the dust to which the infants were subjected. To this end, the ELISA method was used.

Each 96-well microtitre plate was coated with antibodies specific to the antigen being studied. The standard solution and solution containing unknown levels of antigens were then added, followed by a second, labelled antibody.

The standard solutions were obtained by initially diluting the full-strength standard (2500 ng/ml) to the range of interest, that is to 80 ng/ml and then a further seven times by two-fold dilutions down to 0.623 ng/ml. Then, 100 ml of each of these eight standard solutions were placed in two wells of the plate. For the test solutions, an extract was prepared from the dust in homes of participants in the study and 100 ml added to each of two wells of the plate.

Then, the rate of optical density change was measured for each well. Those for detecting *Dermatophagoides pteronyssinus* allergen for the wells from the same plate are given in Table C.22. Each series corresponds to a different column of the plate.

A trained technician manually performed the dilutions. This procedure may be subject to random errors that propagate from the high to the low concentrations. On the other hand, sequences were pipetted in random order to avoid any systematic effect. Independent investigations indicated no systematic effect with column of the plate.

(a) Develop an appropriate regression function to describe the change in response (optical density change) with dilution.

(b) How have you allowed for the propagation of errors due to the manual dilution procedure?

(c) Did you need to allow for the dispersion changing with dilution level?

(d) Is there any indication of a systematic effect among columns of the plate?

(5) The decrease in concentration of the reactant in certain chemical processes can be described by

$$\frac{d\mu(t)}{dt} = -k\mu(t)^\delta \tag{9.23}$$

where δ is usually taken to be an integer. This value is called the order of the process. In assay work, zero- and first-order processes are most important.

    (a) A dilute solution of penicillin G was hydrolysed at pH 1.3 and 37°C. It was assayed repeatedly over 24 hours with results as shown in Table C.23. Fit a model to estimate the order of the process.

    (b) The rate of release of theophylline was studied for 300 mg sustained-release tablets, with the results also shown in Table C.23. Fit a model to estimate the order of this process.

(3) For the pill dissolution data of Section 9.5:

    (a) Does any dynamic model with different distributional assumptions provide a better fit than the multivariate log normal distribution with autoregression?

    (b) Does the variability depend on the mean?

10
Molecular genetics

With the sequencing of the human genome, molecular biology has received a great deal of publicity. It is seen by some to have the potential to provide solutions to most of the problems of human health. However, the availability of the sequence is only the very beginning of the story. Genes must be located within the sequence, their function in the body must be determined, the mechanisms by which they are differentially expressed in different kinds of cells discovered, these must be related to the progression of a disease, and a cure must be found.

10.1 Sequence analysis

Molecular genetics is concerned with three types of rather large molecules that, fortunately, have a fundamentally linear structure. The central molecule in genetics is deoxyribonucleic acid (DNA) which, although helical, is strictly linear in the structure of its most important components. This molecule, in turn, carries codes for all of the polypeptides (proteins) in the body as well as for certain ribonucleic acids (RNA). Although also basically linear, proteins have a more complex three-dimensional structure because they fold up into very specific forms. Many types of RNA also fold but in somewhat less complex ways than proteins. Here, I shall only consider some very simple problems related to the linear structure of DNA as a small taste of the challenges available.

10.1.1 BASIC DNA STRUCTURE

The double-stranded helical form of DNA is well known. Each strand consists of a linear sequence of the four nucleic acid bases, adenine (A), cytosine (C), guanine (G), and thymine (T). Opposite strands contain complementary pairs: adenine with thymine and cytosine with guanine, so that, at least in certain applications, only one of the strands need be studied. Most DNA occurs in the nucleus of the cells but the mitochondria also contain some (Section 10.3.1).

Triplets of bases, called *codons*, code the 20 different amino acids. In a region of DNA containing a protein-coding gene, consecutive, nonoverlapping triplets of bases, called an open reading frame (ORF), code the corresponding sequences consisting of amino acids that make up a protein. These may be on either strand, being read in the opposite direction on each. Thus, most coding regions are read by messenger RNA (mRNA) and spliced to remove noncoding sections, within the nucleus, before being translated, outside the nucleus, by ribosomes into a protein. The others are read directly to create other types of RNA used in the ribosomes and elsewhere.

Because there are 64 possible combinations of the bases and only 20 amino acids, the code is redundant for producing proteins, particularly in the third base, with several triplets often coding the same amino acid. Special three-base codes also signal the initiation (ATG) and termination (TAG, TGA, TAA) of a coding sequence.

However, most bases in a DNA sequence do not code for the amino acids of proteins. Thus, a promoter and enhancer signal region, containing so-called promoter boxes (for example, TATA, CCAAT), generally occurs somewhat before the first exon in a protein-coding section. Some other regions are genes coding for ribosomal (rRNA) or transfer (tRNA) ribonucleic acids. Hence, only selective parts of the strands are actually active; the rest may have unknown functions.

In addition, the bases coding a given protein are not necessarily all consecutive but may be split into several sections. This is why splicing is necessary. The coding sequences of a gene are called the exons, whereas the noncoding sections in between are called introns. Because the set of exons defines a protein, they are subject to natural selection, whereas one may expect the bases in the introns to be more random, although there are some indications that they may play other roles. A mutation in an exon sequence will often result in a code for a nonviable or inappropriate protein, whereas a mutation in an intron does not have this harmful effect (although it may have others).

10.1.2 SEQUENCING METHODS

The first step in sequencing is to divide a chromosome, one very long piece of DNA, in some ordered way into smaller pieces. DNA molecules are digested by restriction endonuclease, cutting them into small fragments. Each specific endonuclease has a target site of cutting defined by a unique sequence of four to eight base pairs. For example, the enzyme *Not*I recognizes the eight base pair sequence, GCGGCCGC. Because such sequences are not distributed randomly and because the four nucleotide bases do not all appear equally frequently in the genome, the length of the fragments produced depends on the target cutting sequence.

These fragments are separated by size using electrophoresis in agarose. They must, then, be multiplied for mapping and sequencing to be possible. Bacteriophage λ, bacteria containing cosmid recombinants, or yeast artificial chromosomes (YACs) can be used to clone the fragments and generate a library of them. Then, the cloned fragments must be positioned in the same linear order as in the chromosome by detecting overlaps, in this way producing a physical map of the chromosome.

One possibility for ordering the fragments is chromosome walking: a clone is chosen and used as a probe to detect other clones with which it will hybridize; these should overlap with it. This is repeated many times, providing a series of steps. Other techniques such as restriction enzyme fingerprinting, marker sequences, and hybridization assays are also used.

The chain terminator or dideoxy method for DNA sequencing developed by Sanger uses two important properties of these molecules: the ability to synthesize a complementary copy from a single strand of DNA and the possibility of using dideoxynucleotides as chain terminators. DNA is synthesized in the presence of the four deoxynucleoside triphosphate bases, one of which is labelled with ^{32}P. Four batches each contain a low concentration of one of the different dideoxynucleotides. Because of the difference in termination, each batch will contain partially synthesized radioactive DNA molecules of different length.

A high-resolution sequencing gel fractionates denatured (single-strand) DNA fragments according to size by electrophoresis; it is capable of distinguishing fragments differing in length by only one base pair. The labelled DNA bands can be examined manually to determine the sequence after autoradiography on X-ray film. The maximum length of DNA that can be sequenced at one pass is between 300 and 500 bases.

However, for the process to be automated, the radioactive tags are replaced by fluorescent ones attached to the terminators, each dideoxynucleotide carrying a different fluorophore. The four bands can then be detected in the same lane of gel and many lanes electronically analysed simultaneously.

The sequenced fragments can be reassembled either by previously constructing a physical map of the genome or by a shotgun approach of matching overlapping ends of fragments to produce the assembly. The latter is a highly computer-intensive procedure. During this process, the partial sequences created are known as contigs (contiguous sequences). The final result of the assembly is a consensus sequence. Roughly 5000 to 10 000 bases must be analysed to produce a sequence of 1000 bases.

10.1.3 ALIGNMENT

DNA sequences coding similar proteins may be expected to be similar. This will be true of two proteins in the same organism but also of those in two closely related organisms. The latter may differ through evolutionary mutations. On the other hand, the noncoding sequences may differ widely. As we have seen, only certain mutations that change an exon, those that still produce a viable protein, are permissible. Mutations of the introns may often be much more random because they do not affect the production of a protein in this way.

In order to compare such sequences, the DNA must be aligned. Then, one can decide if such an alignment would be likely to have arisen by chance or because the sequences are related. Several factors must be taken into account (Durbin *et al.*, 1998, p. 12):

- what alignments should be allowed;
- how they should be ranked;
- what algorithm should be applied to find an optimal alignment;

- what statistical procedure should be used to evaluate significance of the ranked scores.

Simple procedures only perform pairwise alignment.

Two basic types of mutations can change sequences: substitutions of one base for another and insertions or deletions of bases. Some forms of mutations are observed more frequently than others because natural selection generally removes the nonviable ones. For example, because of the redundancy in the third base of a triplet, more variability can often be observed there.

In the alignment of two sequences, a score is assigned to the pair of bases occurring at each site. For DNA bases, there are 16 possible scores but, by symmetry, not all are different. These form a 4×4 score or substitution matrix. To align sequences optimally, gaps may have to be left in some of the sequences, corresponding to insertions and deletions. A penalty is assigned for opening a gap and another (usually smaller) one for widening it. The total ranked score for an alignment, then, consists of a sum of terms for each aligned pair of bases plus those for the gaps. Additivity implies that mutations at different sites have occurred independently.

Various algorithms are used to obtain optimal alignment among two or more sequences. These dynamic programming techniques are guaranteed to find the optimal pairwise alignment. A number of these programs are publicly available; sequences can also be submitted for alignment over the internet. Global alignment of complete sequences is generally performed by the Needleman–Wunsch algorithm, whereas location alignment of subsequences uses the Smith–Waterman algorithm.

Multiple sequence alignments are more complex. Scoring methods must allow for the evolutionary dependence among the sequences, including the fact that some sites may be more conserved than others. Generally, such a complex phylogenetic model is not possible and simplifying assumptions must be made. Once a set of scores has been chosen, multidimensional dynamic programming must be applied.

After a set of sequences from different species and/or different genes has been aligned, one may be interested in constructing an evolutionary tree in an attempt to determine the phylogenetic structure among the species.

10.2 Finding genes and their exons

Once a section of DNA has been sequenced so that its content is known, one of the first questions to be asked is which sections of it are active in coding a protein? In other words, where are (potential) genes located? Evidence for the location of genes in a sequence must be derived from a variety of indications. A protein-coding sequence may have a number of characteristics:

- It should be preceded by known promoter regions such as a TATA box.
- It should start with an initiation codon and end with a termination codon.

10.2. FINDING GENES AND THEIR EXONS

- It may be sufficiently similar to that for another gene in the genome or to the same gene in another genome to be recognizable.
- It can show codon (triplet) regularity.
- It is unlikely to contain major sections of repeats.

Gene finding is particularly difficult when introns are present.

Many types of software are available on the internet for

- integrated gene identification;
- promoter box recognition;
- database searches to find similar gene sequences;
- repeat analysis.

(See Primrose, 1998, pp. 128–129.) Most have been developed by computer scientists, not by statisticians.

Here, I shall not look at such complex methods but only consider one simple, and unrealistic, approach in order to illustrate the ideas. In developing methods to fulfil this aim of finding genes, it is generally useful to work first with genes having known location, which is what I shall do here.

10.2.1 THE β-GLOBIN GENE

The area of the human genome in which the β-globin gene is located is one of the most intensively studied of all loci. This gene is associated with several inherited diseases in the family of hæmoglobinopathies. These include some of the commonest human genetic disorders such as sickle-cell anæmia and β-thalassæmia. Methods are being developed to perform prenatal diagnosis of these diseases using molecular biology.

Genetic studies of sickle-cell anæmia first demonstrated the one-to-one correspondence between genetic constitution and protein synthesis in the late 1940s. One point mutation changes the codon for glutamic acid (GAG) to that for valine (GTG). This was the first hereditary polymorphism to be identified and the first to be shown to cause a human disease. Since then, hundreds of other mutations of hæmoglobin have been discovered.

β-thalassæmia was one of the first human genetic diseases to be studied using recombinant DNA analysis. At least eight different mutations of the β-globin gene are involved in this family of diseases.

In order to study nucleotide polymorphism, Fullerton *et al.* (1994) performed molecular and population genetic analysis on a sample of 36 unrelated Melanesians, 12 of whom were β-thalassæmia heterozygotes. They used polymerase chain reaction (PCR) with allelic-specific amplification for a section of 3007 bases surrounding the human β-globin locus. The gene itself occupies 1424 bases starting at position 871 of this section. It contains two introns of 130 and 850 bases leaving 444 bases, or 148 coding triplets, for the three exons. Here, I shall use one of these sequences to see if hidden Markov models (Section B.5.2) can locate the gene and its exons.

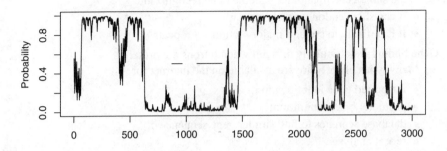

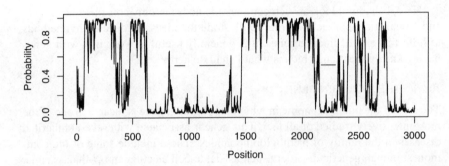

Fig. 10.1. Filtered conditional probabilities of being in state 1 for the complete β-globin sequence. Top graph: simple two-state model; bottom graph: model with two Markov chains. Horizontal bars at height 0.5 indicate the exons of the gene at positions 871–963, 1094–1316, and 2167–2294.

10.2.2 LOCATING THE GENE

I shall first apply hidden Markov models to the complete sequence of 3007 bases to see if any correspondence can be found between the hidden states and the coding sections. Because I am looking for coding and noncoding sections, models with two hidden states will be appropriate. The model for multinomial independence has an AIC of 4091.8, whereas that with two hidden states has 4044.2. The filtered probabilities for the first state are shown in Figure 10.1. We see that the three exons are, with high probability, all completely located in one of the states. The second intron is similar to the sections of the sequence before and after the gene whereas the first intron is indistinguishable from the exons by this method.

The hidden transition matrix is

$$\begin{pmatrix} 0.997 & 0.003 \\ 0.003 & 0.997 \end{pmatrix}$$

with stationary probabilities 0.481 and 0.519. In the first state, the probabilities

10.2. FINDING GENES AND THEIR EXONS

of A, C, G, and T are respectively 0.31, 0.15, 0.14, and 0.40. In the second, they are 0.23, 0.25, 0.26, and 0.27. The second is the state in which the exons occur. Thus, the noncoding regions are CG poor.

Adding a third state reduces the AIC to 4023.8 but does not further aid in distinguishing the gene. One of the states corresponds closely to that shown in Figure 10.1. Allowing the probability of each type of base to cycle through each of the three positions of triplets along the whole sequence with two hidden states does not improve the model; the AIC is 4048.6.

On the other hand, if an ordinary Markov chain is used instead of a hidden one, the AIC is reduced to 3997.0. If the process is allowed to switch between two such Markov chains using a hidden Markov model, the AIC is 3938.6. The hidden transition matrix for this model is

$$\begin{pmatrix} 0.995 & 0.005 \\ 0.004 & 0.996 \end{pmatrix}$$

and the two 'observed' transition matrices are

	A	C	G	T
A	0.338	0.140	0.124	0.399
C	0.365	0.284	0.064	0.288
G	0.141	0.317	0.394	0.148
T	0.193	0.175	0.420	0.212
A	0.240	0.223	0.331	0.206
C	0.288	0.300	0.035	0.377
G	0.254	0.212	0.313	0.222
T	0.164	0.242	0.326	0.268

Notice how rarely G follows C in either state.

10.2.3 LOCATING THE EXONS

Let us now look more closely at the gene itself, ignoring the noncoding regions on each side. The multinomial independence model has an AIC of 1939.3 compared to 1913.2 for the two-state model (obviously, these AICs are not comparable with the previous ones). The filtered probabilities are plotted in the top graph of Figure 10.2. The complete exons still occur in one hidden state. However, we see that the second intron is not so clearly distinguished as when the whole sequence is used. On the other hand, there is some indication of the first intron being similar to the second.

The hidden transition matrix is

$$\begin{pmatrix} 0.976 & 0.024 \\ 0.009 & 0.991 \end{pmatrix}$$

with stationary probabilities 0.265 and 0.735. The probabilities of the four bases in state 2, which contains the exons, are respectively 0.27, 0.20, 0.26, and 0.27,

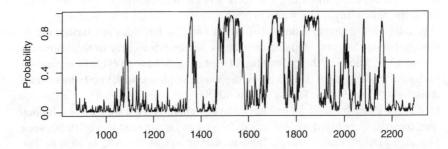

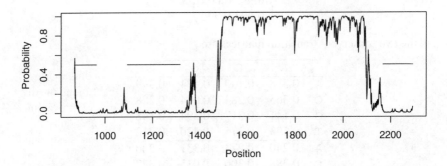

Fig. 10.2. Filtered conditional probabilities of being in state 1 for the gene section of the β-globin sequence. Top graph: simple two-state model; bottom graph: model with dependence on triplet position. Horizontal bars at height 0.5 indicate the exons of the gene at positions 871–963, 1094–1316, and 2167–2294.

whereas they are 0.21, 0.18, 0.06, and 0.54 in state 1. Indeed, 41% of intron 2 consists of T.

If I now allow a different set of probabilities for the four bases at each of the three positions in a triplet, the AIC is reduced to 1912.0. This is rather surprising as only the second exon has a complete set of triplets (these do not correspond to amino acids because the first intron occurs in the middle of a triplet) and neither of the introns does. Thus, as is generally the case, triplets are out of alignment among the three exons.

Nevertheless, the changes of state become much clearer, as can be seen in the lower graph of Figure 10.2. The hidden transition matrix is now

$$\begin{pmatrix} 0.998 & 0.002 \\ 0.001 & 0.999 \end{pmatrix}$$

with stationary probabilities 0.317 and 0.683. The probabilities of the four bases at the three positions of a triplet in the two states are summarized in the following table:

State	Position	A	C	G	T
	1	0.29	0.18	0.10	0.43
1	2	0.31	0.13	0.13	0.43
	3	0.29	0.14	0.11	0.46
	1	0.19	0.21	0.29	0.31
2	2	0.25	0.25	0.27	0.23
	3	0.22	0.23	0.28	0.27

As for the complete sequence, adding a third state improves the model, with an AIC of 1896.9, but does not further help to locate the coding regions.

This example should not be taken as typical of the success with which coding sections of a sequence can be located. It happens that intron 2 of this gene is rather special; this greatly helped in locating the areas of interest.

10.3 Detecting locations of mutations

One important medical application of molecular genetics is to locate regions of the genome having high mutation rates. In certain cases, these may then be linked with hereditary diseases. Here, I shall look at a special part of the human genome, located outside the nucleus.

10.3.1 MITOCHONDRIAL DNA

Mitochondria are bodies in cells that have separate replicating DNA, autonomous from that in the nucleus of the cell. Anderson *et al.* (1981) gave the complete genome sequence for human beings. Human mitochondrial DNA is a 16 569 base-pair, closed, circular molecule. There are no introns, some genes overlap, and almost every base pair belongs to a gene. This DNA encodes 13 proteins for oxidative phosphorylation plus the rRNA and tRNA necessary for its expression.

Since the original sequencing, sections of the mitochondrial genome have been extensively used in studying the genealogical history of human beings. Two reasons for this are that the mitochondrial genome is maternally inherited and that it evolves (that is, mutates) quickly. Here, I shall not attempt a phylogenic analysis but instead study the location of mutations on segments of the genome.

A number of degenerative diseases may be associated with defects in oxidative phosphorylation arising from mitochondrial DNA mutations (Wallace, 1992). Oxidative phosphorylation generates mitochondrial energy for the cell in the form of adenosine triphosphate (ATP). This provides the main source of energy for many organs and tissues including the brain, heart, kidney, liver, and muscles. The process declines with age. Deleterious mutations can occur in both the RNA genes and in the protein-coding genes.

Myoclonic epilepsy and ragged-red fibre disease result from a mutation of the lysine tRNA gene. Leber's hereditary optic neuropathy, a form of central optic nerve death associated with acute bilateral blindness, arises from at least four different mutations of the mitochondrial DNA electron transport gene. Neurogenic muscle weakness, ataxia, and retinitis pigmentosa are associated with seizures, dementia, and development delay, caused by a mutation of the mitochondrial DNA *ATPase* 6 gene. All of these are maternally inherited. Other mitochondrial related diseases included Kearns–Sayre syndrome, chronic external ophthalmoplegia plus, and Pearson's marrow/pancrease syndrome. These are generally spontaneous, probably arising from somatic mutations. Other diseases related to aging, such as Parkinson's, Alzheimer's, and Huntington's, may also be associated with oxidative phosphorylation defects.

Vigilant *et al.* (1991) studied the evolution of two segments of the control region of the mitochondrial genome. This region contains 1122 base pairs that are noncoding DNA. It is believed to be the most rapidly evolving and polymorphic region of the human mitochondrial genome. The segments that they used are respectively of lengths 376 and 387 bases and come from 189 individuals. Of these, 121 are native Africans, 20 from Papua New Guinea, one native Australian, 15 Europeans, 24 Asians, and eight African Americans. In aligning the sequences, a number of gaps had to be introduced.

Of the 376 bases in the first segment, 261 are identical on all subjects; 328 of the 387 bases in the second segment are identical. This does not imply that the rest are all important mutation sites; some correspond to deletions (gaps) and others may only occur very rarely.

When a site is polymorphic, usually only two bases are observed in a sample of sequences. One base may have a low frequency and the other a high one or both may have intermediate frequencies. For the mitochondrial genome, the former case is most often found.

10.3.2 MODELLING MUTATION RATES

Let us look first at the relative frequency of mutation at the various sites. At each position, I shall take the most common base there to be the nonmutated standard and regroup the other three together without distinguishing which mutation has occurred. I shall ignore the gaps rather than include them in the latter as they are not point (single-base) mutations but arise by other mechanisms. Then, it is possible to plot the estimated probability of mutation at each site, as shown in the top panel of Figure 10.3 for the two segments.

The estimated mean probability of a mutation over all sites on the two sequences is 0.0123; it is 0.0152 for the first segment and 0.0095 for the second. The AIC for a model with constant probability of mutation at all sites on the two segments is 4348.6 as compared to 4304.0 for a different constant probability on each segment.

Let us now allow the probability of a mutation to vary along the sequence according to the two unknown states of a hidden Markov model. With a common model for both segments, the AIC is 1500.9 whereas it is 1478.8 if distinct parameters are allowed for each segment. The hidden transition matrices for the two segments are respectively estimated to be

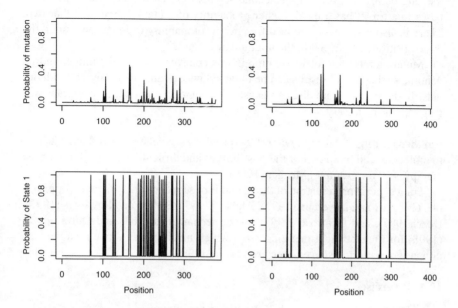

Fig. 10.3. Relative frequencies of mutation (first row) and filtered conditional probabilities of being in the first state (second row) for two segments of the control region of the mitochondrial genome of 189 human beings.

$$\begin{pmatrix} 0.11 & 0.89 \\ 0.09 & 0.91 \end{pmatrix} \text{ and } \begin{pmatrix} 0.21 & 0.79 \\ 0.05 & 0.95 \end{pmatrix}$$

with estimated marginal stationary distributions $(0.09, 0.91)$ and $(0.06, 0.94)$. Although there is a higher estimated probability of being in the first state in the first segment, the probability of staying in it at two consecutive sites is twice as high in the second segment as the first.

State 1 is clearly that where mutations tend to occur. Indeed, in this state, the estimated probability of mutation is 0.136 for the first segment and 0.132 for the second segment, whereas the probabilities of mutation are respectively 0.0027 and 0.00099 in the second state.

The filtered probabilities of being in state 1 at each site of each segment are plotted in the lower panel of Figure 10.3. State 1 points to relative frequencies of mutations being higher than about 0.05 at a site.

These segments contain noncoding DNA so that a triplet structure should not be relevant. It is then interesting to note that the model is improved by allowing the probability of mutation in each state to vary at three consecutive positions. This could have arisen if this region formerly was a gene, but no longer codes because of some mutation. The AIC is reduced to 1456.1. In the first segment, the probabilities of a mutation in state 1 form a cycle of 0.19, 0.13, 0.13, whereas they are 0.25, 0.12, 0.10 in the second segment. In each case, one of the three bases in a triplet has a much higher probability of mutation than the other two. There is also some evidence of difference in probability of mutation among the three positions of a triplet in the nonmutating state 2.

Mutation rates are relatively high in this control region of the mitochondrial genome so that useful results can be obtained with a sample of only 189 individuals. In the study of rare diseases caused by mutations, much larger samples will generally be necessary.

Further reading   Alberts *et al.* (1994) provide an excellent general introduction to molecular cell biology. For the possibilities and difficulties in developing gene therapy, see, for example, Meager (1999).

For a general presentation of the methods of sequence analysis, see, for example, Gribskov and Devereux (1992), Alphey (1997), Bishop and Rawlings (1997), Dear (1997), and Primrose (1998) for the technical methods and Durbin *et al.* (1998) for the statistical methods, from which much of the above material was drawn. For pattern discovery, see Wang *et al.* (1999).

10.4   Exercises

(1) DNA sequences are freely available on the internet.
   (1) Obtain the collection of globin genes for several primates and check if the results obtained in Section 10.2.1 can be reproduced for them.
   (2) What happens with more distantly related animals?
(2) Obtain a collection of sequences of some (nuclear) gene from a number of different individuals.
   (1) If they are not aligned, align them, either over the internet or by obtaining the appropriate software and doing it yourself.
   (2) Perform an analysis of the mutations.
(3) Hidden Markov models have been used to attempt to find CG-rich segments of DNA. Obtain a long sequence of DNA and see if you can detect such regions.

Appendices

Appendices

Appendix A
Data and model examples from R

A.1 Data

Following upon the typology of variables given in Section 2.1, we can ask a number of questions:
- How should we read in such data?
- How should we store them?
- What should we do with missing values?

I shall now describe one solution to some of these problems, mentioning the functions in my R libraries that permit this to be done.

A.1.1 DATA OBJECTS

Recording and reading Each type of variable (Section 2.1) will generally be recorded in a separate file (usually, a maximum of three files, although more may be necessary if several time-varying covariates are measured, each at different times). Such data can create problems as much of the most widely used recording technology (spreadsheets) conforms to the rectangular format. Foolproof ways of making the links among values in the different files must be available, as in database technology.

In simple cases, the data can first be read into the statistical software in rectangular form (for example, the dataframe in R). If the data exist in the classical form, perhaps with inter-unit (time-constant) covariates unnecessarily repeated, they can be transformed directly to the appropriate data objects, described below, using dftorep if the data are in a dataframe or read.rep if they are in one file.

If the data are not in such balanced rectangular form, they will generally have to be read as a list (read.list or read.surv, respectively, for the two examples given in Section 2.1.1) with one element (vector or matrix) in the list per individual. In either case, they will then have to be converted into the data objects to be described next.

Storage In an object-oriented language such as R, data are stored in *objects*. In such a language, the standard data object is the rectangular dataframe. From the arguments and examples in Section 2.1, this is not always appropriate for modern data handling.

The one major innovation of the dataframe structure was the ability to store quantitative and qualitative (factor) variables together without transforming the latter into indicator (dummy) variables. However, this is accompanied by subsequent important inefficiencies as the factor variables do have to be transformed into the appropriate set of indicator variables before a model can be fitted. This contrasts with statistical software such as GLIM where such a matrix containing indicator variables is never actually constructed in the model-fitting process. However, such an approach would generally not be possible for nonlinear models in any case.

Objects contain *slots* in which various items of different types can be stored and have *methods* by which they can be accessed without the user knowing the internal structure. The objects have *classes* so that the language can recognize which methods are appropriate for which objects. They can *inherit* characteristics, including methods, from other similar objects.

Here, in the implementation in R, the objects will simply be constructed internally as lists (as is a dataframe), permitting storage of varying types of information. The methods to access them will be functions specific to the object.

However, lists cannot easily and simply be directly transferred to and efficiently accessed in a lower level language such as C or Fortran where the more complex model construction will often need to be done. Hence, for modelling efficiency, data for all individuals, in an object's slots, will be stored together as vectors or matrices so that these can be directly accessed in the lower level language. This also allows their efficient manipulation by vector and matrix operations in R itself.

Another major inefficiency of Lisp-like languages such as R is that copies of objects are generally made when they are passed between functions. In contrast to Fortran or C, objects cannot be accessed through pointers. In R, this problem can be minimized by using R's scoping rules and function closure; see Ihaka and Gentleman (1996) and Gentleman and Ihaka (2000). (However, this implies that many of the specific procedures developed here for R will not work in S-Plus.)

In the R implementation, three classes of objects are available; they correspond to the types of variables and are called response, tccov for inter-subject/time-constant covariates, and tvcov for intra-subject/time-varying covariates.

Response variables The response class contains all of the relevant available information, discussed in Section 2.1.1, as a set of vectors or matrices; for a given problem, irrelevant slots are NULL. The set of one or more response variables, along with any transformations, is stored in one slot as a matrix.

If there is nesting, the first level defines the unit of observation, called the *individual*. This is especially important in repeated measurements; a vector in a separate slot indicates the number of observations per individual and allows the appropriate observations for each individual to be located. For independent observations, there is one observation per individual.

The unit of measurement and Jacobian are combined in one slot: the unit of measurement is the precision of the instrument used (when different from unity) for that response variable, whereas the Jacobian of its transformation is a set of numerical values. For example, if a transformation, say $\log(y)$, of a response variable is stored in its slot, then its Jacobian is stored as $1/y$ (times the original unit of measurement). An optional slot contains a character vector with the name of the units of each response (metres, hours, ...).

Finally, a slot contains a character vector with the type of each variable: nominal, ordinal, discrete, duration, continuous, or unknown. Unless specified otherwise:

- if a response is not censored and has a unit of measurement/Jacobian, it is assumed to be continuous;
- if it is censored, it is assumed to be a duration;
- if it has a binomial denominator, it is assumed to be nominal.

This information is used to check, as far as possible, if the user is attempting to fit an appropriate model to the data.

Covariates Consider now the tccov and tvcov classes for covariates. These are generally stored as a matrix. However, if factor variables are present among either the intra-unit or inter-unit covariates, the user may choose to store them in the corresponding slot in the object as a dataframe instead of as an ordinary matrix.

In a dataframe, the factor variables remain as such whereas, in a matrix, they are transformed to the appropriate indicator variables. Model-fitting functions need to know how to handle this. If the dataframe approach is chosen, it can lead to serious inefficiencies as a copy of all of the data (not just the indicators for the factor variables) must be made when the indicator variables are constructed in setting up a model. In contrast, when the covariates are stored as a matrix, with the indicator variables already calculated for the factor variables, they can be directly read in the object without making a copy. However, each indicator variable now carries a separate name. Thus, the user must make a choice where the tradeoff is between ease of referencing variables by name (indicator variables must all be specified separately by name) and speed of model fitting.

When the observation times for the response(s) and a time-varying covariate differ, one possible procedure is to bring forward the most recent value of the latter to the response time using the function gettvc. However, care must be taken with ties in the times when the response(s) and the covariate are recorded. If the covariate and the response(s) are measured at the same time, one must decide if the effect begins instantaneously (Section 2.1.2).

The special covariates, times and nesting indicators contained in the response object, can be accessed in model formulæ by keywords: times, individuals (for the first level of nesting), and `nesting` (for clusters within individuals, for example in certain cross-over trials). The latter two are automatically used as factor variables.

In a similar way, if longitudinal multivariate responses are present or graphical models are being fitted, conditioning of one response on other may be required. This can be done using their names, as with intra-subject/time-varying covariates.

Repeated objects Finally, all of the information from a set of one to three objects of classes `response`, `tccov`, and `tvcov` must be combined to produce an object of the new class called `repeated` (using `rmna` or `lvna`), created directly from a dataframe (using `dftorep`), or read directly from a file containing a rectangular table (using `read.rep`). In this way, a given combination of variables in a model is combined, with observations having missing values (NAs) in any variables either removed or simply indicated and left for the model-fitting algorithm to handle. This object provides all of the information that will be required to fit some set of models of interest that will be directly comparable because they are based on the same set of data (for example, with the same missing values removed).

The handling of missing values is a particularly thorny issue. The missing value process will rarely be independent of the process of interest. The only appropriate procedure would seem to be to have a separate slot containing information as to why each particular value is missing so that a model for missingness could be constructed. This would be required in all three classes of objects. Such a structure has not yet been implemented, but such information could, at present, in many cases, simply be stored as extra covariates.

A.1.2 DATA METHODS

Some of the functions and methods required for this approach have already been discussed above. It is now time to look at the required methods in some more detail.

The first basic set of procedures must be able to transform the matrices and/or lists read into the software to create the required objects just described. In simple cases, with all variables in one file, they can be read directly into a `repeated` object using `read.rep`. If they are in a dataframe, they can be transformed to a `repeated` object using `dftorep`. In each case, the class of object to which each variable will belong must be given.

More specialized methods are `restovec` to create `response` objects, `tcctomat` to create inter-subject/time-constant `tccov` objects, and `tvctomat` for intra-subject/time-varying `tvcov` objects. These functions can generally automatically transform vectors, matrices, or lists of data to the appropriate object. For example, if a list of matrices (one for each individual, containing responses as the first column and possibly times as the second column) is supplied to `restovec`, it can automatically detect which other columns contain binomial denominators, censoring, nesting, and/or units of measurement.

Various validity checks are performed, such as ensuring that weights and binomial denominators are not negative, that there are no negative time steps, and so on. Because of the structure of the data objects, model-fitting functions can perform many further checks that are impossible with traditional rectangular data objects.

Once the objects have been created, methods are available to print summary information for each class, not the whole data array, and to plot responses and time-varying covariates. The latter allows

- choice of subsets;
- individual points or profiles;
- if nesting, times starting over at zero in each cluster (for example, in a cross-over design).

Particular types of information can be extracted from the slots in these data objects, either for all individuals or for a specified subset, using the methods response, resptype, units, delta (unit of measurement and/or Jacobian), weights, times, nesting, covariates, and names. A data object can also be coerced to a standard dataframe (as.data.frame), extending inter-subject/time-constant covariates so as to have one value per observation. This is automatically used in standard R modelling functions such as glm.

Methods must also be available to create specific forms of information for a given model.

- As described above, time-varying covariates may need to be carried forward to response times (gettvc).
- The user may want to transform the response, the times, or certain covariates (transform). If a response is transformed, the Jacobian is also automatically updated.
- If the model-fitting procedure does not perform the task itself in constructing the likelihood, inter-unit/time-constant covariates must be matched to individual responses (covind).
- Interactions among intra-subject/time-varying covariates or with inter-unit/time-constant covariates may be required (tvctomat) although generally it is preferable to specify them directly in a model formula.

As discussed above, missing values can only be handled after all information has been joined for a given model. Methods must be available so that, when applicable, this can be coordinated for each given combination of variables (rmna or lvna).

The only general method currently available for handling missing values is the elimination of these recordings (rmna), with the accompanying (generally incorrect) assumption of randomness. The alternative is to leave them for the specific model function to handle (lvna) with an indicator of their position. These methods can only be performed for a given combination of all three types of variables, as otherwise the individual values could no longer be matched up. In the first case, this has the consequence that the number of recorded observations can change with the covariates present in the model and that entire individuals can disappear when the model is changed, for example if an inter-individual covariate value is missing and this covariate is added to the model. However, it would be technically, if not conceptually, easy to develop other general methods for handling missing values to be used in place of the rmna and lvna methods.

A.2 Models

Nonlinear modelling creates special problems in the interaction between human beings and the computer. It is now time to look at these in more detail.

A.2.1 SOFTWARE

In the mid 1970s, statistics was at the forefront of computations using electronic computers with the introduction of the GLIM interactive system for generalized linear models. Later, S (Becker and Chambers, 1984) extended the same basic paradigm to a wider class of statistical operations, the major innovation for modelling being to allow the user to extend the language, something that was rather difficult with GLIM macros. This lead was, however, rather quickly lost as more powerful packages were developed in other areas, such as Matlab for linear algebra and Maple and Mathematica for symbolic algebraic manipulation. For example, the latter packages contain powerful facilities for distinguishing among known and unknown variables, for translating functions directly into C or Fortran, and for exporting formulæ into TEX. These, and other, useful possibilities that would be invaluable aids for statistical modelling have not been made available in standard packages designed specifically for statisticians.

The pioneering software, GLIM, of the 1970s clearly separated specification of the distribution ($yvariate and $error) from the linear structure in the model ($fit) using the Wilkinson and Rogers (1973) notation. Between these is the link function ($link). S (Chambers and Hastie, 1992) obscured this clarity in model construction by combining the first and third GLIM instructions as, in a simple case, y~x1+x2. This structure appears to imply that Y is distributed with mean depending linearly on x_1 and x_2. However, this can only be true when the link function is the identity and hence is generally misleading. Both the GLIM and the S approaches have the additional defect of maintaining the user in a mentality whereby only the mean parameter can possibly depend on covariates.

A.2.2 PROBABILITY DISTRIBUTION

Reasonable selections of density ('d') and cumulative distribution ('p') functions are available in statistical languages such as R. The latter are needed for censored data (Sections 7.1.3 and B.6.1). Additional sets of such functions are available in my rmutil library. All of these functions can easily be combined to build up an appropriate probability model for a given data set (for an example, see Section

A.3.2). The modelling functions in my libraries perform this, providing an interface to many nonlinear models. A choice of well over 30 different distributions is available. Once this is done, the ways in which parameters of the probability distribution change with covariates must be specified by means of regression functions.

A.2.3 COVARIATE DEPENDENCE

Nonlinear function construction In a language such as R, one natural way to specify complex regression functions, not handled by the Wilkinson and Rogers (1973) notation, is to use the built-in function construction abilities of these languages. Let us first look at this approach.

As an example, let us consider an open, first-order, one-compartment model (Section 3.2.1), widely used in pharmacokinetics (Chapter 7). The location parameter over time is assumed to vary as

$$\mu_t = \frac{dk_a}{V(k_a - k_e)} \left(e^{-k_e t} - e^{-k_a t} \right)$$

where time t and dose d are observed and the volume V, the absorption rate k_a, and the elimination rate k_e are unknown parameters. In R, this can be specified as a function of the parameter vector:

```
mu <- function(p){
    dose*p[2]/(p[1]*(p[2]-p[3]))*
    (exp(-p[3]*times)-exp(-p[2]*times))}
```

Note that this is not the best way to set up this equation because there are no constraints to guarantee that the three parameters are positive.

This function does not have, as argument, the times or dose, so that they are not copied when the function is evaluated, but must be found somewhere in the environment, preferably in a specified data object (Section A.1.1). This is how standard R functions such as glm also operate.

In addition, the dispersion parameter depends on time through the location parameter, often assumed to be

$$\sigma^2 = \mu_t^\delta$$

(Section 7.1.3). The corresponding function for the log dispersion, to ensure that the parameter is positive, might be

```
logdisp <- function(p, mu) p[1]*log(mu)
```

Another possibility is that the regression functions for two parameters of the probability distribution may have parameters in common without one being a strict function of the other, as here.

The parameters in such a regression function, k_a, k_e, V, may also depend, in various ways, on other covariates. I next consider this.

Linear (in parameters) part Nonlinear regression functions may often have a linear part (Section 1.3.2). As already mentioned, such a linear part is generally specified by the Wilkinson and Rogers (1973) notation for formulæ. The extensions described here retain this as a subset. On the other hand, link functions are only useful for a (transformed) parameter depending on covariates through a strictly linear model, as shown in Equation (1.2).

To pursue my example, if the dependence of a parameter, say k_a, on the covariates contains a strictly linear part, this might be specified as

```
mu <- function(p, linear){
    ka <- exp(linear)
    dose*ka/(p[1]*(ka-p[2]))*
        (exp(-p[2]*t)-exp(-ka*t))}
```

Here, the absorption parameter depends on the covariates through a linear (in the parameters) part, after application of a log 'link' to ensure that its value is always positive.

Then, a call to some model-fitting function might have the following general form:

```
modelfn(..., mu=mu, linear=~height+gfr,
    dispersion=logdisp, ...)
```

Here, the expression following the tilde is in standard Wilkinson and Rogers (1973) notation and may refer to factor variables. It never contains anything before the tilde and, hence, can be used to specify how *any* parameter of a probability distribution depends on covariates.

The function fnenvir can modify an R function such as the above so that it can read covariates from the data objects described in Section A.1.1. This is called by my model-fitting functions and normally will not be needed by the general user.

A.2.4 GENERAL NONLINEAR SPECIFICATION

The above approach to specifying nonlinear models, through R functions, is powerful and useful, but is certainly not always as intuitively clear and user friendly as it might be.

Let us now consider the requirements to be able to use formulæ instead of functions to specify nonlinear regression functions. In a linear regression function, the positions of the parameter coefficients in the formula do not need to appear explicitly. They can be implicitly assumed, as in the Wilkinson and Rogers (1973) notation. This is no longer possible in any extension to nonlinear regression functions.

For nonlinear user specification to be possible, the software must be able to distinguish between variables and parameters (existing vectors and unknowns) in formulæ (as Maple and Mathematica do). Both variables and parameters can retain their individual names. Thus, for the above example, the user should be able to specify, as an argument to a model-fitting function,

```
mu = ~dose*absorption/
    (volume*(absorption-elimination))*
    (exp(-elimination*times)-exp(-absorption*times))
```
and the model-fitting function should detect automatically which are known covariates (preferably stored in the data objects described above) and which are unknown parameters.

Here, the tilde begins the formula to indicate that it is a formula; again, it is not preceded by the name of the response variable. Thus, it does not have the restrictive S-Plus signification that the response is 'distributed as' the model in the formula. Again, such formulæ can be used to describe how any parameter in a probability distribution depends on covariates.

If the regression function contains a linear part, we can specify it in two steps, using the keyword, `linear`:
```
mu = ~{
    tmp <- exp(linear)
    dose*tmp/(volume*(tmp-elimination))*
    (exp(-elimination*times)-exp(-tmp*times))}
linear = ~height+gfr
```
A more elaborate approach would be required if more than one linear part were present.

Various criteria are required for handling such expressions containing unknowns:

- Existing covariate vectors, located in the place specified by the user, must be detected and only these, so that the data that the user wants are actually used in fitting the models and not some other variables with the same name located elsewhere in memory.
- Conflicts of unknown parameter names with existing (nonvariable) object names, such as functions, must be ignored.
- The formula must be transformed into a function of *one* vector of unknown parameters, if required.
- The resulting function must be substituted into a probability distribution function to construct a likelihood *function* that can be rapidly evaluated by a nonlinear optimizer.
- It must be evaluated, either in the appropriate environment or with respect to the data object(s) supplied to the model-fitting function, if possible without copying the data.

All of the above criteria have been fulfilled in my R implementation: the function `finterp` constructs the appropriate R function from such a model formulation with known covariates and unknown parameters, using function closure to retain the environment in which it was defined. As for Wilkinson and Rogers (1973) formulæ, which `finterp` also recognizes and can also transform into R functions, the formulæ begin with a tilde so that they have class `formula` and are `language` objects.

Note that such a formulation may be inefficient in complex situations, as with the linear part for the dependence of the absorption parameter on covariates above. Here, this would have to be given twice whereas it was only given once above in the R function. Matters quickly become worse in still more complex cases so that the direct use of R functions is then still necessary.

As with fnenvir, the function finterp is called by my model-fitting functions and generally will not be needed by the general user.

A.3 Likelihoods

Once a model has been specified, the construction of the (log) likelihood is usually relatively simple.

A.3.1 A SIMPLE EXAMPLE

The basic ideas of constructing a likelihood function and its nonlinear optimization can easily be illustrated using the formula interpreter described above. Note, however, that this interpreter is not really designed for such an application and that the use of 'd' and 'p' functions is usually preferable.

Thus, although its primary use is to define regression functions, the formulation of nonlinear models described in Section A.2.4 can also be used to construct a complete likelihood function, as the following example for Poisson nonlinear regression shows. Instead of using the built-in density function (dpois), I build the likelihood from scratch.

```
# the regression function
regfn <- finterp(~a+exp(b0+b1*x1+b2*x2))
# the terms of the negative log likelihood function
# .vector=F is specified so that the names are
#    parameters are retained
poisfn <-
      finterp(~-y*theta+exp(theta)+lgamma(y+1),
         .vector=F)
# the null negative log likelihood
poislikefn <- function(p) sum(poisfn(theta=p))
# the regression negative log likelihood
poisreglikefn <-
      function(p) sum(poisfn(theta=regfn(p)))
```

where y is the name of the response variable, and x1 and x2 are covariates.

The latter two assignments yield R functions that can be fed directly into the nonlinear optimizer (nlm). Here, the variables, y, x1, and x2, are searched for in the global environment and theta, a, b0, b1, and b2 are recognized to be unknown parameters (if they do not exist in the specified environment), the latter four being collected together to form one vector argument to the function regfn. If the appropriate data object were instead specified as the environment in an additional argument to finterp, the variables would be sought in that object (and only there).

The preferable approach is, however,
```
# the regression function
regfn <- finterp(~a+exp(b0+b1*x1+b2*x2))
# the null likelihood
poislikefn <- function(p)
    -sum(dpois(y, lambda=p, log=T))
# the regression likelihood
poisreglikefn <-
    function(p) -sum(dpois(y, lambda=regfn(p),
        log=T))
```
Again, these latter two functions can be fed directly into the nonlinear optimizer.

A.3.2 MORE COMPLEX CASES

Suppose that we wish to set up the likelihood for a random effects model that allows one arbitrarily chosen parameter of a nonlinear regression function to have an arbitrary mixing distribution. The user supplies the nonlinear location formula, mu, containing a parameter, here called random, which will have the chosen mixing distribution, here Cauchy. The dispersion formula, disp, must also be given. The response variable, y, has a Weibull distribution and id is the factor variable distinguishing among individuals.

```
# number of initial parameter estimates supplied
np <- length(pinit)
# transform the formulae to functions
# the resulting location function has, as second
#     argument, the random parameter
mu1 <- finterp(mu, .args="random")
disp1 <- finterp(disp)
# the response distribution, here Weibull
respdist <- function(p, r)
    dweibull(y, disp1(p), mu1(p, r))
# the mixing distribution centred on zero,
#     here Cauchy
mixing <- function(p, r) dcauchy(r, 0, p[np])
#     both with the random parameter
#     as second argument
# the negative log likelihood function, where the
#     function int performs numerical integration
likefn <- function(p){
    fn <- function(r)
        mixing(p, r)*
            tapply(respdist(p, r[id]), id, prod)
    -sum(log(int(fn)))}
```
This function can be fed to the nonlinear optimizer. Immediate generalizations

will include allowing a choice of distributions using a `switch` statement and an arbitrary name for the random parameter.

Naturally, this skeleton function requires elaborate development to provide a suitable user interface. It is the basis of my `gnlmix` function.

Appendix B
Stochastic dependence structures

In medical studies where nonlinear models are required, several observations will generally be made on each of several subjects. The set of observations on a given individual will not be independent and this dependence must be taken into account in any models constructed.

Three basic types of dependence may be distinguished in medical studies:

(1) Each subject may have unmeasured inherent characteristics that make him or her more or less susceptible to the phenomenon under study, often called a frailty. This will make observations on the same subject more similar than those on different subjects (Section B.1).
(2) Subjects may have unmeasured characteristics that are varying more or less slowly over time, making observations closer in time on a given individual more similar than those further apart (Section B.2).
(3) An individual may be subject to abrupt changes of state that last some length of time, called spells (Section B.5.2).

I shall briefly look at how to model these various types of dependence here. For more details, see Lindsey (1999a).

B.1 Random effects

Responses on the same subject can often be expected to be more closely related than those across subjects. Indeed, we generally assume the latter to be independent, whereas the former are not. We say that responses are nested within subjects. There may be more than one level of nesting, as in multicentre clinical trials and cross-over designs.

B.1.1 MIXTURE MODELS

A location regression function is used to describe how characteristics of a population vary *systematically*, in observable ways, in subsets of the population, as conditions change (Section 1.1.4). If adequate covariates, distinguishing among subjects, are available, the responses on the same subject will be independent, conditional on these covariates. However, all such conditions may not be observable and, indeed, may not be relevant for a given problem at hand. Thus, a location parameter itself might be thought to have some random distribution across some population, independent of the distribution of the responses. The resulting construction is called a *mixture distribution*.

The distribution of responses on the same subject will have some location parameter that takes values conditional on any subject-specific covariates; this parameter may change in some nonlinear way with them if they are time-varying. On the other hand, the value of this location parameter, or of some parameters in the nonlinear regression function, may vary randomly across subjects. The distribution of the parameter(s) may help to account for the random variability or heterogeneity among subjects that is not relevant to the study at hand and for which, in any case, no covariates are available. In survival studies, the unobserved variable is known as the subject's *frailty*.

Random variation may be introduced in at least two ways:

(1) The location parameter in the probability distribution may be given some distribution. Then, once the resulting mixture distribution is obtained, the location regression function, describing systematic changes, may be introduced into it. This can be called a *population-averaged* model (Zeger et al., 1988), because covariates describing differences among the responses specific to a subject cannot be introduced.

(2) The location model may first be included in the probability distribution, including covariates describing differences among the responses of a subject, and, then, some parameter in it given a distribution. This can be called a *subject-specific* model.

In either case, we construct a joint distribution of the responses and the random parameter.

The (marginal) distribution of the responses, the mixture distribution, is obtained by integration. If $f(y_{ijk}|\lambda_{ij})$ is the probability (density for continuous distributions) of the responses, given the random parameter, λ_{ij}, and $p_j(\lambda_{ij})$ is the *mixing distribution* of that parameter (I shall use $p(\cdot)$ for the probability of an unobservable quantity), then

$$\Pr(y_{ij1},\ldots,y_{ijR}) = \int \prod_{k=1}^{R} f(y_{ijk}|\lambda_{ij}) p_j(\lambda_{ij}) \mathrm{d}\lambda_{ij} \qquad (\text{B.1})$$

where i is the subject, j indexes conditions across subjects, and k those within subjects. Because the 'location parameter', λ_{ij}, having the random distribution, disappears with the integration, it is, in fact, a purely imaginary construct. Thus, we obtain a joint multivariate distribution of all responses having fixed location parameter, those on the same subject. However, except in special cases, this distribution cannot be written in closed form, so that numerical integration must be used.

The next question is the choice of the mixing distribution for the parameter. Hopefully, this might be selected on theoretical grounds, in the context of a specific scientific study. Often, this is not possible. When the location parameter can take on only a restricted range of values, this is another factor that must be taken into account.

B.1.2 CONJUGATE DISTRIBUTIONS

Let us, first, look at cases where we can obtain a closed form for the multivariate distribution. A mixing distribution that yields such a result is said to be *conjugate*. For members of the exponential (dispersion) family, it can be written down in general (see Diaconis and Ylvisaker, 1979; Morris, 1983).

In this family, giving a distribution to the mean, when it is constant for all observations on a subject (a population-averaged model), is equivalent to giving the distribution to the canonical parameter. Recall, from Equation (1.4), that members of this family have the form

$$f(y;\phi|\lambda) = \exp\left\{\frac{yg(\lambda) - b[g(\lambda)]}{a(\phi)} + c(y,\phi)\right\}$$

where $g(\cdot)$ is the canonical link function and λ is now the random mean parameter. Then, the conjugate distribution will have the form

$$p(\lambda;\kappa,v) = \exp\left\{\kappa g(\lambda) - \frac{b[g(\lambda)]}{v} + d(\kappa,v)\right\} \quad (B.2)$$

where $d(\cdot,\cdot)$ is a term not involving λ. The resulting closed-form marginal distribution, for one response, is

$$f(y;\kappa,v,\phi) = \exp\left\{d(\kappa,v) + c(y,\phi) - d\left[\kappa + \frac{y}{a(\phi)}, \frac{va(\phi)}{v+a(\phi)}\right]\right\} \quad (B.3)$$

The expected value of λ can be found from the conjugate distribution, as a function of κ and v. Then, a function of this, most often the same link function as would be used for the original exponential family distribution, can be used to set up a location regression function in the usual way.

B.1.3 OTHER MIXTURES

If we construct a location regression function for the responses and then give a distribution to one of its parameters, we can incorporate changing conditions for the responses on a subject within the location model.

We can add some parameter to the location regression function that indexes the subjects explicitly. In a very simple case, this might be

$$\mu_i = \lambda_i + h(\mathbf{x}_i, \boldsymbol{\beta}) \quad (B.4)$$

In more complex models, one or more nonlinear parameters in $\boldsymbol{\beta}$ may be random. Some of the variables in the vector $\mathbf{x}_i$ may describe changing conditions for the subject, whereas others refer to conditions common to groups of subjects.

Suppose that this parameter, λ_i, is constant for a subject, but varies randomly across subjects. The location is not assumed to remain constant for all responses on a subject; for example, in Equation (B.4), the height of the nonlinear response curve, $h(\cdot)$, varies randomly among subjects. When we integrate to obtain the marginal distribution of the responses, we again obtain a multivariate distribution. However, there is generally no simple closed form, no matter what distribution is chosen for the random parameter, so that estimation must rely on numerical methods.

Because the random parameter can usually take any value on the real line, the mixing distribution has often been assumed to be normal. However, numerical integration must be performed, so that there is frequently no good reason for this.

In the common models using mixture distributions, as just described, the responses on a subject are often all equally interdependent, although this will not generally be the case if a nonlinear parameter is made random. However, an important characteristic of random effects models is that they are *static*: differences among individuals remain constant over time. In other words, they may be thought to allow for missing inter-subject/time-constant covariates that describe inherent constant characteristics of each individual. Modelling such stochastic dependence will often be necessary because of the heterogeneity of subjects, at least when adequate individual (time-constant) covariates are unavailable.

B.2 Time dependence

If the observations arise from a longitudinal study, we can expect that responses on a subject closer together in time may be more similar, more closely related. The model must be *dynamic*, varying over time. An adequate model without such dependence will require the availability of appropriate individual time-varying covariates. Thus, the static stochastic dependence of random effects is usually not the only type that may be present unless there is no ordering of the responses.

B.2.1 ORDERED DEPENDENCE

Our models assume that some specific stochastic mechanism is producing the responses. If adequate time-varying covariates are available, the present response, conditional on them, will be independent of previous responses. If not, the response at a given time point will be related to those already produced: the probability of a given response will be conditional, in some way, on the values generated previously. Present events will depend on the previous history, in contrast to random effects models that account for unobserved immutable characteristics of a subject.

For time dependence, we can set up a hierarchical series of conditional distributions:

$$\Pr(y_t | y_1, \ldots, y_{t-1}) = \frac{\Pr(y_1, \ldots, y_t)}{\Pr(y_1, \ldots, y_{t-1})} \tag{B.5}$$

By means of univariate conditional probabilities, a multivariate distribution of the responses on a subject can be constructed.

To proceed, we may choose a given form either for the conditional distribution, on the left-hand side of Equation (B.5), or for the multivariate distributions, on the right-hand side. In general, the conditional distribution will be different from the multivariate and marginal distributions, because the ratio of two multivariate distributions does not yield a conditional distribution of the same form except in very special circumstances such as the normal distribution. The one or the other will most often be intractable.

The hierarchical relationship among the ordered responses on a subject implies, by recursion, that the conditional probabilities are independent:

$$\Pr(y_1,\ldots,y_t) = \Pr(y_1)\Pr(y_2|y_1)\cdots\Pr(y_t|y_1,\ldots,y_{t-1}) \tag{B.6}$$

so that the likelihood is composed of a product of terms, and univariate analysis may be used. Thus, multivariate distributions with known conditional form are much easier to fit than those with known marginal form. Because few useful non-normal multivariate distributions are available (see, however, Section B.3), suitable models can often only be obtained by direct construction of the conditional distribution.

The formulation of Equation (B.6) highlights some potential problems. Each response depends on a different number of previous responses; this may or may not be medically reasonable. As well, the unconditional distribution of the first response is required. The choice here will depend upon the initial conditions for the process.

If the dependence does not extend very far in time, the random variables Y_t and Y_{t-k} may be assumed (conditionally) independent for $k > M$. This is the property of a *Markov process* of order M.

In constructing general time-dependence models, we may wish to imitate normal theory autoregression. But there, both the marginal and conditional distributions are normal, the AR(1) autoregression coefficient is also an autocorrelation, defining the autocovariances, and successive responses are linearly related. Not all of these characteristics can be simultaneously preserved in generalizations. Thus, perhaps the simplest possibility is to use the earlier responses as covariates, as the name 'autoregression' implies. But, even this is not unique and it is not the only generalization, as we shall now see.

B.2.2 AUTOREGRESSION

A model for the location parameter can incorporate previously generated values of the response, in addition to the other covariates. Thus, in a simple case, it could be

$$\mu_i(t) = \rho_i y_{i,t-1} + h(\boldsymbol{\beta}_i, \mathbf{z}_{it}) \tag{B.7}$$

where z_{it} are time-varying covariates in a nonlinear regression function. This model, with the response entered with M lags, is one way to define an *autoregression process* of order 1, or AR(1). The extension to order M, or an AR(M), is direct, and will not be discussed in what follows. Note that the dependence parameter, ρ_i, may vary among individuals.

State dependence What I have just done is to relate the location parameter directly to the previously observed response values. For the normal distribution, the link function is usually the identity; in some other cases, it might make more sense to transform the responses in the same way as the location parameter:

$$g_i[\mu_i(t)] = \rho_i g_i(y_{i,t-1}) + h(\boldsymbol{\beta}_i, \mathbf{z}_{it}) \qquad (B.8)$$

Note, however, that there are cases where it is impossible to link-transform the lagged response. Two common ones are binary data and count data containing zeros. In neither case could the canonical link, involving a logarithm, be used for the responses, even though there is no problem for the mean because it cannot be zero.

An alternative possible generalization of Equation (B.8) is to work directly in terms of the location parameter:

$$\mu_i(t) = \rho_i y_{i,t-1} + g_i^{-1}[h(\boldsymbol{\beta}_i, \mathbf{z}_{it})] \qquad (B.9)$$

If $h(\cdot)$ is a linear function of $\boldsymbol{\beta}_i$, Equations (B.7) and (B.9) will be different; if it is nonlinear, the two are equivalent. This form is generally more easily interpretable and does not create problems with inappropriate transformations of the observations. Note that Equations (B.7), (B.8), and (B.9) all yield the same model when an identity link is used.

These three autoregression models may be called *state dependence* models because the present location parameter depends directly on the previous state of the subject, as given by the previous responses.

Serial dependence A quite different possibility is to allow the present location parameter to depend, not directly on the previous response, but on the difference between the previous response and its prediction at that time:

$$\mu_i(t) = \rho_h[y_{i,t-1} - h(\boldsymbol{\beta}_i, \mathbf{z}_{i,t-1})] + h(\boldsymbol{\beta}_i, \mathbf{z}_{it}) \qquad (B.10)$$

Dependence among responses is now restricted to a more purely stochastic component, the difference between the previous response and its location regression function. This is more clearly seen by rewriting Equation (B.10) in terms of these differences:

$$\mu_i(t) - h(\boldsymbol{\beta}_i, \mathbf{z}_{it}) = \rho_i[y_{i,t-1} - h(\boldsymbol{\beta}_i, \mathbf{z}_{i,t-1})] \qquad (B.11)$$

Successive differences are related by ρ_i (Lindsey, 1997, pp. 98–102). As in Equations (B.7) and (B.9), the previous observed value, $y_{i,t-1}$, is being used to predict the new expected value, $\mu_i(t)$.

I shall call this autoregression a *serial dependence* model. The present location parameter depends on how far the previous response was from the corresponding location parameter, the previous residual or innovation.

Implementation For non-normal distributions, constructing a model involving state dependence is straightforward: we condition on the previous value of the response at each point in time. The model for extending serial dependence, outside the traditional context of the normal distribution, is slightly more complex because it is necessarily nonlinear even if $h(\cdot)$ is linear. The easiest approach to the problem is to condition on the previous deviation of the observed from the predicted response, the residual or innovation, as in Equation (B.11).

Suppose that a common underlying profile, $\mu(t) = h(\boldsymbol{\beta}, \mathbf{z}_t)$, exists for all subjects under the same observed conditions. We want to obtain individual profiles by predicting the result at time t from the previously available information. Suppose that we use the common profile, corrected by how far individual i was from it at the previous time point. Then, Equation (B.10) can be rewritten as

$$\mu_i(t) = \mu(t) + \rho_i^{\Delta t}[y_{i,t-1} - \mu(t-1)] \quad (B.12)$$

with $0 < \rho_i < 1$ and the initial condition, $y_{i0} = \mu(0)$. Here, $\mu(t)$ represents the common underlying profile for all subjects under the same conditions at time point t, $\mu_i(t)$ is the corresponding predicted individual value, and Δt is the time between observations, to allow for cases where they are unequally spaced. The model must be estimated iteratively because each value depends on that at the previous point in time. It can easily be extended to a higher order autoregression.

B.3 Multivariate distributions with correlation matrices

One reason that the multivariate normal distribution is widely used is because of the ease with which dependency relationships can be modelled in the correlation or covariance matrix. However, a number of other families of multivariate distributions are also available which have such a matrix. I shall review these in this section.

B.3.1 MULTIVARIATE STUDENT t DISTRIBUTION

The best known is the multivariate Student t distribution, defined by

$$f(\mathbf{y};\boldsymbol{\mu},\boldsymbol{\Sigma},\kappa) = \frac{\Gamma\left(\frac{\kappa+R}{2}\right)}{\pi^{\frac{R}{2}}\sqrt{|\boldsymbol{\Sigma}|}\Gamma\left(\frac{\kappa}{2}\right)\kappa^{\frac{R}{2}}\left[1+\frac{1}{\kappa}(\mathbf{y}-\boldsymbol{\mu})^{\mathrm{T}}\boldsymbol{\Sigma}^{-1}(\mathbf{y}-\boldsymbol{\mu})\right]^{\frac{\kappa+R}{2}}} \quad (B.13)$$

where κ is the number of degrees of freedom and R the number of dependent responses. This is a member of the elliptically-contoured family of distributions.

The mean vector and covariance matrix are

$$E(\mathbf{Y}) = \boldsymbol{\mu}, \quad \kappa > 1$$
$$\text{cov}(\mathbf{Y}) = \frac{\kappa}{\kappa-2}\boldsymbol{\Sigma}, \quad \kappa > 2 \qquad (B.14)$$

Note that, as discussed below for the multivariate power-exponential distribution, zero correlation does not imply independence. Here, $\kappa \to \infty$ yields a multivariate normal distribution, whereas $\kappa = 1$ is a multivariate Cauchy distribution. Because of the skewed nature of most medical data, a log transform of the responses will often be necessary.

B.3.2 MULTIVARIATE POWER-EXPONENTIAL DISTRIBUTION

The univariate power-exponential distribution,

$$f(y;\mu,\sigma,\kappa) = \frac{1}{\sigma\Gamma\left(1+\frac{1}{2\kappa}\right)2^{1+\frac{1}{2\kappa}}} \exp\left[-\frac{1}{2}\left|\frac{y-\mu}{\sigma}\right|^{2\kappa}\right] \qquad (B.15)$$

can be generalized to a multivariate distribution:

$$f(\mathbf{y};\boldsymbol{\mu},\boldsymbol{\Sigma},\kappa) = \frac{R\Gamma\left(\frac{R}{2}\right)}{\pi^{\frac{R}{2}}\sqrt{|\boldsymbol{\Sigma}|}\Gamma\left(1+\frac{R}{2\kappa}\right)2^{1+\frac{R}{2\kappa}}}$$
$$\times \exp\left\{-\frac{1}{2}\left[(\mathbf{y}-\boldsymbol{\mu})^T\boldsymbol{\Sigma}^{-1}(\mathbf{y}-\boldsymbol{\mu})\right]^\kappa\right\} \qquad (B.16)$$

This is also a member of the elliptically-contoured family (Lindsey, 1999b).

This multivariate distribution has mean and variance

$$E(\mathbf{Y}) = \boldsymbol{\mu} \qquad (B.17)$$

$$\text{var}(\mathbf{Y}) = \frac{2^{\frac{1}{\kappa}}\Gamma\left(\frac{R+2}{2\kappa}\right)}{R\Gamma\left(\frac{R}{2\kappa}\right)}\boldsymbol{\Sigma} \qquad (B.18)$$

and κ determines kurtosis (Gómez *et al.*, 1998). Thus, the correlation structure can be obtained directly from $\boldsymbol{\Sigma}$ in the usual way. However, when $\kappa \neq 1$, the even cumulants are nonzero, in contrast to the multivariate normal distribution.

When $\kappa = 1$, this is a multivariate normal distribution, when $\kappa = 1/2$, a form of multivariate Laplace (double exponential) distribution, and when $\kappa \to \infty$, a multivariate uniform distribution. Thus, for $\kappa < 1$, the distribution has heavier tails than the multivariate normal and can be useful in providing robustness against 'outliers'. The marginal and conditional distributions are more complex, elliptically-contoured distributions, not of the power-exponential type.

In constructing multivariate normal models, the covariance matrix can be written simultaneously as one large matrix for all observations on all units by setting the appropriate elements to zero so that observations on different units are independent. In other words, this is equivalent to taking a separate multivariate normal distribution for each unit, with a suitable covariance structure, and multiplying them together. This is no longer true once $\kappa \neq 1$. Thus, for example, when Σ is diagonal in Equation (B.16) so that the correlation among observations is zero, this distribution cannot be written as a product of independent univariate distributions, from Equation (B.15), unless $\kappa = 1$. For $\kappa \neq 1$, the multivariate distribution retains a dependence structure among the observations on a unit even though the correlation among them may be zero. Of course, responses on different units can be made independent by multiplying together the multivariate distributions on units in the usual way.

B.3.3 COPULAS

One approach to the construction of multivariate distributions is by the specification of the univariate marginals. This is not sufficient to define completely the distribution and many supplementary conditions have been proposed, usually for specific marginals. Let us look at one general method.

Suppose that the desired univariate marginal distributions are given by their cumulative distribution functions, $F(y_i)$. Then, a multivariate distribution with these marginals can be formed as

$$F_R(y_1,\ldots,y_R) = c[F(y_1),\ldots,F(y_R)] \tag{B.19}$$

where $c(\cdot)$ is a function from $[0,1]^R$ to $[0,1]$. Such a construction is called a copula. Although all of the margins are shown to have the same form here, they can, in principle, be different. Equation (B.19) can be inverted to give

$$c(u_1,\ldots,u_R) = F_R[F^{-1}(u_1),\ldots,F^{-1}(u_R)] \tag{B.20}$$

where $F^{-1}(\cdot)$ is the corresponding quantile function and u_i is a uniform $[0,1]$ variable.

One particularly useful copula is the Gaussian one; Song (2000) presents a special case related to generalized linear models. The general form of the corresponding density can be obtained from the standardized multivariate normal density by transforming the response using a vector of univariate normal quantile functions, $\Phi^{-1}(\mathbf{u})$ (without forgetting the Jacobian):

$$f_R(\mathbf{u};\Sigma) = \frac{1}{\sqrt{|\Sigma|}} e^{-\frac{1}{2}[\Phi^{-1}(\mathbf{u})]^T \Sigma^{-1} \Phi^{-1}(\mathbf{u}) + \frac{1}{2}[\Phi^{-1}(\mathbf{u})]^T \Phi^{-1}(\mathbf{u})} \tag{B.21}$$

where Σ is a correlation matrix (not a covariance matrix as in the previous families). When we substitute in the univariate marginal distributions for $\mathbf{u}$, we obtain the multivariate density

$$f_R(\mathbf{y};\boldsymbol{\theta},\Sigma) = \frac{1}{\sqrt{|\Sigma|}} e^{-\frac{1}{2}[\Phi^{-1}(F(\mathbf{y};\theta))]^T [\Sigma^{-1} - \mathbf{I}_R] \Phi^{-1}(F(\mathbf{y};\theta))} \prod_{i=1}^{R} f(y_i) \tag{B.22}$$

where I_R is an $R \times R$ identity matrix, $F(\mathbf{y})$ is the vector of chosen univariate marginal cumulative distributions, and $f(y_i)$ is the corresponding individual univariate density. Then, as with the multivariate normal distribution, Σ can be structured in any desired way to created dependencies among the responses.

B.4 Dynamic models

B.4.1 DYNAMIC GENERALIZED LINEAR MODELS

Another conditional approach to constructing multivariate distributions for longitudinal data is to have some of the model coefficients evolve over time according to a Markov process. This has similarities both to autoregression and to random effects, and is able to encompass both. Let us first look at what have been called *dynamic generalized linear models*, a special case of a *state space model*. These are usually estimated by a procedure involving the *Kalman filter*. Although originally proposed as the dynamic linear model for normally distributed data, they have been extended to other distributions, notably by West *et al.* (1985), Harvey (1989), and Fahrmeir and Tutz (1994).

The location regression function, now called the *observation* or *measurement equation*, is

$$\mu_{it} = h(\boldsymbol{\lambda}_{it}, \mathbf{v}_{it}) \qquad (B.23)$$

where $\boldsymbol{\lambda}_{it}$ is a random vector of coefficients, defining the *state* of subject i at time t, with a distribution conditional on the previous responses and on $\mathbf{v}_{it}$. In contrast to a random effects model, here coefficients can vary randomly over time on the same subject, as well as across subjects. The state is simply the minimum past and present information necessary to predict a future response.

The state of the system is assumed to evolve over time according to a *state transition equation*,

$$E[\boldsymbol{\lambda}_{it}] = \mathbf{T}_{it} \boldsymbol{\lambda}_{i,t-1} \qquad (B.24)$$

where $\mathbf{T}_{it}$ is a first-order Markovian *state transition matrix* (Section B.5). Note that $\boldsymbol{\lambda}_{it}$ may contain values before time t as well as present values. The distributions of Y_{it} and $\boldsymbol{\lambda}_{it}$ are assumed to be independent. Then, the multivariate probabilities can be obtained by using the recursive relationship of Equation (B.6) above.

The dynamic generalized linear model for an autoregression of order M has measurement and state equations that can be specified by

$$g_i(\mu_{it}) = [1, 0, \ldots] \boldsymbol{\lambda}_{it}$$

$$E\left[\begin{pmatrix} \lambda_{it} \\ \lambda_{i,t-1} \\ \vdots \\ \lambda_{i,t-M+1} \end{pmatrix}\right] = \begin{pmatrix} \rho_{i1} & \cdots & \rho_{i,M-1} & \rho_{iM} \\ 1 & \cdots & 0 & 0 \\ \vdots & \ddots & \vdots & \vdots \\ 0 & \cdots & 1 & 0 \end{pmatrix} \begin{pmatrix} \lambda_{i,t-1} \\ \lambda_{i,t-2} \\ \vdots \\ \lambda_{i,t-M} \end{pmatrix} \qquad (B.25)$$

For a random effects model, the equations are

$$g_i(\mu_{it}) = \mu + \lambda_{it}$$
$$\mathrm{E}[\lambda_{it}] = 0 \qquad (B.26)$$

a special case of Equation (B.4) above. Simple models, such as these, can be combined in any desired way.

Filtering means estimating the current state given responses up to the present. The Kalman filter is a sequential or recursive procedure, yielding new distributions at each time point. From Bayes's formula,

$$p(\lambda_{it}|\mathcal{F}_{it}) = \frac{f(y_{it}|\lambda_{it},\mathcal{F}_{i,t-1})p(\lambda_{it}|\mathcal{F}_{i,t-1})}{f(y_{it}|\mathcal{F}_{i,t-1})} \qquad (B.27)$$

where $\mathcal{F}_{it}$ denotes the history of responses for subject i up to and including time t, that is, the vector of responses $(y_{i1},\ldots,y_{it})^\mathrm{T}$, with all pertinent relationships among them. In Equation (B.27), $p(\lambda_{it}|\mathcal{F}_{it})$ is called the *filtering* or *observation update* and

$$f(y_{it}|\mathcal{F}_{i,t-1}) = \int_{-\infty}^{\infty} f(y_{it}|\lambda_{it},\mathcal{F}_{i,t-1})p(\lambda_{it}|\mathcal{F}_{i,t-1})\mathrm{d}\lambda_{it} \qquad (B.28)$$

a mixture distribution, whereas $f(y_{it}|\lambda_{it},\mathcal{F}_{i,t-1})$ is the usual distribution defined by the observation equation.

The *one-step-ahead prediction* or *time update*,

$$p(\lambda_{it}|\mathcal{F}_{i,t-1}) = \int_{-\infty}^{\infty} p(\lambda_{it}|\lambda_{i,t-1})p(\lambda_{i,t-1}|\mathcal{F}_{i,t-1})\mathrm{d}\lambda_{i,t-1} \qquad (B.29)$$

is defined by the transition equation. Both of these integrals are usually complicated when the distributions are not normal and/or the regression function is nonlinear. The conditional distribution, $f(y_{it}|\mathcal{F}_{i,t-1})$, will be used to calculate the likelihood function.

Two advantages of this Kalman-filter-type approach are that it can be extended to handle unequally spaced time intervals and (randomly) missing observations and that it encompasses many useful models as special cases.

B.4.2 GENERAL DYNAMIC NONLINEAR MODELS

Mixture distributions can be constructed within the exponential dispersion family by means of conjugate distributions (Section B.1). Here, I shall apply a transformation to continuous variables so that their distribution is exponential and thus has, as a conjugate, the gamma distribution. These then can be dynamically updated without producing intractable integrals.

Gamma mixture model Suppose that each subject has some process operating over continuous time, t, although observations will necessarily be made at discrete points to be indexed by k. Associated with each of these will be some recorded value which may be a count of events between t_{k-1} and t_k, say n_k, some continuous measurement, say y_k, or the time since the last event, $y_k = t_k - t_{k-1}$. In the latter two cases, suppose that a cumulative distribution function of interest is

$$F(y_k; \kappa) = 1 - e^{-\Omega(y_k; \kappa)} \tag{B.30}$$

where κ can contain both location and shape parameters. In the context of duration distributions (Section B.6 and Chapter 6), $\Omega(y_k; \kappa)$ is the corresponding integrated intensity function; here, we can think of it as a transformation of the responses, y_k. I shall now develop a multivariate generalization of $F(y_k; \kappa)$ that will allow us to account for longitudinal dependence in longitudinal data or intraclass (frailty) dependence under clustering.

We can see that the transformed response, that is, the integrated intensity function, $\Omega(y_k; \kappa)$, has a unit exponential distribution. To obtain a mixture distribution for it (Hougaard, 1986, 2000; Aalen and Husebye, 1991), suppose that $\Omega(y_k; \kappa)$ varies randomly by a multiplicative factor, z, in the population so that the survival function becomes

$$S(y_k; \kappa | z) = e^{-z\Omega(y_k; \kappa)} \tag{B.31}$$

conditional on the unknown value of z. If Z has the gamma distribution of Equation (7.6), reparametrized as

$$f_g(z; \boldsymbol{\lambda}) = \frac{\lambda_2^{\lambda_1} z^{\lambda_1 - 1} e^{-\lambda_2 z}}{\Gamma(\lambda_1)} \tag{B.32}$$

conveniently, its Laplace transform is $E[\exp\{-z\Omega(y_k; \kappa)\}]$. This has a closed form, yielding a mixture distribution with survival function

$$S_m(y_k; \kappa, \boldsymbol{\lambda}) = \left[\frac{\lambda_2}{\lambda_2 + \Omega(y_k; \kappa)} \right]^{\lambda_1} \tag{B.33}$$

The corresponding density function is

$$f_m(y_k; \kappa, \boldsymbol{\lambda}) = \frac{\lambda_1 \lambda_2^{\lambda_1}}{[\lambda_2 + \Omega(y_k; \kappa)]^{\lambda_1 + 1}} \omega(y_k; \kappa) \tag{B.34}$$

and the intensity function is

$$\omega_m(y_k; \kappa, \boldsymbol{\lambda}) = \frac{\lambda_1}{\lambda_2 + \Omega(y_k; \kappa)} \omega(y_k; \kappa) \tag{B.35}$$

where the intensity function, $\omega(y_k; \kappa) = d\Omega(y_k; \kappa)/dy_k$, is the Jacobian of the transformation, $\Omega(\cdot)$, of y_k. Thus, the density, survival, and intensity functions are all explicitly available, the only integration being that possibly required to obtain

$$\Omega(y_k;\kappa) = -\log[1 - F(y_k;\kappa)] \tag{B.36}$$

the inverse of Equation (B.30).

This construction thus yields a mixture distribution from the original distribution, where the mixing distribution is gamma. The resulting distribution for $\Omega(y_k;\kappa)$ in Equation (B.34) is a type of Pareto distribution. Notice that $F(y_k;\kappa)$ can be *any* continuous distribution function. When it is a Weibull distribution, the mixture is called a Burr distribution.

Interestingly, although I have taken the Y_k to be random, if they are instead fixed time intervals, $y_k = t_k - t_{k-1}$, and the counts of events in these intervals, n_k, are random, then a distribution for counts is produced. Here, if $F(y_k;\kappa)$ is an exponential distribution, the result is a negative binomial distribution.

The parameters, λ_1 and λ_2, arising from the gamma mixing distribution, will now be used to model the dependence among the repeated observations. If they are allowed to vary over time, then, through the mixture, this also implies that the distribution of $\Omega(y_k;\kappa)$ is changing over time, a doubly stochastic process.

Frailty model Suppose, then, that λ_1 and λ_2 are changing over time such that, say,

$$\begin{aligned}\lambda_{1k} &= \lambda_{1,k-1} + n_k \\ \lambda_{2k} &= \lambda_{2,k-1} + \Omega(y_k;\kappa)\end{aligned} \tag{B.37}$$

where, for discrete observation times, n_k is the number of identical tied events observed at that time point. This will generally be unity except for count data; for a right-censored time interval (Section B.6), there is no event and it will be zero.

Then, Equation (B.34) yields the conditional distribution,

$$\begin{aligned}f_m(y_k|y_1,\ldots,y_{k-1};\kappa,\boldsymbol{\lambda}) &= \frac{\lambda_{1,k-1}\lambda_{2,k-1}^{\lambda_{1,k-1}}}{[\lambda_{2,k-1}+\Omega(y_k;\kappa)]^{\lambda_{1,k-1}+1}}\omega(y_k;\kappa) \\ &= \frac{\lambda_{1,k-1}\lambda_{2,k-1}^{\lambda_{1,k-1}}}{\lambda_{2k}^{\lambda_{1k}}}\omega(y_k;\kappa)\end{aligned} \tag{B.38}$$

If, instead, the time intervals are fixed and the counts are random, we have

$$\begin{aligned}f(n_k|n_1,\ldots,n_{k-1};\kappa) &= \frac{\Gamma(\lambda_{1,k-1}+n_k)}{\Gamma(\lambda_{1,k-1})n_k!}\frac{\Omega(y_k;\kappa)^{n_k}\lambda_{2,k-1}^{\lambda_{1,k-1}}}{[\lambda_{2,k-1}+\Omega(y_k;\kappa)]^{\lambda_{1,k-1}+n_k}} \\ &= \frac{\Gamma(\lambda_{1k})}{\Gamma(\lambda_{1,k-1})n_k!}\frac{\Omega(y_k;\kappa)^{n_k}\lambda_{2,k-1}^{\lambda_{1,k-1}}}{\lambda_{2k}^{\lambda_{1k}}}\end{aligned} \tag{B.39}$$

Let the initial conditions $\lambda_{10} = \lambda_{20} = \delta$ be an unknown parameter. (This implies that the mean of the gamma distribution is unity.) Then, the resulting multivariate distributions are respectively

$$f_m(y_1,\ldots,y_R;\kappa,\delta) = \frac{\Gamma(\delta+R)}{\Gamma(\delta)} \frac{\delta^\delta}{[\delta+\sum\Omega(y_k;\kappa)]^{\delta+R}} \prod_{k=1}^R \omega(y_k;\kappa)$$

$$= \frac{\Gamma(\delta+R)}{\Gamma(\delta)} \frac{\delta^\delta}{\lambda_{2R}^{\lambda_{1R}}} \prod_{k=1}^R \omega(y_k;\kappa) \quad \text{(B.40)}$$

and

$$f(n_1,\ldots,n_R;\kappa,\delta) = \frac{\Gamma(\delta+R)}{\Gamma(\delta)} \frac{\delta^\delta}{\lambda_{2R}^{\lambda_{1R}}} \prod_{k=1}^R \frac{\Omega(y_k;\kappa)^{n_k}}{n_k!} \quad \text{(B.41)}$$

When $F(y_k;\kappa)$ is a Weibull distribution, the first is a multivariate Burr distribution and, when it is an exponential distribution, the second is a multivariate negative binomial distribution.

Although the models based on Equation (B.37) were derived from an ordered sequence of observations, the resulting multivariate distributions are invariant to reordering and hence suitable for modelling clusters. Each individual response has a distribution that is conditional on all other responses in the same cluster through the sum of integrated intensities within that cluster. We may, thus, call Equation (B.37) the *frailty update*. This particular distribution can also be derived as a copula (Section B.3.3).

In Equation (B.40), independence occurs when

$$\lim_{\delta \to \infty} f_m(y_1,\ldots,y_R;\kappa,\delta) = \exp\left[-\sum_{k=1}^R n_k\Omega(y_k;\kappa)\right] \prod_{k=1}^R \omega(y_k;\kappa)$$

$$= \prod_{k=1}^R f(y_k;\kappa) \quad \text{(B.42)}$$

This is equivalent to letting the variance of the gamma mixing distribution (from the Laplace transform) go to zero.

Serial dependence models In the context of longitudinal dependence over time, the problem with the functions of time used for λ_1 and λ_2 above is that each new observation depends on all preceding ones to the same extent. One among many other possible ways to update these random parameters is to introduce a new unknown parameter, ρ, such that

$$\lambda_{1k} = \rho^{t_k-t_{k-1}}\lambda_{1,k-1} + (1-\rho^{t_k-t_{k-1}})\delta + n_k$$
$$\lambda_{2k} = \rho^{t_k-t_{k-1}}\lambda_{2,k-1} + (1-\rho^{t_k-t_{k-1}})\delta + \Omega(y_k;\kappa) \quad \text{(B.43)}$$

yielding nonstationary longitudinal dependence, called the *nonstationary update*.

Markov longitudinal dependence can be obtained by changing the second update equation to

$$\lambda_{2k} = \delta + \rho^{t_k - t_{k-1}} \Omega(y_{k-1}; \kappa) + \Omega(y_k; \kappa) \tag{B.44}$$

the *Markov update*. Many other updates are also possible. One of these used in Section 6.2.2 is the *count update*:

$$\begin{aligned}\lambda_{1k} &= \rho \lambda_{1,k-1} + 1 \\ \lambda_{2k} &= \delta + \Omega(y_k)\end{aligned} \tag{B.45}$$

These are new types of longitudinal dependence, in addition to the serial and state dependence of Section B.2.

The conditional distribution of Equation (B.38) remains unchanged, but the multivariate distribution no longer collapses to a simple form as it did in Equations (B.40) and (B.41). For example, for Y_k random, it is

$$f_m(y_1,\ldots,y_R; \kappa, \delta, \rho) = \prod_{k=1}^{R} \frac{\lambda_{1,k-1} \lambda_{2,k-1}^{\lambda_{1,k-1}}}{[\lambda_{2,k-1} + \Omega(y_k; \kappa)]^{\lambda_{1,k-1}+1}} \omega(y_k; \kappa) \tag{B.46}$$

When $\rho = 1$ in the nonstationary update, we obtain the cluster (frailty) model of Equation (B.40). With a Markov update, independence occurs when $\rho = 0$.

A third type of dynamic model will be presented in Section B.5.2 below.

B.5 Markov processes

Any series of observations where

$$f(y_k | y_1, \ldots, y_{k-1}) = f(y_k | y_{k-1}) \tag{B.47}$$

so that each response only depends on the immediately preceding one, is known as a *Markov process* (of order one, i.e. $M = 1$). We have already looked at a number of these in previous sections of this appendix. Here, I shall look more closely at the case where there are a finite number of discrete states.

B.5.1 MARKOV CHAINS

If the response variable for a Markov process can only take discrete values or states, it is known as a *Markov chain*. Usually, there is a finite number of possible discrete states, and observations are made at equally spaced, discrete, time intervals. Thus, a finite number of different types of events, observed at equally spaced time points, defines the *states* of the process. This is an example of a state dependence model (Section B.2). Conditional analysis of categorical longitudinal data can yield models for Markov chains. These may be studied using logistic or log linear models.

Suppose that the individual response, here a state, at a given time point depends only on the state at the immediately preceding point, the hypothesis of a *first-order* Markov chain. Then, the probabilities of change of state from one period to the next can be represented by a square *transition matrix* of non-negative values, with the entries of each line summing to one. This matrix of conditional probabilities, $\mathbf{T}(t)$, of each state given the previous one, may vary in time. If the rows correspond to the states at the previous time point and the columns to the present states, then the row probabilities sum to one. Pre-multiplying this matrix by the vector, $\pi(t)$, of marginal probabilities of the different states at a given time point, t, will give the vector for the next time period, $t+1$:

$$\pi(t+1)^{\mathrm{T}} = \pi(t)^{\mathrm{T}}\mathbf{T}(t) \tag{B.48}$$

Thus, the transition matrix represents the pattern of change.

The transition matrix is stationary if it is the same at all time points:

$$\pi(t+1)^{\mathrm{T}} = \pi(t)^{\mathrm{T}}\mathbf{T} \tag{B.49}$$

Then, the stationary marginal distribution is given by

$$\pi^{\mathrm{T}} = \pi^{\mathrm{T}}\mathbf{T} \tag{B.50}$$

It will arise after the process has run for a sufficiently long time.

When time is continuous, the transition matrix contains intensities, with rows summing to zero; see Section B.6.2. Then, the transition probabilities for a given time interval are obtained by matrix exponentiation; see Equation (1.14).

B.5.2 HIDDEN MARKOV MODELS

A third type of dependence, in addition to those described in Sections B.1 and B.2, may arise in medical data. In longitudinal observations, individuals may be subject to spells at various periods in time. The dynamic models to be described here provide one way to handle such data.

Suppose, for the moment, that a sequence of responses is discrete valued, representing, for example, categories that would appear to be the observed states of some Markov chain. Then, in a hidden Markov model, an underlying, unobserved sequence of states follows a Markov chain, the hidden state at a given time point determining the probabilities of the observed states. Thus, these models are closely related to the dynamic models of Section B.4; one difference is that here the number of possible states is finite whereas there it was infinite. These models are widely used in speech processing (Rabiner, 1989; Juang and Rabiner, 1991) and in molecular biological sequence analysis of nucleic acids in DNA and of amino acids in proteins (Chapter 10 and Durbin *et al.*, 1998).

As a simple example for a binary time series, each event might be generated by one of two Bernoulli distributions. The process switches from the one to the other according to the state of the two-state hidden Markov chain, in this way generating state dependence. Analogous models can be constructed for other discrete distributions, such as the Poisson or binomial distributions.

Suppose that we have an irreducible, homogeneous Markov chain with an $M \times M$ (hidden) transition matrix, $\mathbf{T}$. This gives the probabilities of changing among the hidden states, with marginal stationary distribution, π. The latter can be calculated from the transition matrix and hence does not introduce any new parameters. Then, the probability of the observed response at time t, $\nu_m(t) = f(y_t|m; \kappa_m)$, will depend on the unobserved state, m, at that time. The series of responses on a given unit are assumed to be independent, given the hidden states. Thus, there are $M(M-1)$ unknown parameters in the transition matrix as well as M times the length of κ_m in the probability distributions.

The resulting probability of the observed data is a complex form of mixture distribution. However, it can be written in a recursive form over time:

$$f(\mathbf{y}; \kappa, \mathbf{T}) = \pi^{\mathrm{T}} \prod_{t=1}^{R} [\mathbf{T}\mathbf{F}(t)] \mathbf{J} \qquad (B.51)$$

where $\mathbf{F}(t)$ is an $M \times M$ diagonal matrix containing, on the diagonal, the probabilities, $\nu_m(t)$, of the observed data given the various possible states and $\mathbf{J}$ is a column vector of ones.

To construct the likelihood function from this, the finite mixture distribution given by the marginal probability times the observed probability for each state at time 1, say, $a_m = \pi_m f(y_1|m; \kappa_m)$, is first calculated. At the second time point, the first step is to calculate the observed probability for each state multiplied by this quantity and by the transition probabilities in the corresponding column of $\mathbf{T}$. These are summed yielding, say, $b_m = \sum_h a_h T_{hm} f(y_2|m; \kappa_m)$. This is the new vector of forward recurrence probabilities, but it is divided by its average (to prevent underflow), yielding a new vector, $\mathbf{a}$. This average is also cumulated as a correction to the likelihood function. These steps are repeated at each successive time point. Finally, the sum of these a_m at the last time point is the likelihood defined by Equation (B.51) except that the cumulative correction must be added to it. At each step, the vector, $\mathbf{a}$, divided by its sum gives the (filtered) conditional probabilities of being in the various possible states given the previous observations (Guttorp, 1995, pp. 103–113; MacDonald and Zucchini, 1997, pp. 77–85).

This model can be applied in continuous time (Guttorp, 1995, pp. 176–180; see Section B.6.2) by using a matrix of transition intensities, so that, say, Ω (here not the integrated intensity as elsewhere in this appendix) has rows summing to zero (instead of one), and applying the matrix exponentiation of Equation (1.14) to give the transition probabilities, $\mathbf{T}_{\Delta t} = \exp(\Delta t \Omega)$, where Δt is the time interval between observations.

B.6 Duration data

The construction of models for duration data introduces a number of complications as compared to many other types of data; durations have several important characteristics that distinguish them from most other responses:

(1) They must be non-negative and are usually positive (unless several events can occur simultaneously).
(2) The distribution is usually positively skewed.
(3) Because time and money of the observer are limited and subjects may be susceptible to disappear from observation, measurements may be *censored*: some durations may be only partially recorded, although this still provides useful information.

Duration data can be studied in two closely related ways: by the durations or by the frequency of events in given intervals. In the latter case, when the intervals are allowed to become very small, we obtain the intensity of the event. The function describing this intensity is strictly equivalent to the distribution of the durations; both contain the same information expressed in different ways. Modelling the intensity directly, instead of the probability or density, as in other areas of statistics, is often the most flexible approach, although the risk functions for certain common distributions are relatively complex, having nonlinear form. Many different distributions, and their corresponding intensity functions, exist to model the durations of times until events.

B.6.1 SURVIVAL AND INTENSITY FUNCTIONS

Three important functions for analysis of durations that are related to the density function, $f(y)$, are

- the probability of a duration lasting at least a given time, called the *survival function*,

$$S(y) = \Pr(Y > y) \\ = 1 - F(y) \qquad (B.52)$$

- the instantaneous probability that the event will occur at a given time, so that duration terminates conditional on it having continued until then, or the *intensity* with which termination occurs:

$$\omega(y) = \frac{f(y)}{S(y)} \qquad (B.53)$$

also called the *risk*, the *hazard*, the *failure rate*, or the *mortality rate*, and
- the integrated intensity, used in Section (B.4.2),

$$\Omega(y) = \int_0^y \omega(u) du \\ = -\log[S(y)] \qquad (B.54)$$

from Equation (B.36).

In most cases, any one of the four functions, $f(\cdot)$, $S(\cdot)$, $\omega(\cdot)$, and $\Omega(\cdot)$, defines the (univariate) distributional part of a model completely. However, in certain situations, the density and survival functions will not be defined so that Equation

(B.53) cannot be used and the intensity function must be defined directly. The most important case is when there are endogenous time-varying covariates, that is, covariates that depend on the previous history of the process.

Special families If the intensity function can be written as the product

$$\omega(y_i|\mathbf{x}_i;\boldsymbol{\beta},\boldsymbol{\theta}) = \omega_0(y_i,\boldsymbol{\theta})h(\mathbf{x}_i,\boldsymbol{\beta}) \tag{B.55}$$

where $\omega_0(y_i,\boldsymbol{\theta})$ is a baseline intensity function for $\mathbf{x}_i = 0$ and $h(\mathbf{x}_i,\boldsymbol{\beta})$ is some regression function that may be nonlinear, we have a *multiplicative intensities model*. Generally, the two factors do not have any parameters in common. Intensities for all subjects are proportional, depending on the covariates. If the baseline function, $\omega_0(y_i,\boldsymbol{\theta})$, is left unspecified, generally with $h(\mathbf{x}_i,\boldsymbol{\beta}) = \exp(\mathbf{x}_i^T\boldsymbol{\beta})$, we have a semi-parametric proportional hazards model (Cox, 1972). Unfortunately, this widely employed proportionality assumption is rarely empirically justifiable.

If the intensity function can be written

$$\omega(y_i|\mathbf{x}_i;\boldsymbol{\beta},\boldsymbol{\theta}) = \omega_0(y_ih(\mathbf{x}_i,\boldsymbol{\beta}),\boldsymbol{\theta})h(\mathbf{x}_i,\boldsymbol{\beta}) \tag{B.56}$$

it is called an *accelerated life* or *failure time model*. The effect of covariates is to accelerate or decelerate the time to completion of the duration. It can yield a simple regression model for the log duration if $h(\mathbf{x}_i,\boldsymbol{\beta}) = \exp(\mathbf{x}_i^T\boldsymbol{\beta})$.

Censoring By definition, responses that are measured as a duration occur over time. However, any medical research study must occupy a limited period, so that some durations will, almost invariably, be incomplete or *censored*. If observation must stop because the subject drops out of the study, this may produce differential censoring in the population that can bias the results. Appropriate measures should be taken either to minimize or to model this type of censorship. On the other hand, the general way in which observation is to stop for all subjects will be under the control of the research worker. Thus, an important question involves the nature of the stopping rule.

In the collection of survival data, two types of planned censoring are usually distinguished:

(1) All recording may be stopped after a fixed interval of time, called Type I or time censoring, most often used in medical studies.
(2) Recording may be continued until complete information is available on a fixed number of subjects, that is, until a pre-specified number of events has occurred, called Type II or failure censoring, more often used in engineering studies.

As examples of censoring in event histories (Section 6.1.2), Aalen and Husebye (1991) suggest several possibilities:

(1) Censoring time is fixed in advance, as in Type I above.

(2) Censoring times are random variables, independent of the stochastic process.
(3) Recording of each process stops when it has completed a fixed number of durations, as in Type II above.
(4) Recording of each process stops either when it has completed a fixed number of durations or after a fixed time, whichever comes first.
(5) Recording of each process stops at the first event after a fixed period.

The last three differ from the first two in that they depend on the event history itself. However, because these three depend only on what has already been observed, and not on any as yet incompletely observed data, all five can be treated in the same way. This can be demonstrated using the concept of stopping time (see Section B.6.2 below) from martingale theory.

Suppose now that the last, incomplete, duration in Type I censoring of an event history is ignored, and not recorded. However, to know that the last duration recorded is the last complete one, one must look beyond it up to the fixed endpoint. This differs from the above examples, in that the cutting point depends on information after that point. It is not a martingale stopping time. One can also see that this will bias downwards the average duration time, because long intervals have a higher probability of being incomplete at the end.

The start of observation must also be at a 'stopping time'. Interestingly, this implies that incomplete durations at the beginning can be ignored. This will involve some loss of information, but no bias.

Likelihood function When it exists, the density of a duration is the product of the intensity and the survival function, as can be seen from Equation (B.53). This term will be included in the likelihood function for all complete durations. For a censored duration, we only know that there was no new event up to that point; this is given by the survival function alone. Thus, censored data will contribute to the likelihood function a term that is only the survival function. Then, for independent observations of durations, y_i, the likelihood function will be

$$L(\boldsymbol{\beta},\boldsymbol{\theta};\mathbf{y},\mathbf{x}) = \prod_i \omega(y_i;\boldsymbol{\beta},\boldsymbol{\theta},\mathbf{x})^{I(y_i<t_i)} S(y_i;\boldsymbol{\beta},\boldsymbol{\theta},\mathbf{x}) \qquad (B.57)$$

where t_i is the censoring time for the ith observation and $I(\cdot)$ is the indicator function. When this does not exist, for example when endogenous time-varying covariates are present, the likelihood function must be constructed directly from the intensity function, a subject to which I now turn.

B.6.2 COUNTING PROCESSES

Basic concepts The cumulated number, N_t, of events up to time, t, in a point process is known as a *counting process* with intensity, $\omega_{jk}(t|\mathcal{F}_{t-})$, of transition from state j to state k defined by

$$\omega_{jk}(t|\mathcal{F}_{t-})dt = \Pr(\text{the event in } (t, t+dt)|\mathcal{F}_{t-})$$
$$= \Pr(dN_t = 1|\mathcal{F}_{t-}) \tag{B.58}$$

where $\mathcal{F}_{t-}$ is the complete history up to, but not including, t, called the *filtration*. (Note that, in this formulation, we are implicitly assuming that more than one event cannot occur in the time interval, dt, if it is very small.)

If
$$\begin{aligned} \mathrm{E}[M_t] &< \infty \\ \mathrm{E}[M_{t+k} - M_t|\mathcal{F}_{t-}] &= 0, \quad \forall t; \quad 0 < k < \infty \end{aligned} \tag{B.59}$$

M_t is called a *martingale*. For a counting process, $M_t = N_t - \int_0^t \omega_{jk}(t|\mathcal{F}_{t-})dt$ fulfils this condition. A *stopping* or *Markov time* is a time that depends only on $\mathcal{F}_{t-}$, and not on events after t.

Some simple cases Important simplifications occur when the intensity depends only on the complete history through N_t: $\omega_{jk}(t|N_t)$. Special cases include:

- the ordinary homogeneous *Poisson process*, with

$$\omega(t|N_t) = \omega \tag{B.60}$$

  where the intensity is always the same (the only counting process with stationary independent increments);

- the *nonhomogeneous Poisson process*, with

$$\omega(t|N_t) = \omega(t) \tag{B.61}$$

  where the intensity is a function of time;

- the *pure birth* or *Yule process*, with

$$\omega(t|N_t) = N_t \omega \tag{B.62}$$

  where the intensity is proportional to the number of previous events;

- the *nonhomogeneous birth process*, with

$$\omega(t|N_t) = N_t \omega(t) \tag{B.63}$$

  where the intensity, proportional to the number of previous events, is also a function of time;

- the *renewal process*, with

$$\omega(t|N_t) = \omega(t - t_{N_t}) \tag{B.64}$$

  where the intensity depends on the time since the last recurrent event, starting afresh after each event;

- the *semi-Markov* or *Markov renewal process*, with

$$\omega_{jk}(t|N_t) = \omega_{jk}(t - t_{N_t}) \tag{B.65}$$

where the form of the intensity function depends on the time since the last event, with the process changing state at each event. (For further discussion of Markov processes, see Sections B.2 and B.5.)

Those processes with an intensity depending on time are nonstationary. As we see, this dependence may be on the elapsed time, either total or since the previous event, or on the number of previous events, or both. In more complex cases, it may also depend on other time-varying covariates.

Modelling intensities Construction of a model directly by means of the duration distribution is only straightforward when the conditions for a subject remain constant over each period between events. If there are time-varying covariates that change within the period, then this cannot easily be allowed for in the probability distribution. If the covariates are endogenous, then the density is not even defined. Instead, the intensity of the process should be modelled; of course, this can also be done in other simpler contexts as well.

Models for intensities can easily be constructed in terms of a counting process (Lindsey, 1995b). As its name suggests, N_t is a random variable over time that counts the number of events that have occurred up to time t. As we saw in Equation (B.58), the corresponding intensity of the process is $\omega_{jk}(t|\mathcal{F}_{t-})$. Then, the kernel of the log likelihood function for observation over the interval $(0, T]$ is

$$\log[L(\beta)] = \int_0^T \log[\omega_{jk}(t|\mathcal{F}_{t-}; \beta)]dN_t - \int_0^T \omega_{jk}(t|\mathcal{F}_{t-}; \beta)I(t)dt \tag{B.66}$$

where $I(t)$ is an indicator function, with value one if the process is under observation at time t and zero otherwise. Because the second term on the right is the integrated intensity and dN_t is zero except when there is an event, this is essentially the logarithm of the likelihood function in Equation (B.57).

Now, in any empirical situation, even a continuous-time process will only be observed at discrete time intervals, once an hour, once a day, once a week. Suppose that these are sufficiently small so that at most one event is observed to occur in any interval, although there will be a finite nonzero theoretical probability of more than one, unless the event is absorbing or a transition to another state. With R intervals of observation, not all necessarily the same size, Equation (B.66) becomes, by numerical approximation,

$$\log[L(\beta)] \doteq \sum_{t=1}^{R} \log[\omega_{jk}(t|\mathcal{F}_{t-}; \beta)]\Delta N_t - \sum_{t=1}^{R} \omega_{jk}(t|\mathcal{F}_{t-}; \beta)I(t)\Delta_t \tag{B.67}$$

where Δ_t is the width of the tth observation interval and ΔN_t is the change in the count during that interval, with possible values zero and one. Equation (B.67) is the kernel of the log likelihood for the Poisson distribution of ΔN_t, with mean $\omega(t|\mathcal{F}_{t-};\beta)\Delta_t$. Conditional on the filtration, it is the likelihood for a Poisson process. Any observable counting process is locally a Poisson process, conditional on the filtration, if events cannot occur simultaneously.

The structure that one places on this likelihood will determine what stochastic process is being modelled. If it is multiplicative, we have a log linear model. For example, if the logarithm of the elapsed time since the previous event is included in the Poisson regression, we obtain a Weibull process, whereas, if the intensity is allowed to jump at each event time, we have the semi-parametric proportional hazards model. However, there is no reason why the model should be linear, so that the intensity function for any distribution can be so modelled.

B.6.3 IMPORTANT SPECIAL CASES

Birth processes A simple birth or contagion process is a point process that has the intensity proportional to the number of previous events. It is nonhomogeneous if it is also a function of time in other ways. Consider Equation (B.63),

$$\omega(t|N_t) = N_t \omega(t)$$

where $\omega(t)$ is some arbitrary function, and may depend also on covariates. For example, for a Weibull model, $\omega(t) = \kappa t^{\kappa-1}$. The exponential model yields a pure birth process.

Birth processes can be generalized by replacing N_t by some function of the number of previous events, for example

$$\omega(t|N_t) = N_t^\nu \omega(t) \tag{B.68}$$

This is especially important if time is already measured before the first event, as in many medical studies, because then $N_t = 0$. Several approaches are possible. For example, all values of N_t could be augmented by one, as if time started at an event; N_t could be set to one in the first two periods, until there are two events; or N_t could be replaced by $\exp(\nu N_t)$.

Semi-Markov processes In a semi-Markov or Markov renewal process, as in Equation (B.65), the intensity function depends on the time since the last event, but the form of the function is also changing over time, different in each state. The function may be of any appropriate form; changes might occur, for example, because the intensity is a function of some time-varying covariates.

In the simpler cases, there may be a progression of irreversible states, such as in the advance of incurable diseases, with a final, absorbing, death state. Then, there will be one less transition intensity than the number of states. However, when at least some of the state transitions are reversible, many more different intensity functions may need to be estimated and the problem becomes more difficult. When any one of several states may be entered at a given time point, this is similar to competing risks in the simpler context of survival analysis. For further discussion of some of these simple examples, see Section 6.1.2.

Transition probabilities Consider more closely now the situation where an event marks a change of state. From the transition intensities, the transition probabilities can be found. These are defined as

$$\pi_{jk}(t-,t) = \Pr(Y_t = k | Y_{t-} = j, \mathcal{F}_{t-}) \tag{B.69}$$

the probability of being in state k at time t given the previous history up until that time, including the previous state(s), the immediately preceding one being j. These satisfy

$$\pi_{jk}(t_1,t_3) = \sum_l \pi_{jl}(t_1,t_2)\pi_{lk}(t_2,t_3) \tag{B.70}$$

for $t_1 \leq t_2 \leq t_3$. They can be obtained from the set of differential equations,

$$\frac{d\mathbf{T}(t-,t)}{dt} = \mathbf{T}(t-,t)\mathbf{\Omega}(t) \tag{B.71}$$

where $\mathbf{T}(t-,t)$ is the matrix of transition probabilities, $\pi_{jk}(t-,t)$, to and from all possible states and $\mathbf{\Omega}$ (again not an integrated intensity) is a matrix with elements $\omega_{jk}(t)$, the transition intensity from state j to state k, off diagonal and $-\sum_j \omega_{jk}(t)$ on diagonal. These are the forward recurrence equations.

These equations can only easily be solved for homogeneous Markov processes where none of the transition intensities either vary with time or depend on time-varying covariates. Then, the matrix exponentiation of Equation (1.14) can be used. This means that, if the eigenvalues of $\mathbf{T}$ are all distinct, the solution will be of the form

$$\pi_{jk}(t_1,t_2) = \sum_l \beta_{jkl} e^{-E_l(t_1-t_2)} \tag{B.72}$$

where E_l are the eigenvalues. In such cases,

$$\pi_{jk}(t_1,t_2) = \pi_{jk}(0, t_2 - t_1) \tag{B.73}$$

The boundary conditions are $\pi_{jj}(t,t) = 1$ and $\pi_{jk}(t,t) = 0$ for $j \neq k$.

As an example, suppose that an individual can move in either direction between healthy (1) and sick (2) states with intensities $\omega_{jk} = k_{jk}$, and can die (state 3) while in either other state j with intensities $\omega_{j3} = k_j$. The intensity matrix is

$$\mathbf{\Omega} = \begin{pmatrix} -k_1 - k_{12} & k_{12} & k_1 \\ k_{21} & -k_2 - k_{21} & k_2 \\ 0 & 0 & 0 \end{pmatrix} \tag{B.74}$$

However, the absorbing death state 3 can be deleted without affecting the solution, yielding the intensity matrix in Equation (1.17). Then, the solution is obtained as for that equation in the example in Section 1.4.2. (A model in which the rows of the intensity matrix do not sum to zero, as for the two states here, is called defective because there is a net flow out of those two states.)

Appendix C
Data tables for the exercises

C.1 Gastric half-emptying times

Treatment					
A		B		C	
Period	Response	Period	Response	Period	Response
1	84	2	62	3	58
3	87	2	108	1	38
3	85	1	85	2	96
1	82	3	46	2	61
2	83	1	70	3	46
2	110	3	110	1	66
3	215	2	86	1	42
1	50	3	46	2	34
2	92	3	50	1	80
1	70	2	61	3	55
3	97	1	40	2	78
2	95	1	147	3	57

Table C.1. Gastric half-emptying time (min) for 12 subjects in a cross-over trial. Each line corresponds to the period, treatment, and response of one subject. (Keene, 1995)

C.2 Bacteriuria infections

Group A	Group B
1001010100101	111100011
10001	1111111111111111
1010010010101010	111111111111001
101000101	100011111110111
100011010111111	1111111111010000
1100100010101001	111110011111111
100010101	1000111110111001
1000	111000111011
1001000000100010	111011111111111
1010011	1110
1010110101	1011111111
1001010101	1011111111111111
100110	1111111100000110
10100011010100	100010
10010	1001111011011111
1000101100100100	10011
1010100110110100	111111100000
1000100010000000	1000111111111000
1010001010011001	1111001100011111
101000011011	1001111111111111
101000111011101	1000000000000000
1001000100	1100111111100111
1000101001110001	100100
1010001010010011	11111100000
1010101001001	100111110100
1000101010100010	1111111111
1010001001	1111111110111111
100010110101	1111101110111111
111000	110011
1001000010100010	1100000110010000
10000101001	100001111111111
110011011	100011110101001
100101100010001	1111110011111111
11010011001010	1111000101111111
10010010	1100000111
100100	1111000

Table C.2. Time series of infections (1) with bacteriuria for patients randomized to two treatment groups. (Joe, 1997, p. 353; he imputed 11 missing values.)

C.3 Cases of lung cancer

Years smoking	Cigarettes smoked per day							
	0		1–9		10–14		15–19	
15–19	1	10366	0	3121	0	3577	0	4317
20–24	0	8162	0	2937	1	3286	0	4214
25–29	0	5969	0	2288	1	2546	0	3185
30–34	0	4496	0	2015	2	2219	4	2560
35–39	0	3512	1	1648	0	1826	0	1893
40–44	0	2201	2	1310	1	1386	2	1334
45–49	0	1421	0	927	2	988	2	849
50–54	0	1121	3	710	4	684	2	470
55–59	2	826	0	606	3	449	5	280
	20–24		25–34		35+			
15–19	0	5683	0	3042	0	670		
20–24	1	6385	1	4050	0	1166		
25–29	1	5483	4	4290	0	1482		
30–34	6	4687	9	4268	4	1580		
35–39	5	3646	9	3529	6	1336		
40–44	12	2411	11	2424	10	924		
45–49	9	1567	10	1409	7	556		
50–54	7	857	5	663	4	255		
55–59	7	416	3	284	1	104		

Table C.3. Numbers of lung cancer cases and the corresponding person-years at risk (units of 100 000), by years of smoking (age minus 20 years) and number of cigarettes smoked per day. (Whittemore and Altschuler, 1976)

C.4 Case–control study of asbestos

		Exposure (1000 fibres/cm^3 × days)				
Age		< 1	1–9	10–39	40–99	≥ 100
45–49	Cases	3	2	1	0	0
	Controls	8	9	7	0	0
50–54	Cases	1	2	3	3	1
	Controls	15	14	4	7	0
55–59	Cases	0	0	3	3	0
	Controls	10	8	3	3	0
60–64	Cases	0	1	0	4	1
	Controls	9	4	5	2	0
65–69	Cases	1	3	0	1	1
	Controls	5	6	6	4	3
70–74	Cases	0	2	3	0	0
	Controls	2	2	3	0	1

Table C.4. Deaths from lung cancer (cases) in a case–control study of asbestos exposure. (Checkoway *et al.*, 1989, p. 196)

C.5 Rectal polyps

Sex	Baseline	Month							
		3	6	9	12	15	18	21	24
Placebo									
F	41	22	36	56	34	46	61	56	73	28
M	2	—	3	1	1	3	3	1	4	1
F	2	5	4	10	9	17	8	4	7	22
F	7	1	10	31	31	37	11	15	12	9
F	3	1	3	1	1	4	0	1	0	0
F	8	15	16	17	22	24	36	7	15	20
M	1	4	6	4	3	11	6	3	4	3
M	5	4	1	4	2	0	0	1	1	0
F	11	13	7	4	11	8	8	12	5	17
F	2	2	3	4	4	1	3	2	3	4
M	3	1	5	3	3	3	2	8	5	—
M	10	8	4	1	3	2	1	1	7	1
M	1	0	0	1	3	0	0	2	0	0
M	0	—	0	0	0	0	1	0	1	1
F	3	10	10	13	11	12	6	12	18	12
M	2	1	1	1	3	3	1	3	1	1
M	4	3	3	2	3	5	2	1	1	12
M	26	23	14	33	20	21	32	26	13	22
M	9	14	5	11	11	11	—	9	5	3
F	12	12	15	10	8	11	19	8	4	14
F	5	4	2	7	4	5	3	6	8	7
M	4	7	6	—	—	11	—	—	—	—
Vitamins C and E									
M	5	13	4	6	6	11	16	11	9	12
F	0	0	0	0	0	0	0	0	0	0
F	27	18	15	10	37	32	30	62	63	41
M	6	8	15	9	4	4	2	6	3	4
F	1	12	7	8	5	3	6	8	10	3
F	1	1	2	1	1	1	2	0	0	1
M	10	11	6	3	3	7	9	2	3	6
M	1	17	4	4	10	4	7	7	5	12
M	1	8	3	3	7	6	7	4	6	5
M	7	2	5	7	3	4	4	0	5	—
M	4	5	4	8	17	11	12	11	10	10
M	5	6	5	—	2	6	1	3	3	3
M	0	0	0	0	0	0	0	0	—	0
M	7	19	9	18	10	23	18	11	—	13
F	4	8	11	5	8	4	7	5	3	3
M	1	1	1	1	1	0	1	2	1	0

| | | \multicolumn{8}{c}{Month} |
Sex	Baseline	27	30	33	36	39	42	45	48
				Placebo					
F	41	22	53	28	33	12	46	39	8	21
M	2	—	1	0	1	1	2	0	1	0
F	2	5	23	10	8	10	4	12	6	15
F	7	1	22	5	18	15	5	14	15	3
F	3	1	2	0	2	1	1	0	1	1
F	8	15	22	33	10	21	25	20	34	33
M	1	4	5	14	12	5	3	7	2	12
M	5	4	0	0	2	0	1	1	1	2
F	11	13	20	13	2	9	4	3	5	9
F	2	2	3	4	2	1	2	1	2	1
M	3	1	—	10	—	—	—	8	—	—
M	10	8	4	8	6	3	2	6	1	2
M	1	0	—	0	0	0	0	0	0	0
M	0	—	1	0	2	1	2	2	1	2
F	3	10	7	12	7	13	9	12	14	10
M	2	1	2	1	1	0	0	2	0	1
M	4	3	3	2	4	3	4	3	3	1
M	26	23	16	21	9	14	—	7	20	18
M	9	14	9	1	—	—	—	—	—	—
F	12	12	9	10	8	21	11	10	7	—
F	5	4	4	7	8	6	4	6	4	—
M	4	7	—	—	—	—	—	—	—	—
				Vitamins C and E					
M	5	13	4	12	5	16	4	8	19	5
F	0	0	0	0	0	0	0	0	0	0
F	27	18	32	33	19	23	28	26	50	30
M	6	8	4	6	4	2	5	7	2	7
F	1	12	12	7	9	12	5	3	5	2
F	1	1	1	0	0	2	0	0	0	1
M	10	11	1	1	4	1	1	2	3	4
M	1	17	9	6	4	3	—	9	1	8
M	1	8	3	2	3	1	2	1	3	3
M	7	2	—	—	8	1	3	0	0	2
M	4	5	5	5	13	6	11	10	—	10
M	5	6	6	5	3	2	4	8	6	2
M	0	0	0	1	—	—	—	—	1	1
M	7	19	9	13	—	—	13	—	5	—
F	4	8	2	2	3	6	6	7	12	—
M	1	1	1	0	0	1	1	1	0	—

| | | \multicolumn{8}{c}{Month} |
Sex	Baseline	3	6	9	12	15	18	21	24
\multicolumn{10}{c}{Vitamins C and E and high fibre}
M	4	6	2	2	0	1	1	1	1	0
M	26	7	1	2	0	0	1	1	0	0
F	15	10	13	6	12	6	12	8	6	6
F	9	2	6	2	8	6	4	4	4	5
M	25	7	8	6	8	11	16	18	19	19
F	1	0	0	0	0	0	0	0	0	0
M	4	3	5	2	1	1	2	3	2	1
F	24	6	21	13	14	9	16	15	8	7
F	8	1	1	1	2	2	1	0	0	1
M	3	9	5	5	6	4	1	2	1	0
M	10	19	11	9	9	21	23	20	14	13
M	7	3	3	5	6	13	14	—	—	9
M	1	2	4	2	2	6	7	5	8	5
F	1	1	1	2	2	2	0	2	2	1
M	1	1	4	5	4	5	4	2	1	2
M	1	0	0	0	0	1	1	1	2	0
M	7	6	5	4	3	4	4	3	3	1
M	0	1	2	0	1	2	2	2	2	3
M	18	11	34	15	—	21	11	23	—	5
M	1	1	3	1	2	3	—	—	—	—

		Month							
Sex	Baseline	27	30	33	36	39	42	45	48
Vitamins C and E and high fibre									
M	4	6	0	0	0	0	2	0	0	0
M	26	7	1	1	0	1	2	2	2	1
F	15	10	3	6	3	9	8	4	9	10
F	9	2	1	1	5	3	3	4	6	10
M	25	7	7	14	2	6	6	3	2	—
F	1	0	1	1	0	0	0	0	0	0
M	4	3	2	3	4	4	3	2	1	1
F	24	6	2	6	3	1	1	3	2	5
F	8	1	0	1	0	1	0	0	0	1
M	3	9	1	0	0	0	0	1	3	1
M	10	19	13	23	6	7	12	21	25	30
M	7	3	3	3	2	3	3	2	5	8
M	1	2	3	3	—	5	4	8	—	3
F	1	1	1	2	2	2	2	2	3	2
M	1	1	5	6	3	6	9	1	3	2
M	1	0	1	1	1	0	—	6	5	4
M	7	6	3	2	2	2	7	4	2	2
M	0	1	1	—	0	0	0	0	1	—
M	18	11	16	—	12	—	—	33	30	—
M	1	1	—	—	—	—	—	—	—	—

Table C.5. Counts of rectal polyps at three-month intervals under three treatments, with two baseline counts. (Stukel, 1993)

C.6 Recurrence of kidney infections

Times		Sex	Disease	Age
8	16	M	Other	28
23	13*	F	GN	48
22	28	M	Other	32
447	318	F	Other	31–32
30	12	M	Other	10
24	245	F	Other	16–17
7	9	M	GN	51
511	30	F	GN	55–56
53	196	F	AN	69
15	154	M	GN	51–52
7	333	F	AN	44
141	8*	F	Other	34
96	38	F	AN	35
149*	70*	F	AN	42
536	25*	F	Other	17
17	4*	M	AN	60
185	177	F	Other	60
292	114	F	Other	43–44
22*	159*	F	GN	53
15	108*	F	Other	44
152	562	M	PKD	46–47
402	24*	F	Other	30
13	66	F	AN	62–63
39	46*	F	AN	42–43
12	40	M	AN	43
113*	201	F	AN	57–58
132	156	F	GN	10
34	30	F	AN	52
2	25	M	GN	53
130	26	F	GN	54
27	58	F	AN	56
5	43*	F	AN	50–51
152	30	F	PKD	57
190	5*	F	GN	44–45
119	8	F	Other	22
54*	16*	F	Other	42
6*	78	F	PKD	52
63	8*	M	PKD	60

Table C.6. Times (units not specified) to recurrence of infections in kidney patients. Censored values are indicated by an asterisk. (McGilchrist and Aisbett, 1991)

C.7 Mammary tumours

Rat			Retinoid				
1	182						
2	182*						
3	63	68	182*				
4	152	182*					
5	130	134	145	152	182*		
6	98	152	182				
7	88	95	105	130	137	167	182*
8	152	182*					
9	81	182*					
10	71	84	126	134	152	182*	
11	116	130	182*				
12	91	182*					
13	63	68	84	95	152	182*	
14	105	152	182*				
15	63	102	152	182*			
16	63	77	112	140	182*		
17	77	119	152	161	167	182*	
18	105	112	145	161	182		
19	152	182*					
20	81	95	182*				
21	84	91	102	108	130	134	182*
22	182*						
23	91	182*					

C.7. MAMMARY TUMOURS

Rat	Control								
24	63	102	119	161	161	172	179	182*	
25	88	91	95	105	112	119	119	137	145
		167	172	182*					
26	91	98	108	112	134	137	161	161	179
		182*							
27	71	174	182*						
28	95	105	134	134	137	140	145	150	150
		182*							
29	68	68	130	137	182*				
30	77	95	112	137	161	174	182*		
31	81	84	126	134	161	161	174	182*	
32	68	77	98	102	102	102	182*		
33	112	182*							
34	88	88	91	98	112	134	134	137	137
		140	140	152	152	182*			
35	77	179	182*						
36	112	182*							
37	71	71	74	77	112	116	116	140	140
		167	182*						
38	77	95	126	150	182*				
39	88	126	130	130	134	182*			
40	63	74	84	84	88	91	95	108	134
		137	179	182*					
41	81	88	105	116	123	140	145	152	161
		161	179	182*					
42	88	95	112	119	126	126	150	157	179
		182*							
43	68	68	84	102	105	119	123	123	137
		161	179	182					
44	140	182*							
45	152	182	182						
46	81	182*							
47	63	88	134	182*					
48	84	134	182						

Table C.7. Times (days) of appearance of mammary tumours in female rats under two treatments. Asterisks indicate censoring. (Gail *et al.*, 1980)

C.8 Skin papilloma in mice

							Week							
6	7	8	9	10	11	12	13	14	15	16	17	18	19	20
							Acetone							
0	0	0	0	0	2	2	2	2	2	2	2	2	2	2
0	0	0	0	0	0	0	0	0	1	4	4	4	4	4
0	0	0	0	0	0	0	0	0	0	1	1	1	1	1
0	0	0	0	0	0	0	0	0	0	0	0	0	0	0
0	0	0	0	0	0	0	0	0	0	—	—	—	—	—
							Benzene							
0	0	0	0	0	0	0	0	0	0	0	0	0	0	2
0	0	0	0	0	0	0	0	0	0	0	0	0	0	0
0	0	0	0	0	0	0	0	0	0	0	0	0	0	1
1	1	2	3	4	7	10	13	16	19	22	22	21	21	23
0	0	0	0	0	0	0	0	0	0	0	0	0	0	0
0	0	0	0	0	0	0	0	—	—	—	—	—	—	—
0	0	0	1	1	4	5	7	8	8	8	6	6	6	6
0	0	0	0	0	0	0	0	0	0	1	1	3	3	3
2	4	5	5	5	7	7	7	7	7	7	9	7	7	6
0	0	0	0	0	2	5	8	7	7	15	15	15	21	26

Table C.8. Skin papilloma counts for female Tg.AC mice exposed to acetone or 400 μl benzene. (Dunson and Haseman, 1999)

C.9 Leukæmia clinical trial

Prior treatment		No treatment		Therapy after randomization	
186	197	57	201	380	380
82	201	191	261	277	436
128	226	152	266	501	529
166	247	197	283	571	604
111	272	264	343	396	626
230	304	223	349*	635*	635*
304	333	254	437	688	767
273	334	249	490	358	812
294	342	258	552	506	971
284	347	269	576	1028	1151
304	355	583*	583*	1229*	1229*
117	359	534	687	1145	1237
247	365	510	743	1323*	1323*
341	378	171	1115	1349*	1349*
209	442	642	1447*	1482*	1482*
395	506	1584*	1584*	1492*	1492*
332	517	1812*	1812*	1076	1501
393	546	697	1865*	1553*	1553*
518	620	1908*	1908*	1352	1597*
487	670			1604*	1604*
608	702			736	1648
518	806			1820*	1820*
516	871			1989*	1989*
270	946				
1160	1355				
955	1392				
2182*	2182*				
2270*	2270*				
2331*	2331*				

Table C.9. Times (days) from remission to relapse and from remission to death for leukæmia patients in three treatment groups. Asterisks indicate censoring. (Matthews, 1988, from Glucksberg *et al.*)

C.10 Leukæmia patients

Relapse	Death
238	571
72	179
99	100
140	204
294	67
937	21
517	159
126	123
783	63*
56	11
889*	—
246	151
951*	—
931*	—
146	40

Table C.10. Times (days) from remission to relapse and to death for leukæmia patients, with censored values indicated by an asterisk. (Clayton, 1988, with corrections)

C.11 Breast cancer

Initial	0	3	6	12	24	60
2	2	2	2	2	2	0
2	2	2	2	0		
1	1	0				
1	2	1	2	2	2	0
2	2	2	2	2	1	0
2	2	2	2	0		
2	2	1	2	2	0	
1	2	1	0			
2	2	2	2	2		
1	1	0				
1	1	0				
2	2	2	2	0		
1	1	0				
1	2	2	2	0		
1	1					
1	1	0				
2	2	2	2	0		
1	1	1	0			
2	2	0				
2	2	1	1	1	0	
1	1	0				
1	2	2	2	2	2	
1	2	0				
2	2	1	—	0		
2	2	2	2	2	0	
1	1	1	1	1	0	
1	2	1	1	1	0	
1	2	2	2	2	0	
1	2	1	1	0		
1	2	2	1	0		
1	2	1	1	1		
2	2	2	1	1	0	
1	2	1	1	0		
2	2	2	2	0		
2	2	2	0			
1	1	0				
1	1	0				

Table C.11. Ambulatory status of 37 breast cancer patients over a five-year period (months). 0, dead; 1, unable to walk; 2, able to walk. (de Stavola, 1988)

C.12 Prednisolone concentrations

				Hours					
0.25	0.5	1	2	3	4	6	8	12	24
				Tablet A					
103.0	194.0	254.0	170.0	149.0	127.0	64.8	41.6	8.6	11.8
228.0	345.0	290.0	225.0	203.0	158.0	67.2	40.4	8.0	0.0
5.4	57.8	181.0	204.0	142.0	149.0	106.0	34.6	21.9	0.0
10.3	70.8	214.0	179.0	170.0	173.0	68.9	32.3	23.9	9.8
209.0	288.0	266.0	210.0	218.0	121.0	48.8	53.1	25.3	0.0
81.0	202.0	263.0	209.0	200.0	220.0	130.0	62.1	25.4	0.0
3.0	138.0	390.0	310.0	305.0	222.0	142.0	73.0	31.6	11.3
0.0	73.0	194.0	189.0	152.0	148.0	63.0	34.2	19.4	0.0
14.5	125.0	201.0	209.0	228.0	129.0	82.5	47.0	3.9	1.3
81.1	217.0	222.0	206.0	169.0	123.0	76.2	25.0	22.8	0.0
19.0	96.1	114.0	165.0	148.0	146.0	94.6	46.6	23.4	0.0
6.2	30.0	173.0	202.0	168.0	135.0	95.6	69.9	20.4	9.4
				Tablet B					
62.3	268.0	249.0	192.0	190.0	129.0	53.2	23.5	11.4	11.2
116.0	178.0	205.0	219.0	161.0	116.0	32.2	17.2	7.3	0.0
29.8	138.0	224.0	196.0	192.0	158.0	105.0	70.2	22.5	0.9
28.5	79.2	173.0	286.0	305.0	229.0	126.0	79.5	25.2	15.7
21.6	154.0	244.0	246.0	357.0	222.0	119.0	58.5	26.8	1.7
76.6	253.0	267.0	242.0	211.0	164.0	98.4	57.2	22.5	2.3
0.0	50.8	168.0	289.0	255.0	170.0	109.0	67.1	26.2	8.3
6.7	160.0	184.0	197.0	246.0	165.0	103.0	69.0	2.0	0.0
22.4	125.0	222.0	166.0	134.0	148.0	52.9	19.0	26.3	12.2
0.0	77.5	163.0	174.0	199.0	170.0	102.0	84.4	27.4	2.3
8.3	56.0	149.0	174.0	130.0	153.0	83.1	39.1	22.0	0.0
25.0	63.4	145.0	148.0	143.0	140.0	95.6	45.9	11.2	24.0

Table C.12. Plasma concentrations (ng/ml) following ingestion of a 5 mg tablet of prednisolone in two different formulations. (Sullivan *et al.*, 1974)

C.13 Indomethicin concentrations

					Hours					
0.25	0.5	0.75	1	1.25	2	3	4	5	6	8
1.50	0.94	0.78	0.48	0.37	0.19	0.12	0.11	0.08	0.07	0.05
2.03	1.63	0.71	0.70	0.64	0.36	0.32	0.20	0.25	0.12	0.08
2.72	1.49	1.16	0.80	0.80	0.39	0.22	0.12	0.11	0.08	0.08
1.85	1.39	1.02	0.89	0.59	0.40	0.16	0.11	0.10	0.07	0.07
2.05	1.04	0.81	0.39	0.30	0.23	0.13	0.11	0.08	0.10	0.06
2.31	1.44	1.03	0.84	0.64	0.42	0.24	0.17	0.13	0.10	0.09

Table C.13. Plasma concentrations (μg/ml) following intravenous injection of indomethicin for six human subjects. (Davidian and Giltinan, 1995, p. 18, from Kwan *et al.*)

C.14 Ephedrine concentrations

					Hours					
0.25	0.5	0.75	1	2	3	4	6	8	10	24
2.5	5.1	14.3	17.1	20.5	21.6	23.3	16.2	14.6	12.0	4.7
1.9	10.8	21.1	28.5	30.9	30.9	30.2	20.0	17.3	13.5	3.5
2.4	11.5	18.1	31.2	35.7	36.4	30.6	24.2	20.0	12.2	2.4
4.9	9.8	18.2	20.1	31.2	27.5	26.0	22.6	15.5	13.4	2.7
3.3	14.7	25.6	38.0	35.6	29.8	29.7	24.6	20.5	16.0	2.5
3.9	13.5	17.8	21.0	22.8	23.0	19.1	14.4	11.8	9.8	1.1
0.5	9.0	15.5	20.9	24.7	24.3	22.8	18.0	14.4	8.9	3.2
2.0	5.3	16.2	21.7	25.4	28.0	23.0	21.0	13.6	10.0	1.2

Table C.14. Blood concentrations of ephedrine (ng/ml) in eight healthy male volunteers after an oral dose of Sho-seiryu-to. (Yafune, 1999)

C.15 Blood glucose levels

−15	0	30	60	90	Time (min) 120 2:00	180	240	300	360	420
5.03	4.99	9.10	10.03	9.20	8.31	7.92	4.86	4.63	3.52	4.17
4.51	4.50	8.74	8.80	7.10	8.20	7.42	5.79	4.85	4.94	2.07
4.87	5.12	6.32	9.48	9.88	6.28	5.58	5.26	4.10	4.25	4.55
4.55	4.44	5.56	8.39	7.85	7.40	6.23	4.59	4.31	3.96	4.05
4.79	4.82	9.29	8.99	8.15	5.71	5.24	4.95	5.06	5.24	4.74
4.33	4.48	8.06	8.49	4.50	7.15	5.91	4.27	4.78	—	5.72
					6:00					
4.22	4.92	8.09	6.74	4.30	4.28	4.59	4.49	5.29	4.95	4.34
4.52	4.22	8.46	9.12	7.50	6.02	4.66	4.69	4.26	4.29	4.47
4.47	4.47	7.95	7.21	6.35	5.58	4.57	3.90	3.44	4.18	4.32
4.27	4.33	6.61	6.89	5.64	4.85	4.82	3.82	4.31	3.81	2.92
4.81	4.85	6.08	8.28	5.73	5.68	4.66	4.62	4.85	4.69	4.86
4.61	4.68	6.01	7.35	6.38	6.16	4.41	4.96	4.33	4.54	4.81
					10:00					
4.90	4.50	7.84	5.46	5.08	4.32	3.91	3.99	4.15	4.41	
4.61	4.65	7.90	6.13	4.45	4.17	4.96	4.36	4.26	4.13	
5.37	5.35	7.94	5.64	5.06	5.49	4.77	4.48	4.39	4.45	
5.10	5.22	7.20	4.95	4.45	3.88	3.65	4.21	—	4.44	
5.34	4.91	5.69	8.21	2.97	4.30	4.18	4.93	5.16	5.54	
5.24	5.04	8.72	4.85	5.57	6.33	4.81	4.55	4.48	5.15	

					Time (min)					
−15	0	30	60	90	120	180	240	300	360	420
					14:00					
4.91	4.18	9.00	9.74	6.95	6.92	4.66	3.45	4.20	4.63	
4.16	3.42	7.09	6.98	6.13	5.36	6.13	3.67	4.37	4.31	
4.95	4.40	7.00	7.80	7.78	7.30	5.82	5.14	3.59	4.00	
3.82	4.00	6.56	6.48	5.66	7.74	4.45	4.07	3.73	3.58	
3.76	4.70	6.76	4.98	5.02	5.95	4.90	4.79	5.25	5.42	
4.13	3.95	5.53	8.55	7.09	5.34	5.56	4.23	3.95	4.29	
					18:00					
4.05	3.78	8.71	7.12	6.17	4.22	4.31	3.15	3.64	3.88	
3.94	4.14	7.82	8.68	6.22	5.10	5.16	4.38	4.22	4.27	
4.19	4.22	7.45	8.07	6.84	6.86	4.79	3.87	3.60	4.92	
4.31	4.45	7.34	6.75	7.55	6.42	5.75	4.56	4.30	3.92	
4.30	4.71	7.44	7.08	6.30	6.50	4.50	4.36	4.83	4.50	
4.45	4.12	7.14	5.68	6.07	5.96	5.20	4.83	4.50	4.71	
					22:00					
4.60	4.72	9.53	10.02	10.25	9.29	5.45	4.82	4.09	3.52	3.92
4.33	4.10	4.36	6.92	9.06	8.11	5.69	5.91	5.65	4.58	3.79
4.42	4.07	5.48	9.05	8.04	7.19	4.87	5.40	4.35	4.51	4.66
4.38	4.54	8.86	10.01	10.47	9.91	6.11	4.37	3.38	4.02	3.84
5.06	5.04	8.86	9.97	8.45	6.58	4.74	4.28	4.04	4.34	4.35
4.43	4.75	6.95	6.64	7.72	7.03	6.38	5.17	4.71	5.14	5.19

Table C.15. Blood glucose levels (mg/10 l) of six volunteers after meals at various times. (Crowder and Hand, 1990, p. 14)

C.16   Theophylline concentrations

Id											
1	0	0.27	0.58	1.15	2.03	3.57	5.00	7.00	9.22	12.10	23.85
	0	1.29	3.08	6.44	6.32	5.53	4.94	4.02	3.46	2.78	0.92
2	0	0.25	0.50	1.02	2.02	3.48	5.00	6.98	9.00	12.05	24.22
	0.15	0.85	2.35	5.02	6.58	7.09	6.66	5.25	4.39	3.53	1.15
3	0	0.25	0.52	0.98	2.02	3.53	5.05	7.15	9.07	12.10	24.12
	0	3.05	3.05	7.31	7.56	6.59	5.88	4.73	4.57	3.00	1.25
4	0	0.25	0.50	0.98	1.98	3.60	5.02	7.03	9.03	12.12	24.08
	0	4.86	7.24	8.00	6.81	5.87	5.22	4.45	3.62	2.69	0.86
5	0	0.27	0.58	1.02	2.02	3.62	5.08	7.07	9.00	12.15	24.17
	0	4.40	6.90	8.20	7.80	7.50	6.20	5.30	4.90	3.70	1.05
6	0	0.27	0.52	1.00	1.92	3.50	5.02	7.03	9.00	12.00	24.30
	0	1.72	7.91	8.31	8.33	6.85	6.08	5.40	4.55	3.01	0.90
7	0	0.35	0.60	1.07	2.13	3.50	5.02	7.02	9.02	11.98	24.65
	0	1.89	4.60	8.60	8.38	7.54	6.88	5.78	5.33	4.19	1.15
8	0	0.30	0.63	1.05	2.02	3.53	5.02	7.17	8.80	11.60	24.43
	0	7.37	9.03	7.14	6.33	5.66	5.67	4.24	4.11	3.16	1.12
9	0	0.25	0.50	1.00	2.00	3.52	5.07	7.07	9.03	12.05	24.15
	0	1.25	3.96	7.82	9.72	9.75	8.57	6.59	6.11	4.57	1.17
10	0	0.37	0.77	1.02	2.05	3.55	5.05	7.08	9.38	12.10	23.70
	0.24	2.89	5.22	6.41	7.83	10.21	9.18	8.02	7.14	5.68	2.42
11	0	0.25	0.57	1.12	2.02	3.82	5.10	7.03	9.05	12.12	24.37
	0.74	2.84	6.57	10.50	9.66	8.58	8.36	7.47	6.89	5.94	3.28
12	0	0.30	0.52	1.00	2.02	3.50	5.02	7.02	9.10	12.00	24.35
	0	2.02	5.63	11.40	9.33	8.74	7.56	7.09	5.90	4.37	1.57

1	2	3	4	5	6	7	8	9	10	11	12
4.02	4.40	4.53	4.40	5.86	4.00	4.95	4.53	3.10	5.50	4.92	5.30
79.6	72.4	70.5	72.7	54.6	80.0	64.6	70.5	86.4	58.2	65.0	60.5

Table C.16. Top panel: times (h, first line) from oral administration and corresponding serum theophylline concentrations (mg/l, second line) over 24 hours for 12 subjects. Bottom panel: their doses (mg/kg, first line) and weights (kg, second line). (Davidian and Giltinan, 1995, pp. 145–147, from Upton)

C.17 Declomycin concentrations

Hours	Fasting	No dairy products	Whole milk	Aluminium hydroxide
0	0.0	0.0	0.0	0.0
1	0.7	1.0	0.1	0.2
2	1.1	1.2	0.3	0.3
3	1.4	1.7	0.4	0.4
4	2.1	2.0	0.4	0.5
5	2.0	—	0.4	0.5
6	1.8	2.1	0.4	0.5
12	1.4	1.8	0.3	0.4
18	—	—	0.2	0.3
24	0.8	1.1	0.1	0.2
48	0.4	0.7	0.0	0.1
72	0.2	0.3	—	0.0
96	0.1	0.2	—	—

Table C.17. Average serum concentrations of Declomycin over time under four experimental conditions. (Notari, 1987, p. 186)

C.18 Propoxyphene concentrations

1/12	1/4	1	3	6	9	24=0
\multicolumn{7}{c}{Subject 1}						
0	0	20	41	28	30	0
9	0	22	52	28	23	12
364	406	384	248	77	78	30
48	76	153	178	117	77	24
40	63	160	136	120	44	27
533	490	336	129	128	60	36
37	36	49	150	83	39	0
18	14	82	33	25	6	7
\multicolumn{7}{c}{Subject 2}						
12	13	56	48	15	10	20
64	108	288	252	142	36	14
16	47	104	120	76	37	22
396	534	445	244	114	90	33
422	392	330	184	117	61	12
17	16	84	73	23	19	15
62	236	252	136	157	61	25
27	28	90	97	53	47	14
\multicolumn{7}{c}{Subject 3}						
117	353	220	138	75	49	8
0	6	8	41	29	16	10
35	132	234	122	100	84	26
33	42	126	179	95	73	32
2	3	14	94	60	33	27
84	174	294	158	117	97	23
30	18	131	114	74	74	32
486	286	172	200	107	118	40
\multicolumn{7}{c}{Subject 4}						
33	88	167	114	92	61	16
283	243	230	67	60	34	4
10	7	6	60	32	23	16
16	12	28	51	24	21	3
0	0	25	16	8	2	0
10	10	10	20	12	13	0
295	269	310	163	65	36	10
136	237	254	124	84	55	15

Table C.18. Concentrations of propoxyphene (μg/l) in the plasma of four normal male volunteers, each in two four-day periods. See Table 7.9 for details of the design. (Rodda *et al.*, 1971)

C.19 Phenylbiguanide and blood pressure

		Dose			
6.25	12.5	25	50	100	200
		Placebo			
1.50	1.50	5.0	16	20	18
0.75	3.00	3.0	14	22	24
1.00	1.25	4.0	12	27	29
1.25	1.50	6.0	19	33	33
0.50	4.50	10	26	37	32
		MDL 72222			
2.40	2.50	1.5	2.0	9.0	19
0.75	2.30	3.0	5.0	26	25
1.40	1.70	1.0	2.0	15	28
2.60	1.20	2.0	3.0	11	22
1.25	0.75	4.0	9.0	25	37

Table C.19. Change in blood pressure in a study involving five rabbits subjected to increasing doses of phenylbiguanide under two treatments. (Pinheiro and Bates, 2000, pp. 438–439)

C.20 ELISA for anticoronavirus

				Dilution			
Month	1/30	1/90	1/270	1/810	1/2430	1/7290	1/21 869	1/65 609
May	1.909	1.856	1.838	1.579	1.057	0.566	0.225	0.072
	1.956	1.876	1.841	1.584	1.072	0.561	0.229	0.114
June	1.886	1.853	1.747	1.424	0.781	0.377	0.153	0.053
	1.880	1.870	1.772	1.406	0.759	0.376	0.138	0.058

Table C.20. Two pairs of ELISAs for anticoronavirus antibodies in the serum of a cow performed in each of May and June. (Huet *et al.*, 1996, p. 7)

C.21 Cortisol radioimmunological assay

0	0	0.02	0.04	0.06	0.08	0.1	0.2
2868	2779	2615	2474	2152	2114	1862	1364
2785	2588	2651	2573	2307	2052	1935	1412
2849	2701	2506	2378	2101	2016	1800	1377
2805	2752	2498	2494	2216	2030	1871	1304

0.4	0.6	0.8	1	1.5	2	4	∞
910	702	586	501	392	330	250	131
919	701	596	495	358	351	261	135
855	689	561	478	399	343	244	134
875	696	562	493	394	333	242	133

Table C.21. Radioimmunological assay of cortisol: counts/min with doses measured in ng/0.1 ml. (Huet *et al.*, 1996, p. 4)

C.22 ELISA for allergens

Concentration (ng/ml)							
80	40	20	10	5	2.5	1.25	0.625
378.414	283.358	170.452	77.009	33.525	16.392	9.355	3.787
361.661	243.582	136.202	59.745	26.648	13.107	8.315	3.798
352.349	235.732	121.814	53.743	23.763	12.528	7.831	3.359
372.952	279.671	166.034	71.845	32.336	15.638	8.933	4.442
366.361	258.437	153.757	70.436	30.486	14.875	9.055	3.362
373.120	271.553	154.617	68.633	29.353	14.964	8.964	3.428
373.930	262.321	142.475	61.374	27.711	13.473	8.947	3.263
353.675	244.266	130.652	57.912	25.404	13.036	7.926	3.234
360.148	259.249	144.234	66.141	29.338	15.467	8.717	3.187
373.587	256.040	144.486	64.300	29.367	13.537	8.325	3.376
380.598	269.563	161.302	70.112	30.697	15.663	8.902	3.281
339.111	253.164	141.192	62.941	27.308	13.442	8.165	3.523

Table C.22. ELISA immunoassay for use in determining allergic asthma in relation to house dust from 12 microtitre plates measured in optical density change/sec. Each row of the table corresponds, in order, to one column of the plate. (Higgins *et al.*, 1998)

C.23 Penicillin G and theophylline

Hour	Penicillin G concentration 10^2 M	Theophylline concentration mg
0.0	9.00	300
1.0	7.40	278
2.0	6.05	246
3.0	5.00	—
4.0	4.08	205
5.0	3.34	—
6.0	2.75	146
7.0	2.25	—
8.0	1.85	105
10.0	1.25	50
12.0	—	6
24.0	0.00	—

Table C.23. Assay of penicillin G and rate of release of theophylline. (Notari, 1987, pp. 8, 14)

Bibliography

1. Aalen, O.O. and Husebye, E. (1991) Statistical analysis of repeated events forming renewal processes. *Statistics in Medicine* **10**, 1227–1240.
2. Aitkin, M.A. and Clayton, D.G. (1980) The fitting of exponential, Weibull, and extreme value distributions to complex censored survival data using GLIM. *Applied Statistics* **29**, 156–163.
3. Aitkin, M.A., Francis, B., Hinde, J., and Anderson, D. (1989) *Statistical Modelling in GLIM*. Oxford: Oxford University Press.
4. Akaike, H. (1973) Information theory and an extension of the maximum likelihood principle. In Petrov, B.N. and Csàki, F. (eds) *Second International Symposium on Inference Theory*, Budapest: Akadémiai Kiadó, pp. 267–281.
5. Alberts, B., Bray, D., Lewis, J., Raff, M., Roberts, K., and Watson, J.D. (1994, 3rd edn.) *Molecular Biology of the Cell*. New York: Garland Publishing.
6. Alphey, L. (1997) *DNA Sequencing. From Experimental Methods to Bioinformatics*. Oxford: BIOS Scientific Publishers.
7. Altham, P.M.E. (1978) Two generalizations of the binomial distribution. *Applied Statistics* **27**, 162–167.
8. Altman, D.G. (1991) *Practical Statistics for Medical Research*. London: Chapman & Hall.
9. Anderson, R.M. and May, R.M. (1991) *Infectious Diseases of Humans. Dynamics and Control*. Oxford: Oxford University Press.
10. Anderson, S., Bankier, A.T., Barrell, B.G., de Bruijn, M.H.L., Coulson, A.R., Drouin, J., Eperon, I.C., Nierlich, D.P., Roe, B.A., Sanger, F., Schreier, P.H., Smith, A.J.H., Staden, R., and Young, I.G. (1981) Sequence and organization of the human mitochondrial genome. *Nature* **290**, 457–465.
11. Andrews, D.F. and Herzberg, A.M. (1985) *Data. A Collection of Problems from Many Fields for the Student and Research Worker*. Berlin: Springer-Verlag.
12. Armstrong, B.K., White, E., and Saracci, R. (1992) *Principles of Exposure Measurement in Epidemiology*. Oxford: Oxford University Press.
13. Bartlett, M.S. (1960) *Stochastic Population Models in Ecology and Epidemiology*. London: Methuen.
14. Bates, D.M. and Watts, D.G. (1988) *Nonlinear Regression Analysis and its Applications*. New York: John Wiley.
15. Bauer, L.A. (1983) Primer on clinical pharmacokinetics. *American Journal of Hospital Pharmacology* **40**, 1637–1641.
16. Becker, R.A. and Chambers, J.M. (1984) *S: An Interactive Environment for Data Analysis and Graphics*. Monterey: Wadsworth.

17. Bishop, M.J. and Rawlings, C.J. (1997, eds.) *DNA and Protein Sequence Analysis.* Oxford: Oxford University Press.
18. Box, G.E.P. (1950) Problems in the analysis of growth and wear curves. *Biometrics* **6**, 362–389.
19. Box, G.E.P. and Hunter, W.G. (1962) A useful method for model-building. *Technometrics* **4**, 301–318.
20. Braun, M. (1983) *Differential Equations and their Applications.* Berlin: Springer-Verlag.
21. Bunke, H. and Bunke, O. (1989) *Nonlinear Regression, Functional Relations, and Robust Methods.* New York: John Wiley.
22. Chambers, J.M. and Hastie, T.J. (1992) *Statistical Models in S.* Monterey: Wadsworth.
23. Checkoway, H., Pearce, N.E., and Crawford-Brown, D.J. (1989) *Research Methods in Occupational Epidemiology.* Oxford: Oxford University Press.
24. Clayton, D.G. (1988) The analysis of event history data: a review of progress and outstanding problems. *Statistics in Medicine* **7**, 819–841.
25. Clayton, D.G. and Hills, M. (1993) *Statistical Models in Epidemiology.* Oxford: Oxford University Press.
26. Cox, D.R. (1972) Regression models and life tables. *Journal of the Royal Statistical Society* **B34**, 187–220.
27. Crowder, M.J. (1996) Keep timing the pills: statistical analysis of pill dissolution rates. *Applied Statistics* **45**, 323–334.
28. Crowder, M.J. and Hand, D.J. (1990) *Analysis of Repeated Measures.* London: Chapman & Hall.
29. Davidian, M. and Giltinan, D.M. (1993) Some simple methods for estimating intraindividual variability in nonlinear mixed effects models. *Biometrics* **49**, 59–73.
30. Davidian, M. and Giltinan, D.M. (1995) *Nonlinear Models for Repeated Measurement Data.* London: Chapman & Hall.
31. Day, N.E. (1966) Fitting curves to longitudinal data. *Biometrics* **22**, 276–291.
32. de Stavola, B.L. (1988) Testing departures from time homogeneity in multistate Markov processes. *Applied Statistics* **37**, 242–250.
33. Dear, P.H. (1997, ed.) *Genome Mapping.* Oxford: Oxford University Press.
34. Dennis, J.E. and Schnabel, R.B. (1983) *Numerical Methods for Unconstrained Optimization and Nonlinear Equations.* New York: Prentice Hall.
35. Dettman, J.W. (1986) *Introduction to Linear Algebra and Differential Equations.* New York: Dover.
36. Diaconis, P. and Ylvisaker, D. (1979) Conjugate priors for exponential families. *Annals of Statistics* **7**, 269–281.
37. Dobson, A.J. (1990) *An Introduction to Generalized Linear Models.* London: Chapman & Hall.
38. Dunson, D.B. and Haseman, J.K. (1999) Modeling tumor onset and multiplicity using transition models with latent variables. *Biometrics* **55**, 965–970.

39. Durbin, R., Eddy, S., Krogh, A., and Mitchison, G. (1998) *Biological Sequence Analysis. Probabilistic Models of Proteins and Nucleic Acids.* Cambridge: Cambridge University Press.
40. Efron, B. (1986) Double exponential families and their use in generalized linear regression. *Journal of the American Statistical Association* **81**, 709–721.
41. Ekholm, B.P., Fox, T.L., and Bolognese, J.A. (1989) Dose-response: relating doses and plasma levels to efficacy and adverse experiences. In Berry, D.A. *Statistical Methodology in the Pharmaceutical Sciences.* Basle: Marcel Dekker, pp. 117–138.
42. Fahrmeir, L. and Tutz, G. (1994) *Multivariate Statistical Modelling Based on Generalized Linear Models.* Berlin: Springer-Verlag.
43. Farewell, V.T. (1982) The use of mixture models for the analysis of survival data with long-term survivors. *Biometrics* **38**, 1041–1046.
44. Finney, D.J. (1978) *Statistical Method in Biological Assay.* Edinburgh: Griffin.
45. Fisher, R.A. (1937) The wave of advance of advantageous genes. *Annals of Eugenics* **7**, 255–369.
46. Fisher, R.A. (1955) Statistical methods and scientific induction. *Journal of the Royal Statistical Society* **B17**, 69–78.
47. Frome, E.L. (1983) The analysis of rates using Poisson regression models. *Biometrics* **39**, 665–674.
48. Fullerton, S.M., Harding, R.M., Boyce, A.J., and Clegg, J.B. (1994) Molecular and population genetic analysis of allelic sequence diversity at the human β-globin locus. *Proceedings of the National Academy of Science, USA* **91**, 1805–1809.
49. Gail, M.H., Santner, T.J., and Brown, C.C. (1980) An analysis of comparative carcinogenesis experiments based on multiple times to tumor. *Biometrics* **36**, 255–266.
50. Gallo, B.V., Hinson, J.L., and Weidler, D.J. (1993) Pharmacokinetic profile of flosequinan in patients with compromised renal function. *Journal of Pharmaceutical Sciences* **82**, 282–285.
51. Gentleman, R. and Ihaka, R. (2000) Lexical scope and statistical computing. *Journal of Computational Graphics and Statistics* **9**, 491–508.
52. Gibaldi, M. and Perrier, D. (1982) *Pharmacokinetics.* Basle: Marcel Dekker.
53. Gómez, E., Gómez-Villegas, M.A., and Marin, J.M. (1998) A multivariate generalization of the power exponential family of distributions. *Communications in Statistics* **A27**, 589–600.
54. Gribskov, M. and Devereux, J. (1992, eds.) *Sequence Analysis Primer.* Oxford: Oxford University Press.
55. Guest, P.B. (1991) *Laplace Transforms and an Introduction to Distributions.* New York: Ellis Horwood.
56. Gutfreund, H. (1995) *Kinetics for the Life Sciences. Receptors, Transmitters, and Catalysts.* Cambridge: Cambridge University Press.
57. Guttorp, P. (1995) *Stochastic Modeling of Scientific Data.* London: Chapman & Hall.
58. Harvey, A.C. (1989) *Forecasting, Structural Time Series Models and the Kalman Filter.* Cambridge: Cambridge University Press.

59. Heitjan, D.F. (1991a) Generalized Norton–Simon models of tumour growth. *Statistics in Medicine* **10**, 1075–1088.
60. Heitjan, D.F. (1991b) Nonlinear modeling of serial immunologic data: a case study. *Journal of the American Statistical Association* **86**, 891–898.
61. Henderson, R. and Matthews, J.N.S. (1993) An investigation of changepoints in the annual number of cases of hæmolytic uræmic syndrome. *Applied Statistics* **42**, 461–471.
62. Higgins, K.M., Davidian, M., Chew, G., and Burge, H. (1998) The effect of serial dilution error on calibration inference in immunoassay. *Biometrics* **54**, 19–32.
63. Hinson, J.L., Hind, I.D., and Weidler, D.J. (1994) Pharmacokinetics, safety, and tolerability of flosequinan in patients with hepatic dysfunction. *Journal of Pharmaceutical Sciences* **83**, 382–385.
64. Hopper, J.L. and Young, G.P. (1988) A random walk model for evaluating clinical trials involving serial observations. *Statistics in Medicine* **7**, 581–590.
65. Hougaard, P. (1986) A class of multivariate failure time distributions. *Biometrika* **73**, 671–678.
66. Hougaard, P. (1999) Multi-state models: a review. *Lifetime Data Analysis* **5**, 239–264.
67. Hougaard, P. (2000) *Analysis of Multivariate Survival Data*. Berlin: Springer-Verlag.
68. Huet, S., Bouvier, A., Gruet, M.A., and Jolivet, E. (1996) *Statistical Tools for Nonlinear Regression*. Berlin: Springer-Verlag.
69. Ihaka, R. and Gentleman, R. (1996) R: a language for data analysis and graphics. *Journal of Computational Graphics and Statistics*, **5**, 299–314.
70. Joe, H. (1997) *Multivariate Models and Dependence Concepts*. London: Chapman & Hall
71. Jones, R.H. (1993) *Longitudinal Data Analysis with Serial Correlation: A State-space Approach*. London: Chapman & Hall.
72. Jørgensen, B. (1987) Exponential dispersion models. *Journal of the Royal Statistical Society* **B49**, 127–162.
73. Juang, B.H. and Rabiner, L.R. (1991) Hidden Markov models for speech recognition. *Technometrics* **33**, 251–272.
74. Kahn, H.A. and Sempos, C.T. (1989) *Statistical Methods in Epidemiology*. Oxford: Oxford University Press.
75. Kamali, F. and Edwards, C. (1995) Possible role of metabolite in flosequinan-related mortality. *Clinical Pharmacokinetics* **29**, 396–403.
76. Kay, R. (1986) A Markov model for analyzing cancer markers and disease states in survival studies. *Biometrics* **42**, 855–865.
77. Keene, O.N. (1995) The log transformation is special. *Statistics in Medicine* **14**, 811–819.
78. Kelsey, J.L., Thompson, W.D., and Evans, A.S. (1986) *Methods in Observational Epidemiology*. Oxford: Oxford University Press.
79. Khoury, M.J., Beaty, T.H., and Cohen, B.H. (1993) *Fundamentals of Genetic Epidemiology*. Oxford: Oxford University Press.
80. Klein, J.P., Klotz, J.H., and Grever, M.R. (1984) A biological marker model for predicting disease transition. *Biometrics* **40**, 927–936.

81. Krewski, D., Leroux, B.G., Bleuer, S.R., and Broekhoven, L.H. (1993) Modeling the Ames *Salmonella*/microsome assay. *Biometrics* **49**, 499–510.
82. Laird, N.M. and Ware, J.H. (1982) Random-effects models for longitudinal data. *Biometrics* **38**, 963–974.
83. Lambert, D. (1992) Zero-inflated Poisson regression, with an application to defects in manufacturing. *Technometrics* **34**, 1–14.
84. Lambert, P. and Lindsey, J.K. (1999) Analysing financial returns using regression models based on non-symmetric stable distributions. *Applied Statistics* **48**, 409–424.
85. Lilienfeld, D.E. and Stolley, P.D. (1994) *Foundations of Epidemiology*. Oxford: Oxford University Press.
86. Lindsey, J.K. (1995a) *Introductory Statistics. A Modelling Approach*. Oxford: Oxford University Press.
87. Lindsey, J.K. (1995b) Fitting parametric counting processes by using log linear models. *Applied Statistics* **44**, 201–212.
88. Lindsey, J.K. (1996) *Parametric Statistical Inference*. Oxford: Oxford University Press.
89. Lindsey, J.K. (1997) *Applying Generalized Linear Models*. Berlin: Springer-Verlag.
90. Lindsey, J.K. (1998) A study of interval censoring in parametric regression models. *Lifetime Data Analysis* **4**, 329–354.
91. Lindsey, J.K. (1999a, 2nd edn.) *Models for Repeated Measurements*. Oxford: Oxford University Press.
92. Lindsey, J.K. (1999b) Multivariate elliptically-contoured distributions for repeated measurements. *Biometrics* **56**, 1277–1280.
93. Lindsey, J.K. (1999c) Some statistical heresies (with discussion). *The Statistician* **48**, 1–40.
94. Lindsey, J.K., Jones, B., and Ebbutt, A.F. (1997) Simple models for repeated ordinal responses with an application to a seasonal rhinitis clinical trial. *Statistics in Medicine* **16**, 2873–2882.
95. Lindsey, P.J. (2001) Time alignment of repeated measurements in the analyses of several veterinary clinical trials. *Journal of Agricultural, Biological, and Environmental Studies* **6**, (in the press).
96. MacDonald, I.L. and Zucchini, W. (1997) *Hidden Markov and Other Models for Discrete-Valued Time Series*. London: Chapman & Hall.
97. Marks, J., Shaw, J.P., and Shen, C.K.J. (1986) Sequence organization and genomic complexity of primate θ_1 globin gene, a novel α-like gene. *Nature* **321**, 785–788.
98. Marshall, A.W. and Olkin, I. (1988) Families of multivariate distributions. *Journal of the American Statistical Association* **83**, 834–841.
99. Matis, J.H. and Kiffe, T.R. (2000) *Stochastic Population Models. A Compartmental Perspective*. Berlin: Springer-Verlag.
100. Matthews, D.E. (1988) Likelihood-based confidence intervals for functions of many parameters. *Biometrika* **75**, 139–144.
101. Matthews, J.N.S. (2000) *An Introduction to Randomized Controlled Clinical Trials*. London: Edward Arnold.

102. McCullagh, P. and Nelder, J.A. (1989, 2nd edn.) *Generalized Linear Models*. London: Chapman & Hall.
103. McGilchrist, C.A. and Aisbett, C.W. (1991) Regression with frailty in survival analysis. *Biometrics* **47**, 461–466.
104. Meager, A. (1999, ed.) *Gene Therapy Technologies, Applications and Regulations From Laboratory to Clinic*. New York: John Wiley.
105. Meinert, C.L. (1986) *Clinical Trials - Design, Conduct, and Analysis*. Oxford: Oxford University Press.
106. Mellen, B.G. (1999) Modeling epidemiologic typing data and likelihood inference for disease spread. *Journal of the American Statistical Association* **94**, 1015–1024.
107. Millqvist, E. (2000) Cough provocation with capsaicin is an objective way to test sensory hyperreactivity in patients with asthma-like symptoms. *Allergy* **55**, 546–550.
108. Morris, C.N. (1983) Natural exponential families with quadratic variance functions: statistical theory. *Annals of Statistics* **11**, 515–529.
109. Murray, J.D. (1993) *Mathematical Biology*. Berlin: Springer-Verlag.
110. Nelder, J.A. (1961) The fitting of a generalization of the logistic curve. *Biometrika* **17**, 89–100.
111. Nelder, J.A. (1962) An alternative form of a generalized logistic equation. *Biometrics* **18**, 614–616.
112. Nelder, J.A. (1966) Inverse polynomials, a useful group of multi-factor response functions. *Biometrics* **22**, 128–141.
113. Nelder, J.A. and Wedderburn, R.W.M. (1972) Generalized linear models. *Journal of the Royal Statistical Society* **A135**, 370–384.
114. Notari, R.E. (1987) *Biopharmaceutics and Clinical Pharmacokinetics. An Introduction*. Basle: Marcel Dekker.
115. Oldham, P.D. and Newell, D.J. (1977) Fluoridation of water supplies and cancer—a possible association? *Applied Statistics* **26**, 125–135.
116. Passaribu, U.S., Hawkes, A.G., and Wainwright, S.J. (1999) Statistical assumptions underlying the fitting of the Michaelis–Menten equation. *Journal of Applied Statistics* **26**, 327–341.
117. Pinheiro, J.C. and Bates, D.M. (2000) *Mixed-effects Models in S and S-Plus*. Berlin: Springer-Verlag.
118. Pocock, S.J. (1983) *Clinical Trials: A Practical Approach*. New York: John Wiley.
119. Potthoff, R.F. and Roy, S.N. (1964) A generalized multivariate analysis of variance model useful especially for growth curve problems. *Biometrika* **51**, 313–326.
120. Primrose, S.B. (1998) *Principles of Genome Analysis. A Guide to Mapping and Sequencing DNA from Different Organisms*. Oxford: Blackwell Science.
121. Rabiner, L.R. (1989) A tutorial on hidden Markov models and selected applications in speech recognition. *Proceedings of the IEEE* **77**, 257–286.
122. Rodda, B.E., Scholz, N.E., Gruber, C.M., and Wolen, R.L. (1971) Evaluation of plasma concentration of propoxyphene utilizing a hybrid principal components–analysis of variance technique. Case I—equimolar doses. Case II—equipotent doses. *Toxicology and Applied Pharmacology* **19**, 554–571.
123. Ross, G.J.S. (1990) *Nonlinear Estimation*. Berlin: Springer-Verlag.

124. Sandland, R.L. and McGilchrist, C.A. (1979) Stochastic growth curve analysis. *Biometrics* **35**, 255–271.
125. Schmidt, P. and Witte, A.D. (1988) *Predicting Recidivism using Survival Models.* Berlin: Springer-Verlag.
126. Seber, G.A.F. and Wild, C.J. (1989) *Nonlinear Regression.* New York: John Wiley.
127. Selvin, S. (1991) *Statistical Analysis of Epidemiological Data.* Oxford: Oxford University Press.
128. Senn, S. (1997) *Statistical Issues in Drug Development.* New York: John Wiley.
129. Shaw, J.P., Marks, J., and Shen, C.K.J. (1987) Evidence that the recently discovered θ_1-globin gene is functional in higher primates. *Nature* **326**, 717–720.
130. Shigesada, N. and Kawasaki, K. (1997) *Biological Invasions: Theory and Practice.* Oxford: Oxford University Press.
131. Skellam, J.G. (1951) Random dispersal in theoretical populations. *Biometrika* **38**, 196–218.
132. Song, P.X.K. (2000) Multivariate dispersion models generated from Gaussian copulas. *Scandinavian Journal of Statistics* **27**, 305–320.
133. Stukel, T.A. (1993) Comparison of methods for the analysis of longitudinal interval count data. *Statistics in Medicine* **12**, 1339–1351.
134. Sullivan, T.J., Still, R.G., Sakmar, E., Blair, D.C., and Wagner, J.G. (1974) *In vitro* and *in vivo* availability of some commercial prednisolone tablets. *Journal of Pharmacokinetics and Biopharmaceutics* **2**, 29–41.
135. Tweedie, M.C.K. (1947) Functions of a statistical variate with given means, with special reference to Laplacian distributions. *Proceedings of the Cambridge Philosophical Society* **43**, 41–49.
136. Vigilant, L., Stoneking, M., Harpending, H., Hawkes, K., and Wilson, A.C. (1991) African populations and the evolution of human mitochondrial DNA. *Science* **253**, 1503–1507.
137. Voit, E.O. and Knapp, R.G. (1997) Derivation of the linear-logistic model and Cox's proportional hazard model from a canonical system description. *Statistics in Medicine* **16**, 1705–1729.
138. Vonesh, E. and Chinchilli, V. (1997) *Linear and Nonlinear Models for the Analysis of Repeated Measurements.* Basle: Marcel Dekker.
139. Wakefield, J. (1996) The Bayesian analysis of population pharmacokinetics models. *Journal of the American Statistical Association* **91**, 62–75.
140. Wakefield, J. and Racine-Poon, A. (1995) An application of Bayesian population pharmacokinetic/pharmacodynamic models to dose recommendations. *Statistics in Medicine* **14**, 971–986.
141. Wallace, D.C. (1992) Mitochondrial genetics: a paradigm for aging and degenerative diseases? *Science* **256**, 628–632.
142. Wang, J.T.L., Shapiro, B.A., and Shasha, D. (1999, eds.) *Pattern Discovery in Biomolecular Data. Tools, Techniques, and Applications.* Oxford: Oxford University Press.
143. Wang, P., Puterman, M.L., Cockburn, I., and Le, N. (1996) Mixed Poisson regression models with covariate dependent rates. *Biometrics* **52**, 381–400.
144. Watson, D.G. (1999) *Pharmaceutical Analysis. A Textbook for Pharmacy Students and Pharmaceutical Chemists.* Edinburgh: Churchill Livingstone.

145. West, M., Harrison, P.J., and Migon, H.S. (1985) Dynamic generalized linear models and Bayesian forecasting. *Journal of the American Statistical Association* **80**, 73–97.
146. Whitehead, J. (1980) Fitting Cox's regression model to survival data using GLIM. *Applied Statistics* **29**, 268–275.
147. Whittemore, A.S. and Altschuler, B. (1976) Lung cancer incidence in cigarette smokers: further analysis of Doll and Hill's data for British physicians. *Biometrics* **32**, 805–816.
148. Wilkinson, G.N. and Rogers, C.E. (1973) Symbolic description of factorial models for analysis of variance. *Applied Statistics* **22**, 392–399.
149. Wynne, R.D., Crampton, E.L., and Hind, I.D. (1985) The pharmacokinetics and haemodynamics of BTS 49465 and its major metabolite in healthy volunteers. *European Journal of Clinical Pharmacology* **28**, 659–664.
150. Yafune, A. (1999) Application to pharmacokinetic analysis. In Akaike, H. and Kitagawa, G. (eds.) *The Practice of Time Series Analysis*. Berlin: Springer-Verlag, pp. 153–162.
151. Zeger, S.L., Liang, K.Y., and Albert, P.S. (1988) Models for longitudinal data: a generalized estimating equation approach. *Biometrics* **44**, 1049–1060.

Author index

Aalen, O.O., 216, 223, 255
Aisbett, C.W., 237, 260
Aitkin, M.A., 12, 21, 255
Akaike, H., 34, 255
Albert, P.S., 262
Alberts, B., 190, 255
Alphey, L., 190, 255
Altham, P.M.E., 11, 255
Altman, D.G., 27, 255
Altschuler, B., 231, 262
Anderson, D., 255
Anderson, R.M., 69, 255
Anderson, S., 187, 255
Andrews, D.F., 88, 255
Armstrong, B.K., 69, 255

Bankier, A.T., 255
Barrell, B.G., 255
Bartlett, M.S., 64, 65, 69, 255
Bates, D.M., v, 17, 21, 32, 155, 251, 255, 260
Bauer, L.A., 135, 255
Beaty, T.H., 258
Becker, R.A., 198, 255
Bishop, M.J., 190, 256
Blair, D.C., 261
Bleuer, S.R., 259
Bolognese, J.A., 257
Bouvier, A., 258
Box, G.E.P., 21, 37, 256
Boyce, A.J., 257
Braun, M., 21, 256
Bray, D., 255
Broekhoven, L.H., 259
Brown, C.C., 257
Bunke, H., 47, 256
Bunke, O., 47, 256
Burge, H., 258

Chambers, J.M., 198, 255, 256
Checkoway, H., 69, 232, 256
Chew, G., 258
Chinchilli, V., v, 21, 261
Clayton, D.G., 12, 69, 99, 242, 255, 256
Clegg, J.B., 257
Cockburn, I., 261
Cohen, B.H., 258
Coulson, A.R., 255
Cox, D.R., 223, 256

Crampton, E.L., 262
Crawford-Brown, D.J., 256
Crowder, M.J., 171–173, 247, 256

Davidian, M., v, 21, 111, 162, 163, 245, 248, 256, 258
Day, N.E., 51, 52, 256
de Bruijn, M.H.L., 255
de Stavola, B.L., 243, 256
Dear, P.H., 190, 256
Dennis, J.E., 14, 29, 256
Dettman, J.W., 21, 256
Devereux, J., 190, 257
Diaconis, P., 207, 256
Dobson, A.J., 21, 256
Drouin, J., 255
Dunson, D.B., 240, 256
Durbin, R., 181, 190, 220, 257

Ebbutt, A.F., 259
Eddy, S., 257
Edwards, C., 113, 119, 258
Efron, B., 11, 257
Ekholm, B.P., 142, 144, 146, 257
Eperon, I.C., 255
Evans, A.S., 258

Fahrmeir, L., 214, 257
Farewell, V.T., 12, 257
Finney, D.J., 174, 257
Fisher, R.A., 3, 44, 257
Fox, T.L., 257
Francis, B., 255
Frome, E.L., 70, 257
Fullerton, S.M., 183, 257

Gail, M.H., 239, 257
Gallo, B.V., 113, 257
Gentleman, R., vi, 194, 257, 258
Gibaldi, M., 135, 257
Giltinan, D.M., v, 21, 111, 162, 163, 245, 248, 256
Gómez, E., 212, 257
Gómez-Villegas, M.A., 257
Grever, M.R., 258
Gribskov, M., 190, 257
Gruber, C.M., 260
Gruet, M.A., 258

Guest, P.B., 21, 257
Gutfreund, H., 21, 43, 135, 257
Guttorp, P., 221, 257

Hand, D.J., 247, 256
Harding, R.M., 257
Harpending, H., 261
Harrison, P.J., 262
Harvey, A.C., 214, 257
Haseman, J.K., 240, 256
Hastie, T.J., 198, 256
Hawkes, A.G., 260
Hawkes, K., 261
Heitjan, D.F., 12, 42, 75, 76, 79, 258
Henderson, R., 58, 258
Herzberg, A.M., 88, 255
Higgins, K.M., 252, 258
Hills, M., 69, 256
Hind, I.D., 258, 262
Hinde, J., 255
Hinson, J.L., 113, 257, 258
Hopper, J.L., 94, 258
Hougaard, P., 99, 216, 258
Huet, S., 251, 252, 258
Hunter, W.G., 21, 256
Husebye, E., 216, 223, 255

Ihaka, R., vi, 194, 257, 258

Joe, H., 230, 258
Jolivet, E., 258
Jones, B., 259
Jones, R.H., 258
Jørgensen, B., 11, 258
Juang, B.H., 220, 258

Kahn, H.A., 69, 258
Kamali, F., 113, 119, 258
Kawasaki, K., 69, 261
Kay, R., 91, 258
Keene, O.N., 229, 258
Kelsey, J.L., 69, 258
Khoury, M.J., 69, 258
Kiffe, T.R., 135, 259
Klein, J.P., 90, 258
Klotz, J.H., 258
Knapp, R.G., 38, 261
Krewski, D., 164, 168, 169, 259
Krogh, A., 257

Laird, N.M., 37, 259
Lambert, D., 12, 259
Lambert, P., 14, 259
Le, N., 261
Leroux, B.G., 259
Lewis, J., 255
Liang, K.Y., 262
Lilienfeld, D.E., 69, 259

Lindsey, J.K., v, 9, 12–14, 21, 24, 25, 36, 76, 79,
  82, 99, 205, 210, 212, 226, 259
Lindsey, P.J., 38, 259

MacDonald, I.L., 221, 259
Marin, J.M., 257
Marks, J., 259, 261
Marshall, A.W., 11, 259
Matis, J.H., 135, 259
Matthews, D.E., 241, 259
Matthews, J.N.S., 58, 82, 258, 259
May, R.M., 69, 255
McCullagh, P., 21, 260
McGilchrist, C.A., 38, 237, 260, 261
Meager, A., 190, 260
Meinert, C.L., 82, 260
Mellen, B.G., 68, 69, 260
Migon, H.S., 262
Millqvist, E., 147, 260
Mitchison, G., 257
Morris, C.N., 207, 260
Murray, J.D., 44, 46, 47, 69, 171, 260

Nelder, J.A., 9, 21, 38, 41, 260
Newell, D.J., 56, 260
Nierlich, D.P., 255
Notari, R.E., 135, 249, 253, 260

Oldham, P.D., 56, 260
Olkin, I., 11, 259

Passaribu, U.S., 159, 260
Pearce, N.E., 256
Perrier, D., 135, 257
Pinheiro, J.C., 155, 251, 260
Pocock, S.J., 82, 260
Potthoff, R.F., 37, 260
Primrose, S.B., 183, 190, 260
Puterman, M.L., 261

Rabiner, L.R., 220, 258, 260
Racine-Poon, A., 113, 261
Raff, M., 255
Rawlings, C.J., 190, 256
Roberts, K., 255
Rodda, B.E., 133, 250, 260
Roe, B.A., 255
Rogers, C.E., 28, 198–201, 262
Ross, G.J.S., v, 21, 30, 260
Roy, S.N., 37, 260

Sakmar, E., 261
Sandland, R.L., 38, 261
Sanger, F., 255
Santner, T.J., 257
Saracci, R., 255
Schmidt, P., 12, 261
Schnabel, R.B., 14, 29, 256

AUTHOR INDEX

Scholz, N.E., 260
Schreier, P.H., 255
Seber, G.A.F., v, 17, 21, 35, 47, 261
Selvin, S., 69, 261
Sempos, C.T., 69, 258
Senn, S., 82, 261
Shapiro, B.A., 261
Shasha, D., 261
Shaw, J.P., 259, 261
Shen, C.K.J., 259, 261
Shigesada, N., 69, 261
Skellam, J.G., 45, 261
Smith, A.J.H., 255
Song, P.X.K., 213, 261
Staden, R., 255
Still, R.G., 261
Stolley, P.D., 69, 259
Stoneking, M., 261
Stukel, T.A., 236, 261
Sullivan, T.J., 244, 261

Thompson, W.D., 258
Tutz, G., 214, 257
Tweedie, M.C.K., 11, 261

Vigilant, L., 188, 261
Voit, E.O., 38, 261
Vonesh, E., v, 21, 261

Wagner, J.G., 261

Wainwright, S.J., 260
Wakefield, J., 111, 113, 261
Wallace, D.C., 187, 261
Wang, J.T.L., 190, 261
Wang, P., 12, 261
Ware, J.H., 37, 259
Watson, D.G., 174, 261
Watson, J.D., 255
Watts, D.G., v, 17, 21, 32, 255
Wedderburn, R.W.M., 9, 260
Weidler, D.J., 257, 258
West, M., 214, 262
White, E., 255
Whitehead, J., 12, 262
Whittemore, A.S., 231, 262
Wild, C.J., v, 17, 21, 35, 47, 261
Wilkinson, G.N., 28, 198–201, 262
Wilson, A.C., 261
Witte, A.D., 12, 261
Wolen, R.L., 260
Wynne, R.D., 113, 262

Yafune, A., 245, 262
Ylvisaker, D., 207, 256
Young, G.P., 94, 258
Young, I.G., 255

Zeger, S.L., 206, 262
Zucchini, W., 221, 259

Subject index

absorbing barrier, 60, 86, 96, 226–228
absorption rate, 19, 43, 107–138, 199–201
accelerated failure time, 223
ACE, 147
acetone, 101–102, 240
acid phosphatase assay, 159–161
adenosine deaminase, 90–93, 102
adenosine triphosphate, 187
adjacent categories model, 88, 95
adverse effect, 74, 99, 142, 146
AIC, 15, 34–36
alignment, 181–182, 186
all subsets regression, 28
allergen assay, 176, 252
allergy, 97, 150, 152, 155
allometry, 41, 45
Alzheimer's disease, 188
ambulatory status, 102, 243
Ames microsome assay, 164–169
amino acid, 179–180, 186
analysis of variance, 6, 15, 18, 22
antacid, 93
antibody, 157
anticoronavirus assay, 174–176, 251
antihistamine, 96–99
apparent volume of distribution, 43, 107–135, 199–201
AR(1), 52–54, 209, 210
AR(M), 210, 214
area under the curve, 18, 107
arithmetic mean, 5, 17, 39, 111, 114, 116, 127, 147
asbestos, 71, 232
assay, 2, 74, 113, 157–169
    acid phosphatase, 159–161
    allergens, 176
    Ames microsome, 164–169
    anticoronavirus, 174–176, 251
    colorimetric enzyme, 159–161
    cortisol, 176, 252
    direct, 157
    DNase, 161–164, 174
    ELISA, 158–159, 161–164, 174
    enzyme-linked immunosorbent, 158–159
    high-pressure liquid chromatography, 158
    hybridization, 181
    indirect, 157
    penicillin G, 176–177, 253
    radioimmuno-, 158
    RIA, 158
asthma, 88, 138, 147, 252
    childhood, 176
asymptote, 31, 37–40, 42, 56, 75, 76, 79, 82, 150, 160, 165
ataxia, 188
ATP, 187
AUC, 18, 107, 121–123, 130
autocorrelation, 42, 209
autocovariance, 209
autoimmune disease, 75–83
autoregression, 36, 131, 132, 138, 143, 146, 155, 208–211, 214
    gamma, 135, 136
        generalized, 126–130
    log Cauchy, 135
    log logistic, 135
    log normal, 53, 54, 129, 135, 146, 172, 174, 177
    negative binomial, 79–81, 149–155
    normal, 53, 82, 209
    Poisson, 151, 152
    Weibull, 135
azathioprine, 75–83

barrier
    absorbing, 60, 86, 96, 226–228
    reflecting, 96
baseline, 24, 83, 96–99, 113, 118, 150–153, 233
baseline intensity function, 223
Bateman equation, 43
Bayes's formula, 215
benzene, 101–102, 240
Bernoulli distribution, 220
beta binomial distribution, 36
β-thalassæmia, 183
bias, 74, 223, 224
binomial distribution, 11, 68, 220
bioassay, 101, 157, 174
bioavailability, 18, 107, 124, 130, 131, 135, 169
birth intensity, 225
    nonhomogeneous, 225
birth process, 86, 88–90, 135, 227
    generalized, 227
    nonhomogeneous, 225
    pure, 225, 227
birth rate, 64

SUBJECT INDEX

blinding, 74, 76, 148
    double, 75, 83, 93, 97
blindness, 187
blood pressure, 26, 113, 251
    diastolic, 150–153
    systolic, 150, 152
bolus, 106, 108, 137, 245
Burr distribution, 217
    multivariate, 89, 218

C, 28, 194, 198
cancer, 74
    breast, 102, 243
    leukæmia, 102, 242
        myeloid, 90–93, 102
        nonlymphoblastic, 102, 241
    lung, 70–71, 231–232
    mammary, 101, 238–239
    neoplasms, 55–56, 69
    papilloma, 101–102, 240
    rectal polyps, 83, 233–236
canonical link function, 11, 14, 16, 207, 210
canonical parameter, 16, 207
capsaicin, 146–155
capsule, 107, 171
carbenoxolone, 93–96
carcinogenesis, 70, 101
carry-over effect, 132, 135
case–control design, 50
    asbestos, 71, 232
    lung cancer, 71, 232
Cauchy distribution, 36
    mixing, 53, 203
    multivariate, 212
censoring, 6, 12, 24, 101, 102, 195, 196, 198, 222–224, 237, 239, 241, 242
    failure, 223
    interval, 12
    left, 112, 118–119, 126, 127
    right, 12, 113, 217
    time, 223
    Type I, 223
    Type II, 223
centring, 30
chain terminator method, 181
change point, 46, 57–60
chemotherapy, 75–83, 88, 102
chicken pox, 65–67, 71
chromosome walking, 180
chronic external ophthalmoplegia, 188
class, 194
    data, 194–197
    formula, 201
clearance, 107
    creatinine, 118, 121, 124, 129
clinical trial, v, 42, 73–83, 85, 102, 146–155
    bladder cancer, 88–90
    double-blind, 75–83, 93, 96–99

ephedrin, 137
leukæmia, 102
    nonlymphoblastic, 102, 241
multiple sclerosis, 75–83
peptic œsophagitis, 93–96, 102–103
phases, 74
rectal polyps, 83, 233–236
rhinitis, 96–99
clustering, 13, 24, 26, 28, 67–69, 149, 153, 196, 197, 216, 218, 219
$C_{\max}$, 107, 121, 123
codon, 179, 183
    initiation, 180, 182
    termination, 180, 182
coefficient of dispersion, 142
coefficient of variation, 39
cohort design, 50, 71
colorimetric enzyme assay, 159–161
compartment model, 16, 18, 20, 33, 42–44, 46, 63, 64, 143
    first-order, 42–44, 106–139, 199–201
    zero-order, 44, 107, 132–135
competing risks, 86, 227
complementary log log link function, 41
compliance, 75
conclusions, 74
conditional distribution, 7, 23, 206, 208, 209, 212, 214, 215, 217–219
confounding, 50
conjugate distribution, 207
    mixing, 207, 215
consensus sequence, 181
constraint
    parameter, 30, 35
        conventional, 116
Consul distribution, 168
contagion process, 227
contagious, 63
contig, 181
continuation ratio model, 88, 95, 97–99
continuous time, 46, 215, 220, 221, 226
control group, 50, 68, 74, 93, 96, 101, 168
convergence, 30, 32–33
COPD, 147
copula, 213–214
    Gaussian, 143–146, 213–214
correlation matrix, 146, 211–214
cortisol assay, 176, 252
cost, 27
cough, 146–155
count update, 89–91, 219
counting process, 12, 224–228
counts, 6–7
    zero, 210
covariance matrix, 146, 211–213
covariate, 7, 25–26
    inter-subject, 25, 26, 193, 194, 196, 197, 208

SUBJECT INDEX

intra-subject, 26, 194, 196, 197, 208, 210, 228
time-constant, 25, 26, 193, 194, 196, 197, 208
time-varying, 12, 25–26, 91–93, 102, 194–197, 206, 208, 210, 226–228
endogenous, 79, 223, 224, 226
cross-over design, 22, 74, 105, 113–135, 142, 155, 196, 197, 205, 229, 250
  capsaicin, 146–155
  flosequinan, 113–131
  gastric half-emptying, 22, 229
  gastric pH, 142–146
  phenylbiguanide, 155
  propoxyphene, 131–135, 138–139, 250
cube-root law, 171
cumulant, 212
cumulative distribution function, 14, 47, 92, 113, 118, 198, 213, 214, 216
curvature
  intrinsic, 17
  relative, 17
cyclic function, 45–46

damping, 64–67
data, 23–26
  acid phosphatase, 159–161
  allergen, 176, 252
  Ames assay, 168–169
  anticoronavirus, 174–176, 251
  asbestos, 71, 232
  assay
    acid phosphatase, 159–161
    allergens, 176, 252
    Ames, 168–169
    anticoronavirus, 174–176, 251
    cortisol, 176, 252
    DNase, 161–164, 174
    penicillin G, 176–177, 253
  β-globin, 183–187
  blood glucose, 137–138, 246–247
  breast cancer, 102, 243
  cancer
    breast, 102, 243
    leukæmia, 102, 241–242
    lung, 70–71, 231–232
    myeloid leukæmia, 90–93, 102
    neoplasms, 55–56, 69
    papilloma, 101–102, 240
    rectal polyps, 83, 233–236
  capsaicin, 146–155
  case–control
    asbestos, 71, 232
  chicken pox, 65–67, 71
  clinical trial
    bladder cancer, 88–90
    ephedrin, 137
    leukæmia, 102, 241–242

multiple sclerosis, 75–83
peptic œsophagitis, 93–96, 102–103
rectal polyps, 83, 233–236
rhinitis, 96–99
cortisol, 176, 252
cross-over
  capsaicin, 146–155
  flosequinan, 113–131
  gastric half-emptying, 22, 229
  gastric pH, 142–146
  phenylbiguanide, 155
  propoxyphene, 131–135, 138–139, 250
Declomycin, 138, 249
dissolution
  pills, 172–174
  theophylline, 177, 253
DNA
  β-globin, 183–187
  mitochondrial, 187–190
DNase, 161–164, 174
ephedrine, 137, 245
flosequinan, 113–131
gastric half-emptying, 22, 229
gastric pH, 142–146
hæmolytic uræmia, 58–60, 70
indomethicin, 137, 245
kidney infection, 101, 237
leukæmia, 102, 241–242
  myeloid, 90–93, 102
lung cancer, 70–71, 231–232
measles, 65–67, 71
mitochondrial, 187–190
multiple sclerosis, 75–83
myeloid leukæmia, 90–93, 102
neoplasms, 55–56, 69
papilloma, 101–102, 240
PD
  capsaicin, 146–155
  gastric pH, 142–146
  phenylbiguanide, 155, 251
penicillin G, 176–177, 253
peptic œsophagitis, 93–96, 102–103
phenylbiguanide, 155, 251
pills, 172–174
PK
  blood glucose, 137–138, 246–247
  Declomycin, 138, 249
  ephedrine, 137, 245
  flosequinan, 113–131
  indomethicin, 137, 245
  prednisolone, 135, 244
  propoxyphene, 131–135, 138–139, 250
  theophylline, 138, 248
prednisolone, 135, 244
pregnant women, 52–55, 69
propoxyphene, 131–135, 138–139, 250
rectal polyps, 83, 233–236
rhinitis, 96–99

theophylline, 138, 177, 248, 253
tuberculosis, 69
tumour
   bladder cancer, 88–90
   mammary, 101, 238–239
   urinary infections, 22, 230
data file, 27
data-generating mechanism, v, 1–9, 18, 34
   deterministic, 3
   probabilistic, 3, 5
data management, 27
data method, 194, 196–198
data object, 193–198
data storage, 26, 193–196
data structures, 23–26, 193–198
dataframe, 193–197
death rate, 55–56
Declomycin, 138, 249
degenerative disease, 187
delay parameter, 46
density function, 14, 36, 47, 92, 113, 198, 202, 206, 214, 216, 222, 224, 226
   multivariate, 213
deoxyribonucleic acid, 179–190
dependent variable, *see* response variable
descriptive model, 18–19
design, 3–4, 7, 50, 74–75
   case–control, 50, 71, 232
   cohort, 50, 71
   cross-over, 22, 74, 105, 113–135, 142–155, 196, 197, 205, 229, 250
   longitudinal, 13, 23, 24, 28, 37, 50, 142, 146, 153, 196, 208, 214, 216, 219, 220
   parallel, 74, 106
   rising-dose, 142
   sample, 4
   split-plot, 13
design matrix, 7, 10
design space, 7
deterministic data-generating mechanism, 3
deterministic model, 7
deviance, 14–15, 34
deviance residuals, 35
diary cards, 96–99
dideoxy method, 181
differential equation, vi, 19–21, 41–44, 63, 106, 108, 172, 228
   nonlinear, 19
diffusion process, 44–45, 171–174
discrete time, 46, 216, 217, 219, 226
dispersion parameter, 5, 11, 13–14
dispersion regression function, 8, 13, 17, 28, 29, 37, 79, 111–112, 115–116, 119, 128, 132, 135, 136, 146, 176, 199
dissolution rate, 169–177
   pills, 172–174
   theophylline, 177, 253

distribution, 5–7, 10–12, 28, 110
   Bernoulli, 220
   beta binomial, 36
   binomial, 11, 68, 220
      multiplicative, 11
   Burr, 217
      multivariate, 89, 218
   Cauchy, 36
      mixing, 53, 203
      multivariate, 212
   conditional, 7, 23, 206, 208, 209, 212, 214, 215, 217–219
   conjugate, 207
      mixing, 207, 215
   Consul, 168
   double exponential, 212
   duration, 216
   elliptically-contoured, 211, 212
   exponential, 15, 215–218
   gamma, 11, 15, 38, 39, 110, 114–123, 125–129, 132, 215, 216
      generalized, 12, 110, 126–130, 138
      mixing, 53, 88, 90, 217, 218
      multivariate, 146
   inverse Gaussian, 11, 15
      generalized, 12
      multivariate, 146
   Laplace, 12
      multivariate, 212
   log Cauchy, 92, 110, 115, 120, 132
      multivariate, 146
   log gamma, 39
   log Laplace, 110, 115, 116, 120
      multivariate, 146
   log logistic, 92, 146, 147
      multivariate, 146
   log normal, 15, 17, 39, 52, 54, 69, 89, 110, 111, 114–116, 118, 120–123, 125–129, 146, 147
      mixing, 112
      mixture, 89, 91
      multivariate, 146, 160, 163, 172, 177
   log power-exponential
      multivariate, 146
   log Student t
      multivariate, 146, 160
   logistic
      generalized, 12
   marginal, 206–209, 212, 213
      gamma, 146
      inverse Gaussian, 146
      log Cauchy, 146
      log Laplace, 146
      log logistic, 146
      normal, 146
      stationary, 96, 189, 220, 221
      Weibull, 146
   mixing, 112, 206

SUBJECT INDEX

Cauchy, 53, 203
conjugate, 207, 215
gamma, 53, 88, 90, 217, 218
log normal, 112
nonparametric, 117
normal, 53, 117, 208
mixture, 12, 13, 89, 205–208, 215–217, 221
finite, 221
log normal, 89, 91
Weibull, 89, 217, 218
multinomial, 86
multivariate, v, 1, 11, 13, 206–209, 211–214
Burr, 89, 218
Cauchy, 212
elliptically-contoured, 211, 212
gamma, 146
inverse Gaussian, 146
Laplace, 212
log Cauchy, 146
log Laplace, 146
log logistic, 146
log normal, 146, 160, 163, 172, 177
log power-exponential, 146
log Student t, 146, 160
negative binomial, 218
normal, v, 13, 21, 44, 146, 160, 163, 172, 211–214
power-exponential, 172, 212–213
Student t, 160, 172, 211–212
uniform, 212
Weibull, 146
negative binomial, 56, 65–67, 79, 81–83, 146, 150–155, 168, 169, 217
multivariate, 218
normal, 4, 6, 8, 10–17, 29, 35, 36, 39, 52, 76, 79, 82, 114–117, 119–121, 135, 142, 208–211, 214
mixing, 53, 117, 208
multivariate, v, 13, 21, 44, 146, 160, 163, 172, 211–214
Pareto, 217
Poisson, 11, 12, 49, 55–58, 65–67, 70, 76, 150, 168, 202, 220, 227
zero-inflated, 12
power-exponential, 212
multivariate, 172, 212–213
stable, 12, 14
Student t, 12
multivariate, 160, 172, 211–212
uniform, 213
multivariate, 212
Weibull, 11, 15, 28, 89, 110, 115, 116, 119–121, 128, 132, 203
generalized, 12
mixture, 89, 217, 218
multivariate, 146

disturbance, 64
DNA
β-globin, 183–187
mitochondrial, 187–190
DNA sequence analysis, 179–182, 220
DNase assay, 161–164, 174
dose proportionality, 106, 113
dose–response curve, 151–153, 155, 157, 163
dose–response model, 50, 166
double blinding, 75, 83, 93, 97
double exponential distribution, 212
double exponential family, 11
doubly stochastic process, 217
drift, 45, 95
dropouts, 75, 83
drug delivery, 169
dummy variable, *see* indicator variable
duration, 6, 7, 12, 22, 24, 50, 75, 85–103, 195, 221–228
duration distribution, 216
dynamic generalized linear model, 214–215
dynamic linear model, 214
dynamic model, 13, 60, 88, 138, 177, 208, 214–221
dynamic programming, 182
multidimensional, 182

EC_{50}, 160, 163, 165
ecological regression, 50–51
ecology, 39
efficacy, 74, 75, 93, 169
eigenvalue, 20, 228
eigenvector, 20
electrophoresis, 180, 181
elimination rate, 19, 43, 44, 107–138, 199–201
ELISA, 158–159, 251–252
elliptically-contoured distribution, 211, 212
endogenous covariate, 79, 223, 224, 226
endoscopy, 93
enzyme, 157
enzyme kinetics, 16
enzyme-linked immunosorbent assay, 158–159
ephedrine, 137, 245
epidemic, 46
recurrent, 60–67
epidemiology, v, 49–71
epilepsy
myoclonic, 187
epileptic fit, 85, 88
equilibrium, 64–67
error
measurement, 2, 4, 17
estimation, 14
event, 6–7
recurrent, 25, 85, 86, 88–90, 101
repeated, *see* recurrent
event history, 42, 85–103, 223, 224
evolution, 181, 182, 188

SUBJECT INDEX

evolutionary tree, 182
exon, 180–187
expense, 27
experimental trial, 74, 105, 138, 158
    animal, 74
explanatory variable, *see* covariate
exponential dispersion family, 10–11, 14, 16, 22, 207, 215
exponential distribution, 15, 215–218
exponential family, 11, 207
exponential growth curve, 19, 38–39, 41, 42, 45, 55, 56
exponential intensity, 91–93, 227
exponential link function, 172
exponential passage time, 135
exposure, 49, 50, 70, 71
external validity, 74

factor
    risk, 50, 101
    variable, 194–196, 200
failure censoring, 223
failure rate, 222
failure time
    accelerated, 223
family
    double exponential, 11
    exponential, 11, 207
    exponential dispersion, 10–11, 14, 16, 22, 207, 215
Fick's law of diffusion, 44, 171
filter
    Kalman, 13, 28, 214, 215
filtering, 184, 186, 189, 215, 221
filtration, 225, 227
first-order kinetics, 106
first-pass metabolism, 108–110, 122–124, 129, 131
fitted value residuals, 35
fixed effects, 25, 53, 112, 116–128
flosequinan, 113–131
formation rate, 107
formulation, 74, 169–174
Fortran, 28, 194, 198
forward recurrence equations, 228
forward recurrence probability, 221
frailty, 89, 101, 205, 206, 216, 219
frailty update, 218
function
    cyclic, 45–46
    exponential, 19, 38–39, 41, 42, 45, 55, 56
    Gompertz, 40–42, 56, 79
    link, 8–11, 22, 198, 200, 207
        canonical, 11, 14, 16, 207, 210
        complementary log log, 41
        identity, 15–17, 39, 198, 210
        log, 15, 38, 51, 200
        log log, 40
        logit, 40, 86–88
        reciprocal, 16
    logistic, 16, 31, 40–41, 44, 45, 52, 56, 98, 150, 161, 164, 174
        generalized, 41–42, 79, 82
    Mitscherlich, 42, 79
    monomolecular, 39, 41
    polynomial, 37–38, 79–82
    power, 45
    quantile, 213
        normal, 213
    regression, 7–9, 12–13, 15–16, 18–21, 28–29, 143, 150, 199–202
        log linear, 51
    Richards, 41, 51–55
    sigmoidal, 39–42, 45, 51, 55, 150
    sums of exponentials, 32–33, 42–45, 47, 143
    von Bertalanffy, 39, 41
function closure, 194, 201

gamma autoregression, 135, 136
gamma distribution, 11, 15, 38, 39, 110, 114–123, 125–129, 132, 215, 216
    generalized, 12, 110, 126–130, 138
    mixing, 53, 88, 90, 217, 218
    multivariate, 146
gamma intensity, 91, 93
gastric half-emptying, 22, 229
gastric pH, 142–146
Gaussian copula, 143–146, 213–214
genealogy, 187
generalized estimating equations, 142
generalized gamma autoregression, 126–130
generalized gamma distribution, 12, 110, 126–130, 138
generalized inverse Gaussian distribution, 12
generalized linear model, 9–14, 21, 40, 213
    dynamic, 214–215
generalized logistic distribution, 12
generalized logistic growth curve, 41–42, 79, 82
generalized Weibull distribution, 12
genetic engineering, 101
genetic toxicology, 101–102, 164
genetics, 179–190
genome, 179–181, 183, 187
    mitochondrial, 187–190
Genstat, 10, 11
geometric mean, 5, 17, 39, 54, 111, 114, 116, 127, 147
GLIM, 11, 15, 194, 198
glucose, 137–138, 246–247
Gompertz growth curve, 40–42, 56, 79
goodness of fit, 34–36
graphical model, 196
graphics, 27
grid search, 29, 35, 58
growth curve, 32, 37–42, 51–55

SUBJECT INDEX

exponential, 19, 38–39, 41, 42, 45, 55, 56
Gompertz, 40–42, 56, 79
logistic, 16, 31, 40–41, 44, 45, 52, 56, 98, 150, 161, 164, 174
  generalized, 41–42, 79, 82
Mitscherlich, 42, 79
polynomial, 37–38, 79–82
Richards, 41, 51–55, 176
sigmoidal, 39–42, 45, 51, 55, 150
von Bertalanffy, 39, 41
growth profile, 37
growth rate, 37–42

H_2 receptor antagonist, 142–146
hæmoglobinopathy, 183
hæmolytic uræmia, 58–60, 70
half-life, 114, 169
hazard function, 222
healthy volunteer, 74, 105, 113, 124, 130, 137, 148, 151, 245
heterogeneity, 206, 208
heteroscedasticity, 29
heterozygote, 183
hidden Markov chain, 46, 60, 62, 63, 93, 96–99, 103, 183–190, 220–221
high-pressure liquid chromatography, 158
histidine, 164–168
homogeneous Markov process, 228
HPLC, 158
Huntington's disease, 188
hypothesis, 74

identifiability, 33, 108
identity link function, 15–17, 39, 198, 210
ill conditioning, 33
immigration rate, 64
immunoglobulin, 75, 157
incidence, 50, 57, 90
independent variable, *see* covariate
index case, 67–69
indicator variable, 194
individual profile, 35, 54, 63, 79–81, 125, 128–130, 135, 136, 146, 153, 154, 175, 211
indomethicin, 137, 245
infection, 6, 64, 85, 88, 157
  bacteriuria, 22, 230
  chicken pox, 65–67
  kidney, 101, 237
  measles, 65–67
  post-viral, 147
  urinary, 22, 230
infectious disease, 49, 60–69
infective, 63–67
inference, 14, 33–36
information
  prior, 3
infusion, 42, 44, 76, 106, 169

ingestion, 42–44, 108, 169–174
inhalation, 146–155, 169
inheritance, 194
initial conditions, 19, 39, 41, 44, 64, 96, 159, 167, 171, 209, 211, 218
initial estimates, v, 11, 14, 30–32, 34
initiation codon, 180, 182
injection, 42, 44, 106, 169
innovations, 37, 211
integral equation, 19
integrated intensity, 216, 218, 221, 222, 226, 228
integro-differential equation, 46
intensity, 6, 12, 50, 92, 93, 102, 216, 222–228
  birth, 225
    nonhomogeneous, 225
  exponential, 91–93, 227
  gamma, 91, 93
  integrated, 216, 218, 221, 222, 226, 228
  log Cauchy, 91–93
  log logistic, 91–93
  log normal, 89–93
  Markov renewal, 226
  multiplicative, 92, 223
  Poisson, 225
    nonhomogeneous, 225
  renewal, 225
  transition, 220, 221, 227, 228
  Weibull, 89, 91–93, 227
intensity function
  baseline, 223
intention-to-treat, 97
inter-subject covariate, 25, 26, 193, 194, 196, 197, 208
internal validity, 74
intra-class dependence, 216
intra-subject covariate, 26, 194, 196, 197, 208, 210, 228
intravenous, 130, 132, 139
  bolus, 106, 137, 245
  infusion, 76, 106
intrinsic curvature, 17
intrinsic nonlinearity, 17–18, 35
intron, 180–187
inverse Gaussian distribution, 11, 15
  generalized, 12
  multivariate, 146
inverse polynomial, 38
investigator, 74
iterated weighted least squares, 10, 11, 16, 28
IWLS, 10, 11, 14, 16, 28

Jacobian, 24, 82, 195, 197, 213, 216

Kalman filter, 13, 28, 214, 215
Kaplan–Meier curve, 88, 89, 91–93
Kearns–Sayre syndrome, 188
kernel density estimation, 18, 117, 120
kidney infection, 101, 237

SUBJECT INDEX

kinetics
    enzyme, 16
    first-order, 106
    single-hit, 167
knockout mice, 101
knowledge
    prior, 3
kurtosis, 212

lag, 82, 141, 210
Laplace distribution, 12
    multivariate, 212
Laplace transform, 20–21, 216, 218
law
    scientific, 2
least squares, 15, 18
    iterated weighted, 10, 11, 16, 28
    nonlinear, 111
Leber's optic neuropathy, 187
leukæmia, 102, 242
    myeloid, 90–93, 102
    nonlymphoblastic, 102, 241
likelihood, 29–33, 202–204
    multimodal, 29–30
    profile, 33–36, 69, 70, 135, 137, 152, 153, 160, 163–165, 172, 173
    region, 34–35
    shape, 29–31, 35
likelihood function, 34, 209, 215, 221, 224, 226, 227
likelihood ratio, 34
linear model, 6, 50
    dynamic, 214
linear predictor, 9–11, 39
linear structure, 9, 40
link function, 8–11, 22, 198, 200, 207
    canonical, 11, 14, 16, 207, 210
    complementary log log, 41
    exponential, 172
    identity, 15–17, 39, 198, 210
    log, 15, 38, 51, 200
    log log, 40
    logit, 40, 86–88
    reciprocal, 16
Lisp, 194
location parameter, 5, 8, 10, 13, 14, 17, 216
    random, 206
location regression function, 10, 11, 28, 199, 205–207, 210, 214
locus, 183
log Cauchy autoregression, 135
log Cauchy distribution, 92, 110, 115, 120, 132
    multivariate, 146
log Cauchy intensity, 91–93
log gamma distribution, 39
log Laplace distribution, 110, 115, 116, 120
    multivariate, 146

log linear model, 49, 55–56, 58, 70, 92, 150, 219, 227
log linear regression function, 51
log link function, 15, 38, 51, 200
log log link function, 40
log logistic distribution, 92, 146, 147
    multivariate, 146
log logistic intensity, 91–93
log normal autoregression, 53, 54, 129, 135, 146, 172, 174, 177
log normal distribution, 15, 17, 39, 52, 54, 69, 89, 110, 111, 114–116, 118, 120–123, 125–129, 146, 147
    mixing, 112
    multivariate, 146, 160, 163, 172, 177
log normal intensity, 89–93
log normal mixture distribution, 89, 91
log power-exponential distribution
    multivariate, 146
log Student t distribution
    multivariate, 146, 160
logistic autoregression, 135
logistic distribution
    generalized, 12
logistic growth curve, 16, 31, 40–41, 44, 45, 52, 56, 98, 150, 161, 164, 174
    generalized, 41–42, 79, 82
logistic regression, 49, 50, 86, 219
logit link function, 40, 86–88
logit transformation, 30
longitudinal dependence, 216, 218
    Markov, 219
    nonstationary, 218
longitudinal study, 13, 23, 24, 28, 37, 50, 142, 146, 153, 196, 208, 214, 216, 219, 220

Maple, 198, 200
marginal distribution, 206–209, 212, 213
    gamma, 146
    inverse Gaussian, 146
    log Cauchy, 146
    log Laplace, 146
    log logistic, 146
    normal, 146
    stationary, 96, 189, 220, 221
    Weibull, 146
marker, 90
marker sequence, 181
Markov chain, 93, 95, 185, 219–220
    first-order, 220
    hidden, 46, 60, 62, 63, 93, 96–99, 103, 183–190, 220–221
    irreducible, 221
Markov process, 209, 214, 219–221
    first-order, 214
    homogeneous, 228
Markov renewal intensity, 226

SUBJECT INDEX

Markov renewal process, 226–227
Markov time, 225
Markov update, 89–91, 219
Markovian transition probability, 86
martingale, 224, 225
matching, 50, 76
    incidence density, 71
Mathematica, 198, 200
Matlab, 198
matrix exponentiation, 19–20, 220, 221, 228
maximum likelihood estimates, 14–16, 29, 31, 34
MD_5-antagonist, 155
mean
    arithmetic, 5, 17, 39, 111, 114, 116, 127, 147
    geometric, 5, 17, 39, 54, 111, 114, 116, 127, 147
mean value parameter, 8
measles, 65–67, 71
measurement equation, 214
measurement error, 2, 4, 17
measurement precision, 4
mechanistic model, v, 9, 18–19, 38, 42, 47, 55, 56, 73, 76, 82, 106, 141, 143, 164, 166–168
methylprednisolone, 75–83
Michaëlis–Menten model, 16, 38, 159–161, 164, 174
    generalized, 161–164
micro-organism subtyping, 67–69
microtitration, 159, 176
migraine, 74, 85
missing values, 13, 27, 75, 83, 97, 193, 196–198
    randomly, 98, 197, 215
mitochondria, 179, 187–190
Mitscherlich growth curve, 42, 79
mixing distribution, 112, 206
    Cauchy, 53, 203
    conjugate, 207, 215
    gamma, 53, 88, 90, 217, 218
    log normal, 112
    nonparametric, 117
    normal, 53, 117, 208
mixture distribution, 12, 13, 89, 205–208, 215–217, 221
    finite, 221
    log normal, 89, 91
    Weibull, 89, 217, 218
model, 1–9, 198–202
    adjacent categories, 88, 95
    analysis of variance, 6, 15, 18, 22
    change-point, 46, 57–60
    compartment, 16, 18, 20, 33, 42–44, 46, 63, 64, 143
        first-order, 42–44, 106–139, 199–201
        zero-order, 44, 107, 132–135
    continuation ratio, 88, 95, 97–99

descriptive, 18–19
deterministic, 7
dose–response, 50, 166
dynamic, 13, 60, 88, 138, 177, 208, 214–221
dynamic linear, 214
fixed-effects, 25, 53, 112, 116–128
generalized linear, 9–14, 21, 40, 213
    dynamic, 214–215
graphical, 196
linear, 6, 50
log linear, 49, 55–56, 58, 70, 92, 150, 219, 227
longitudinal dependence, 216, 218
    Markov, 219
    nonstationary, 218
mechanistic, v, 9, 18–19, 38, 42, 47, 55, 56, 73, 76, 82, 106, 141, 143, 164, 166–168
Michaëlis–Menten, 16, 38, 159–161, 164, 174
    generalized, 161–164
ordinal, 86–88, 95, 97, 103
population-averaged, 206, 207
probability, 3–7, 10, 198–199
proportional odds, 88, 95, 97–99
random coefficients, 126–127, 214
random effects, 13, 28, 112, 126–127, 205–208, 214, 215
random walk, 44, 95–96
regression, 7
    linear, 6, 8–14, 50
    robust, 212
serial dependence, 13, 28, 79–81, 89, 126–130, 132–135, 172, 210–211, 219
SIR
    closed, 63, 64
    open, 64
state dependence, 210–211, 219, 220
state space, 214
statistical, 11
stochastic, 3, 7
subject-specific, 206
survival, 49, 221–227
transport, 171–174
typing, 68–69
model components, 27–28
model formula, 195, 197, 199–202
model matrix, 10
model selection, 3, 34
model specification, 27–29
molecular biology, 67, 179–190
monitoring, 74, 82
monomolecular function, 39, 41
mortality rate, 222
    cancer, 55–56
mRNA, 179
multinomial distribution, 86

multiple regression, 18
multiple sclerosis, 75–83
multiplicative binomial distribution, 11
multiplicative intensities, 92, 223
multivariate distribution, v, 1, 11, 13, 206–209, 211–214, 218, 219
    Burr, 89, 218
    Cauchy, 212
    elliptically-contoured, 211, 212
    gamma, 146
    inverse Gaussian, 146
    Laplace, 212
    log Cauchy, 146
    log Laplace, 146
    log logistic, 146
    log normal, 146, 160, 163, 172, 177
    log power-exponential, 146
    log Student t, 146, 160
    negative binomial, 218
    normal, v, 13, 21, 44, 146, 160, 163, 172, 211–214
    power-exponential, 172, 212–213
    Student t, 160, 172, 211–212
    uniform, 212
    Weibull, 146
mutation, 164–168, 180–182, 187–190
    point, 183, 188
myoclonic epilepsy, 187

ND, 112, 118, 119
Needleman–Wunsch algorithm, 182
negative binomial autoregression, 79–81, 149–155
negative binomial distribution, 56, 65–67, 79, 81–83, 146, 150–155, 168, 169, 217
    multivariate, 218
nesting, 24, 143, 146, 149, 194–197, 205
neurogenic muscle weakness, 188
Newton–Raphson method, 29
nlme, 126
nominal response, 6, 86, 195
nondetectable value, 112–114, 118–120, 126, 127
nonlinearity, 12, 15–18
    intrinsic, 17–18, 35
    parameter-effects, 17–18
    transformable, 16–17
nonparametrics, 18
nonstationary update, 218, 219
normal autoregression, 53, 82, 209
normal distribution, 4, 6, 8, 10–17, 29, 35, 36, 39, 52, 76, 79, 82, 114–117, 119–121, 135, 142, 208–211, 214
    mixing, 53, 117, 208
    multivariate, v, 13, 21, 44, 146, 160, 163, 172, 211–214
normalizing constant, 11
nucleus, 179, 180, 187
numerical derivatives, 14

numerical integration, 13, 28, 107, 203, 206, 208

object
    class, 194
        data, 194–197
        formula, 201
    data, 193–198
    inheritance, 194
    method, 194, 196–198
    slot, 194–197
observation equation, 214
observation update, 215
offset, 55, 70
oncogene, 101
open reading frame, 179
optimization
    constrained, 30
    nonlinear, 12, 14, 29–33, 35, 57, 201–203
oral dose, 76, 106, 113, 130, 132, 137, 138, 148, 169, 245, 248
order, 177
ordinal model, 86–88, 95, 97, 103
ordinal response, 6, 85, 86, 93–99, 142, 195
ORF, 179
orthogonal polynomial, 31
oscillation, 64–67
outlier, 14, 36, 212
overdispersion, 13, 56, 65, 70, 79, 142, 146, 149–155, 168
overflow, 30
oxidative phosphorylation, 187–188

parallel design, 74, 106
parameter, 4–5
    canonical, 16, 207
    delay, 46
    dispersion, 5, 11, 13–14
    location, 5, 8, 10, 13, 14, 17, 216
        random, 206
    mean value, 8
    shape, 5, 7–9, 13, 28, 29, 92, 93, 216
        constant, 7
parameter constraint, 30, 35
    conventional, 116
parameter-effects nonlinearity, 17–18
parameter redundancy, 33
parameter transformation, 16–17, 30–31, 43
    log, 30
parametrization, 30–31
    stable, 31, 35
Pareto distribution, 217
Parkinson's disease, 188
PCR, 183
Pearson's marrow/pancrease syndrome, 188
peeling, 32
penicillin G assay, 176–177, 253
peptic œsophagitis, 93–96, 102–103
period, 64–67

pharmacodynamics, 74, 131, 141–155
    capsaicin, 146–155
    gastric pH, 142–146
    phenylbiguanide, 155, 251
pharmacokinetics, 13, 18, 42, 43, 74, 105–139,
        141, 143, 149, 157, 199
    blood glucose, 137–138, 246–247
    Declomycin, 138, 249
    ephedrine, 137, 245
    flosequinan, 113–131
    indomethicin, 137, 245
    population, 106
    prednisolone, 135, 244
    propoxyphene, 131–135, 138–139, 250
    theophylline, 138, 248
pharmacology, 74
phenylbiguanide, 155, 251
phylogenetic analysis, 182, 187
physical genome map, 181
pill, 107, 171–174, 177
    vitamin, 88
point process, 224, 227
Poisson autoregression, 151, 152
Poisson distribution, 11, 12, 49, 55–58, 65–67,
        70, 76, 150, 168, 202, 220, 227
    zero-inflated, 12
Poisson intensity, 225
    nonhomogeneous, 225
Poisson process, 57–60, 225, 227
    nonhomogeneous, 225
polymerase chain reaction, 183
polymorphism, 183, 188
polynomial
    growth curve, 37–38, 79–82
    inverse, 38
polypeptide, *see* protein
polyposis
    familial, 83, 233–236
population, 4, 5, 7
population-averaged model, 206, 207
population frequencies, 4
population pharmacokinetics, 106
power-exponential distribution
    multivariate, 172, 212–213
power function, 45
precision
    measurement, 4
pre-clinical trial, 74, 101–102, 238–240
predicted profile, 63, 125, 128–130, 135, 136,
        146, 211
prediction, 2, 7, 39, 60, 79, 96, 106, 116, 127,
        131, 153, 210, 211, 214
    one-step-ahead, 215
prednisolone, 135, 244
prevalence, 50
prior information, 3
prior knowledge, 3
probabilistic data-generating mechanism, 3, 5

probability
    forward recurrence, 221
    transition, 93–96, 102, 228
probability model, 3–7, 10, 198–199
process
    autoregression, 36, 131, 132, 138, 143, 146,
        155, 208–211, 214
    gamma, 135, 136
    generalized gamma, 126–130
    log Cauchy, 135
    log logistic, 135
    log normal, 53, 54, 129, 135, 146, 172,
        174, 177
    negative binomial, 79–81, 149–155
    normal, 53, 82, 209
    Poisson, 151, 152
    Weibull, 135
    birth, 86, 88–90, 135, 227
        generalized, 227
        nonhomogeneous, 225
        pure, 225, 227
    contagion, 227
    counting, 12, 224–228
    diffusion, 44–45, 171–174
    doubly stochastic, 217
    Markov, 209, 214, 219–221
        first-order, 214
        homogeneous, 228
    Markov chain, 93, 95, 185, 219–220
        first-order, 220
        hidden, 46, 60, 62, 63, 93, 96–99, 103,
            183–190, 220–221
        irreducible, 221
    Markov renewal, 226–227
    point, 224, 227
    Poisson, 57–60, 225, 227
        nonhomogeneous, 225
    random walk, 44, 95–96
    renewal, 225
        Markov, 226–227
    semi-Markov, 86, 226–227
    stochastic, 1, 4, 135, 224, 227
    Weibull, 227
    Yule, 225
profile, 76, 80, 81, 105, 113, 119, 132, 134, 143,
        145, 197
    growth, 37
    individual, 35, 54, 63, 79–81, 125, 128–
        130, 135, 136, 146, 153, 154, 175,
        211
    predicted, 63, 125, 128–130, 135, 136, 146,
        211
    underlying, 35, 54, 79–81, 135, 136, 146,
        147, 153, 154, 161, 164, 165, 169,
        170, 172, 174, 211
profile likelihood, 33–36, 69, 70, 135, 137, 152,
        153, 160, 163–165, 172, 173
promoter box, 180, 182, 183

proportional hazards
    semi-parametric, 223, 227
proportional odds model, 88, 95, 97–99
propoxyphene, 131–135, 138–139, 250
protein, 157, 179–183, 187
pyridoxine, 88

quality of life, 74, 85–103, 146
quantile function, 213
    normal, 213

R, v, 10, 11, 23, 28, 29, 193–204
radioimmunoassay, 158
ragged-red fibre disease, 187
random coefficients, 126–127, 214
random component, 1–2, 5, 7, 8, 10
random effects, 13, 28, 42, 112, 126–127, 205–208, 214, 215
random walk, 44, 95–96
randomization, 4, 24, 26, 74, 75, 88, 93, 230
randomness, 3–4, 197
rate, 19, 30, 32, 35, 42, 49, 50, 57, 75, 82
    absorption, 19, 43, 107–138, 199–201
    birth, 64
    death, 55–56
    dissolution, 169–177
    elimination, 19, 43, 44, 107–138, 199–201
    failure, 222
    formation, 107
    growth, 37–42
    immigration, 64
    mortality, 222
        cancer, 55–56
    mutation, 187–190
    release, 177
rate constant, 16, 19, 65
rate equations, 19–21
reaction velocity, 16, 159, 160
reciprocal link function, 16
recombinant DNA, 161–164, 180, 183
rectal polyps, 83, 233–236
recurrent events, 25, 85, 86, 88–90, 101
recursive update, 28
reflecting barrier, 96
regression, 7
    all subsets, 28
    linear, 6, 8–14, 50
    log linear, 49, 55–56, 58, 70, 92, 150, 219, 227
    logistic, 49, 50, 86
    multiple, 18
    stepwise, 28
regression function, 7–9, 12–13, 15–16, 18–21, 28–29, 143, 150, 199–202
    dispersion, 8, 13, 17, 28, 29, 37, 79, 111–112, 115–116, 119, 128, 132, 135, 136, 146, 176, 199

location, 10, 11, 28, 199, 205–207, 210, 214
    log linear, 51
relapse, 75, 76, 102, 241–242
relative curvature, 17
release rate, 177
renewal intensity, 225
renewal process, 225
    Markov, 226–227
repeated dosing, 131–135
repeated events, *see* recurrent events
residuals, 10, 211
    deviance, 35
    fitted value, 35
response transformation, 5, 15, 17, 24, 30, 111, 194, 210
    integrated intensity, 215, 216
    log, 15, 17, 111
    reciprocal, 17
    square-root, 76, 79–82
response variable, 3, 5–7, 23–25, 142
    continuous, 6
    count, 6–7
    nominal, 6, 86, 195
    ordinal, 6, 85, 86, 93–99, 142, 195
    positive, 6
restriction endonuclease, 180
restriction enzyme fingerprinting, 181
retinitis pigmentosa, 188
retinyl acetate, 101, 238–239
rhinitis, 96–99
RIA, 158
ribonucleic acid, 179–180
ribosome, 180
Richards growth curve, 41, 51–55, 176
rising-dose trial, 142
risk, 88, 93, 101, 102
    competing, 86
risk factor, 50, 101
risk function, 222
RNA, 179, 187
    messenger, 179
    ribosomal, 180, 187
    transfer, 180, 187
robust model, 212
robustness, 14, 36, 82
rRNA, 180, 187

S, 198
S-Plus, 10, 11, 194, 201
S-shaped growth curve, 39–42, 45, 51, 55, 150
safety, 74
Salmonella, 164–169
sample
    design, 4
sample size, 3–4
sample survey, 74
SAS, 10, 28

SUBJECT INDEX

scaling, 17, 30
scientific law, 2
scoping rules, 194
score equations, 15, 29
score matrix, 182
semi-Markov process, 86, 226–227
semi-parametric proportional hazards, 223, 227
sequence analysis, 179–182
serial dependence, 13, 28, 79–81, 89, 126–130, 132–135, 172, 210–211, 219
shape
    likelihood, 29–31, 35
shape parameter, 5, 7–9, 13, 28, 29, 92, 93, 216
    constant, 7
shotgun method, 181
shrinkage estimate, 112
sickle-cell anæmia, 183
side effect, 74, 85
sigmoidal growth curve, 39–42, 45, 51, 55, 150
single-hit kinetics, 167
SIR model
    closed, 63, 64
    open, 64
skew, 6, 14, 15, 17, 52, 110, 116, 120, 146, 160, 212, 222
skin painting, 101–102
slot, 194–197
Smith–Waterman algorithm, 182
smoothing, 3, 5
software, 27, 198
    choice, 27
space
    design, 7
spectral decomposition, 20
spells, 93, 96–99, 205, 220
spinal metastases, 102
splicing, 179, 180
spline, 18
split-plot design, 13
SPSS, 28
stable distribution, 12, 14
stable parametrization, 31, 35
standard deviation, 39
standard treatment, 74
starting values, *see* initial estimates
Stata, 10, 11
state, 205, 210, 214–221, 224, 226–228
    hidden, 60, 96–99, 183–190, 220–221
state dependence, 210–211, 219, 220
state equation, 214
state space, 91, 219
state space model, 214
state transition equation, 214, 215
state transition matrix, 214
stationarity, 37, 38, 89, 96, 189, 218–221, 226
stationary independent increments, 225
statistical model, 11
steady state, 20, 75, 96, 141

stepwise regression, 28
stochastic component, 1–2, 5, 7, 8, 10, 30, 210
stochastic dependence structure, 1, 27, 28, 38, 208
stochastic model, 3, 7
stochastic process, 1, 4, 135, 224, 227
stopping rule, 223
stopping time, 224, 225
Student t distribution, 12
    multivariate, 160, 172, 211–212
study validity
    external, 74
    internal, 74
subcutaneous, 106
subject-specific model, 206
substitution matrix, 182
sufficient statistics, 14
sums of exponentials, 32–33, 42–45, 47, 143
surrogate endpoint, 105
surveillance, 74
survey, 74
survival, 50, 75, 86, 102, 113, 206, 223, 227
survival function, 92, 93, 216, 222–228
survival model, 49, 221–227
survival time, 102
susceptible, 63–65, 101
sustained-release tablet, 177
systematic component, 1–2, 4, 7–9, 11, 30, 206

tablet, 97, 107, 135, 171
    sustained-release, 177
tachyphylaxis, 148
Taylor series, 37
termination codon, 180, 182
TeX, 198
theophylline, 138, 177, 248, 253
thiotepa, 88
time
    continuous, 46, 215, 220, 221, 226
    discrete, 46, 216, 217, 219, 226
time censoring, 223
time-constant covariate, 25, 26, 193, 194, 196, 197, 208
time series, 23–25, 37, 52, 57, 76, 219
    binary, 22, 220
time update, 215
time-varying covariate, 12, 25–26, 91–93, 102, 194–197, 206, 208, 210, 226–228
    endogenous, 79, 223, 224, 226
T_{max}, 107, 121, 123
total symptom score, 97
toxicity, 74, 76, 83, 105, 131, 166, 167
toxicology, 74
    genetic, 101–102, 164
transdermal, 169
transfer matrix, 19
transformable nonlinearity, 16–17
transformation

SUBJECT INDEX

logit, 30
  parameter, 16–17, 30–31, 43
    log, 30
  response, 5, 15, 17, 24, 30, 111, 194, 210
    integrated intensity, 215, 216
    log, 15, 17, 111
    reciprocal, 17
    square-root, 76, 79–82
transgenic mice, 101
transition, 85–86, 90, 91, 93, 224, 226
transition intensity, 220, 221, 227, 228
transition matrix, 95–96, 185, 219–220
  hidden, 60, 184–186, 188, 220–221
  intensity, 220, 221, 228
  stationary, 220
transition probability, 93–96, 102, 228
  Markovian, 86
transport model, 171–174
treatment
  control, 74, 93, 96, 101, 168
  standard, 74
trial, 74
  animal, 74
  clinical, v, 42, 73–83, 85, 88–90, 93–99, 102, 146–155
  phases, 74
  pre-clinical, 74, 101–102, 238–240
triplet, 179, 182, 183, 185, 186, 189, 190
tRNA, 180, 187
TSS, 97
tuberculosis, 69
tumour
  bladder cancer, 88–90
  mammary, 101, 238–239
tussive agent, 146–155
typing model, 68–69

underlying profile, 35, 54, 79–81, 135, 136, 146, 147, 153, 154, 161, 164, 165, 169, 170, 172, 174, 211
uniform distribution, 213
  multivariate, 212
unit of measurement, 4, 24, 195–197
update, 153
  count, 89–91, 219
  frailty, 218
  Markov, 89–91, 219
  nonstationary, 218, 219

observation, 215
  recursive, 28
  time, 215
urinary infections, 22, 230

validity, 74–75
  study
    external, 74
    internal, 74
variability, 5
variable
  dependent, *see* response
  dummy, *see* indicator
  explanatory, *see* covariate
  factor, 194–196, 200
  independent, *see* covariate
  indicator, 194
  response, 3, 5–7, 23–25, 142
    continuous, 6
    count, 6–7
    nominal, 6, 195
    ordinal, 6, 85, 93–99, 142, 195
    positive, 6
vasodilator, 113
vitamin, 83, 88
volume of distribution
  apparent, 43, 107–135, 199–201
von Bertalanffy growth curve, 39, 41

washout period, 113, 132, 135, 142, 148–150
Weibull autoregression, 135
Weibull distribution, 11, 15, 28, 89, 110, 115, 116, 119–121, 128, 132, 203
  generalized, 12
  multivariate, 146
Weibull intensity, 89, 91–93, 227
Weibull mixture distribution, 89, 217, 218
Weibull process, 227

XLisp-Stat, 10, 11

YAC, 180
yeast artificial chromosome, 180
Yule process, 225

zero counts, 210